SQUARING
THE
CIRCLE

Normal birth research, theory and practice in a technological age

SQUARING
THE
CIRCLE

Normal birth research, theory and practice in a technological age

Edited by
Soo Downe and Sheena Byrom

pinter
&
martin

Squaring the Circle: Normal birth research, theory and practice in a technological age

First published by Pinter & Martin Ltd 2019
reprinted 2021

ISBN 978-1-78066-440-8
Also available as ebook

British Library Cataloguing-in-Publication Data
A catalogue record for this book is available from the British Library.

Layout: Thorsten Knaub
Index: Helen Bilton

Set in Adobe Garamond

Printed and bound by Hussar

Pinter & Martin Ltd
6 Effra Parade
London SW2 1PS

pinterandmartin.com

Contents

FOREWORD

In 2019, women and their families want more from childbirth than simply emerging from the process unscathed. A global consensus exists on the need to ensure that, for every woman, newborn and family, pregnancy and childbirth is not only safe, but is a memorable and rewarding experience filled with love and joy. However, it is a sobering statistic that every day an estimated 380 women die as a result of pregnancy and childbirth, and 7,000 newborns die as a result of being born. It is of great concern that more than half these deaths arise not from an absence of care, but from poor quality of care provided in facilities. This is unconscionable in the 21st century.

We are immediately faced with a challenge: how do we address the tension of providing quality, compassionate care for the vast majority of healthy women and newborns experiencing normal physiological birth, while ensuring the survival of women and newborns who urgently require advanced interventions? This is of particular importance in a decade of dramatic escalation in the use of new technology and intervention in pregnancy and childbirth, around the globe.

Squaring the Circle asks different questions, challenges assumptions to existing knowledge, behaviour and practice. It opens up a groundbreaking approach to finding a range of solutions. Key to most of the chapters is the agency of women and newborns, and the impact of the relationship between the woman and her care provider. The book explores the amazing interconnections between the complex psychological, emotional and physical processes of physiological childbirth with companionship and why place of birth is important. It highlights emerging knowledge on the positive, and negative, impacts of (over-) intervention. The text raises a fundamental precautionary issue about the risk of disrupting millions of years of finely tuned evolution as a result of the rapid escalation to most women and babies of 'just in case' clinical and pharmacological interventions that were originally designed only for those with complications. It brings together new science on endocrinology, epigenetics and the microbiome, and digs deep into current assumptions on how to best care for women and their newborns.

The anthology includes perspectives from researchers around the world, based in a range of professional and academic disciplines. It seeks a critical shift in the development and use of evidence in policy and practice. It resets goals for one of the most important events in the lives of all humans: childbirth. This book must be read, and used widely to ensure that all women and newborns everywhere are given the best quality of care and that they not only survive, but thrive and live long and healthy lives enabling them to transform our societies and our world.

Fran McConville, WHO

Neel Shah, MD, Assistant Professor of Obstetrics, Harvard Medical School

CHAPTER 1

Squaring the circle: why physiological labour and birth matter in a technological world

Soo Downe, Sheena Byrom and *Anastasia Topalidou*

Introduction

The childbirth agenda has changed dramatically over the last decade. In 2004, it was largely taken for granted that both improving the safety and wellbeing of mothers and babies and minimising unnecessary intervention in childbirth were important goals (Downe 2004). However, at the same time as survival rates of women and babies have improved in most (though not all) countries around the world, concern about safety has increased in the public debate, particularly in high-income countries with low rates of maternal and infant deaths. This has occurred in parallel with technological innovation that has brought measuring and monitoring of physical signs closer to individuals, through smartphones and fitness devices. This combination offers the seductive promise of personalised/precision medicine. The argument goes as follows: *if only measurement and monitoring can take place at the individual level, from the genetic to the physical, it will be possible to predict, prevent and treat any or all risks and actual pathologies, and reduce harms to zero.* Such thinking promotes technical solutions as superior to simple physiology. It can even create an environment where it becomes a moral duty for each individual to submit to assessment of their current health status, to establish their risk for a whole range of future illnesses, and to accept prophylactic treatment of these potential future illnesses. The promise is that this will ensure the optimum health of the population, and especially a healthy old age, even if the identification of potential (but not actual) risk is associated with an increase in anxiety and a reduction in social, psychological, and/or emotional wellbeing.

However, acting on the promise of perfect health without clear evidence that it can indeed be fulfilled comes at a price. If health surveillance and treatment becomes a standard or even a morally expected norm, in the absence of concern for human experience and fulfilment, there is a risk that life choices will be determined only by assumptions about physical risk and pathology. In 2012 the front cover of the *BMJ* framed this as a slide from 'Arming the health' to 'Alarming the Healthy' to, eventually, 'Harming the healthy' if it is taken too far.* Beyond this, Nietzsche realised that hope (without knowledge of what will actually happen) is a fundamental characteristic of human optimism for life, saying *Let your love of life be a love for your highest hope*. (Nietzsche (transl Common) 1999, p29)

It is clear from qualitative studies of what women want and need around the world that both safety and human flourishing matter to childbearing women and their families. The pursuit of the best possible maternity care needs to keep both of these things in balance. Most women and babies in all countries of the world are able to give birth with supportive expert care, without needing treatments or technologies. However, the vast majority of the research and evidence produced in this area is still focused on complications, tests and treatments, and very little is known, still, about the nature and outcomes of physiological labour and birth, and how to enable women to experience it.

Indeed, as fewer women who take part in research studies experience physiological labour and birth, it becomes more and more likely that solutions that work in the context of interventions become generalised to all. For example, a recent study recommended the use of IV rather than IM oxytocin for managed third stage of labour, even though sub-analyses of the data, presented in the paper, imply that there was no benefit of this for women who had spontaneous onset of labour, or who were multiparous (Adnan 2018). There is also an implicit assumption that interventions that are now held to be overused can only be reduced by the introduction of different interventions, rather than by increased support for physiological birth. For example, anecdotally, the results of the recent ARRIVE trial (Grobman 2018) are being widely implemented, resulting in routine induction of all nulliparous women in some hospitals after 39 weeks gestation to reduce caesarean section rates. This demonstrates a very rapid translation of results from a study carried out in one healthcare context (the USA) to other healthcare contexts that vary in a range of ways. In contrast, there has been evidence for some years from studies carried out in a range of countries and contexts that continuous support in labour reduces caesarean section by a greater percentage than that resulting from the ARRIVE trial (Bohren 2017). However, this solution, which requires a reduction in technical support and an increase in human contact and relationships, has not been widely rolled out. The widespread introduction of induction of labour for healthy women and babies also carries the risk of as yet unknown long-term consequences for babies born after labour induction, as is suggested in a recent large population cohort study of almost half a million Australian mothers and babies (Peters 2018). This is in contrast to the introduction of labour support, which has no known short or longer term adverse effects. The

---

* www.bmj.com/content/344/bmj.e3783/rr/588178

paradox of the rapid introduction of technical solutions in maternity care, and the slow or minimal rollout of equally or more effective relationship-based solutions, is the context in which this book is set.

Focusing on solutions

For everyone working in this field, the goal is the same: to understand, to contextualise and to facilitate physiological labour and birth. But all those engaging with this topic do not speak the same scientific language. They do not use common methodologies throughout their daily practice. They may not even have the same views about the importance of this topic, or about the nature of its parameters. Within multinational multidisciplinary collaborations, the experiences and cultural history of each researcher add a particular flavour to the mix (Klein 1990; Frost and Jean 2003; Aram 2004). Getting there requires a kind of suspension of disbelief among all the participants.

The question asked in this book, from our various disciplinary and cultural perspectives, is '*can we move from risk-disease-orientation to health-orientation in our research endeavours?*'. And, in so doing, can we ensure the identification of true pathology while ensuring that false positives don't render physiological labour and birth obsolete? This approach authentically meets the Alma-Ata definition of health as *a state of complete physical, mental and social wellbeing, and not merely the absence of disease or infirmity* (Declaration of Alma-Ata, 1978).

To do this, we have set the goal of squaring the circle of our multiple perspectives, beliefs and experiences. We conceptualise this geometrically in Figure 1. Assume that there is a square, each corner of which represents one scientific group. Let's say that the angle A is the group of obstetrics, midwifery, medicine and neurosciences, the angle B is biomechanics and bioengineering, at the angle C is the group of psychology, sociology, and public health and at the angle D the group of philosophy and activism. Based on Euclidean definition, a circle is '*a plane figure bounded by one line, and such that all right lines drawn from a certain point within it to the bounding line, are equal. The bounding line is called its circumference and the point its centre*' (Hazewinkel, 2001). We assume that we have a circle where the circumference is health-oriented and welfare practice, and the centre is the pregnant woman and the foetus, who are in any direction always equidistant from the health-oriented circumference (Figure 1). The following questions then arise: Can we round these corners? Can a scientific solution, a scientific square be created, with the same area as the given circle using only a finite number of steps with compass (scientific techniques) and straight-edge ruler (physiological birth)?

All we needed was to find pi (π). π is the ratio of the circumference of a circle to the diameter. For this book it was defined as *authentic, trusting, relationship-based inter-disciplinary cooperation.* In our model, this inter-disciplinary cooperation must always be equal to health-orientated practice divided by the wellbeing of the pregnant woman and the foetus.

Figure 1.
Squaring the circle

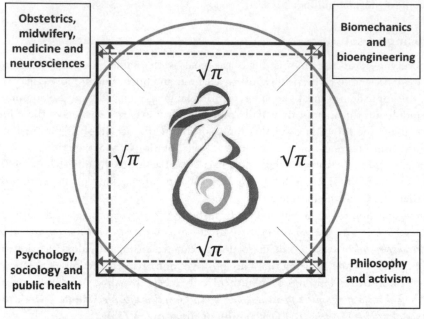

—— **Circle circumference: health-oriented practice**

Conclusion

Reframing maternity services and practices depends on a clear analysis of the current issues, and on proposing new solutions that are exciting, feasible and acceptable. This book brings some of the evidence and debate about normal, physiological labour and birth up to date, from a multidisciplinary perspective. The chapters cover topics from architecture to epigenetics, and from organisational analysis to theory and philosophy. In the process, the authors engage with some of the key questions that are outstanding in this area. They all also offer insights into possible solutions and ways forward.

For the sake of the future health of mothers, babies, families and societies, we have to better understand childbirth physiology and how to support it, both to promote it where it is possible and desirable, and to identify and deal with true pathology. Squaring the interdisciplinary circle is probably the best and only way to achieve this. We hope that readers of this book find our attempt useful and enlightening.

References

Adnan, N. Conlan-Trant, R., McCormick, C., Boland, F., Murphy, D.J. (2018) 'Intramuscular versus intravenous oxytocin to prevent postpartum haemorrhage at vaginal delivery: randomised controlled trial' *BMJ* 2018; 362 doi: https://doi.org/10.1136/bmj.k3546

Aram, J.D. (2004) 'Concepts of Interdisciplinarity: Configurations of Knowledge and Action' *Human Relations* 57(4):379–412.

Bohren MA, Hofmeyr GJ, Sakala C, Fukuzawa RK, Cuthbert A. Continuous support for women during childbirth. Cochrane Database of Systematic Reviews 2017, Issue 7. Art. No.: CD003766. DOI: 10.1002/14651858. CD003766.pub6.

Declaration of Alma-Ata. (1978) International Conference on Primary Health Care, Alma-Ata, USSR, 6-12 September 1978.

Downe, S. (Ed) (2004) *Normal Childbirth, Evidence and Debate*, Churchill Livingston.

Frost, S.H. and Jean, P.M. (2003) 'Bridging the Disciplines—Interdisciplinary Discourse and Faculty Scholarship' *Journal of Higher Education* 74(2):119–149.

Grobman, W.A., Rice, M.M., Reddy, U.M., Tita, A.T.N., Silver, R.M., Mallett, G. et al (2018) 'Labor Induction versus Expectant Management in Low-Risk Nulliparous Women (the ARRIVE trial)'. *N Engl J Med*; 379:513-523

Hazewinkel, M. (Ed) (2001), 'Circle', *Encyclopedia of Mathematics,* Springer, ISBN 978-1-55608-010-4

Klein, J.T. (1990) *Interdisciplinarity: history, theory and practice,* the Wayne State University Press, Detroit.

Nietzsche, F. (transl Common, T.) (1999) *Thus Spake Zarathustra,* Dover Publications, New York.

Peters, L.L., Thornton, C., de Jonge, A., Khashan, A., Tracy, M., Downe, S., Feijen-de Jong, E.I., Dahlen, H.G. (2018) 'The effect of medical and operative birth interventions on child health outcomes in the first 28 days and up to 5 years of age: A linked data population-based cohort study' *Birth* 45(4):347-357. doi: 10.1111/birt.12348. Epub 2018 Mar 25.

Illustrations

Figure 1: With permission from Olga Gouni (www.cosmoanelixis.gr): we also acknowledge that the central logo is used for EU COST Action IS1407 BIRTH (Building Intrapartum Research Through Health) eubirthresearch.eu, also with permission from Olga Gouni.

PART I

The nature and context of normal birth

CHAPTER 2

Nature and consequences of oxytocin and other neuro-hormones during the perinatal period

Sarah Buckley and *Kerstin Uvnäs Moberg*

Introduction

Childbearing is an amazing and biologically complex process. From pregnancy through to the early postpartum period, reproduction-related hormonal and neuro-hormonal systems facilitate adaptive physiological processes in both mother and foetus/baby that promote survival and safety for both.[1, 2]

Over millions of years of mammalian evolution, these hormonal processes have also supported successful lactation and maternal-infant bonding/attachment, both essential to species survival for all mammals, and biologically 'intertwined and continuous' with the processes of labour and birth.[1, 2]

Clinicians and researchers are increasingly acknowledging the importance and influence of the intricate neurohormonal orchestration of physiological birth, including long-term positive effects for mothers and babies.[1-5] However, fewer women and babies are experiencing the full hormonal orchestration of physiological birth, due to rising rates of interventions worldwide.[6]

There is currently limited understanding of the impacts of interventions during and immediately after childbirth on these delicate, adaptive, organising processes. Current biological knowledge predicts that these positive effects could be disrupted by interventions, with possible longer-term consequences.[7-9]

This chapter summarises key knowledge and research findings in this area, focusing on the oxytocin system, the hypothalamic-pituitary-adrenal (HPA) axis (including cortisol), the autonomic nervous system (ANS) and other neurogenic and hormonal systems that mediate stress adaptations in childbearing.

Hormonal systems of physiologic childbearing

Oxytocin

Oxytocin is a hormone (a messenger substance that circulates in the blood) produced in the supraoptic and the paraventricular nuclei, two cell groups within the hypothalamus, an old part of the brain. The 'magnocellular' (big-cell) neurons in these centres connect to the posterior pituitary, from where oxytocin is released into the circulation, including during labour, birth and breastfeeding. Oxytocin is also produced in 'parvocellular' (small-cell) neurons in the paraventricular nucleus, which connect to important regulatory areas within the brain.[2]

Oxytocin released into the brain from the paraventricular nucleus can influence behavioural and physiological processes, including activating pain-relief and dopamine-associated pleasure and reward pathways. Acting via neurogenic mechanisms, oxytocin stimulates social interactions, reduces fear, decreases stress and induces calm and relaxation.[2]

In addition, oxytocin influences the hypothalamic-pituitary-adrenal axis and the autonomic nervous system, activating the parasympathetic nervous system, and inhibiting the hypothalamic-pituitary-adrenal axis as well as the sympathetic nervous system ('fight-or-flight' system). This results in anti-stress and relaxation effects. In addition, oxytocin enhances growth and healing.[2]

Another important oxytocin connection in relation to labour and birth is from the paraventricular nucleus to parasympathetic areas in the lower spinal cord. Oxytocin nerves from the brain activate the parasympathetic 'sacral plexus', which increases uterine contractions and blood flow.[2]

Oxytocin is a polypeptide hormone, made from small protein building-blocks. Oxytocin consists of nine amino acids and, like other polypeptide hormones, does not easily penetrate biological membranes, including the placental membrane and blood-brain barrier. Studies estimate that, when a high dose of synthetic oxytocin is administered into the circulation, only about one-thousandth reaches the brain.[10] This means that infusions of synthetic oxytocin administered during labour, birth or the postpartum period are not likely to reach the brain in biologically significant amounts.

Synthetic oxytocin is biochemically identical to endogenous (naturally produced) oxytocin. When synthetic oxytocin is administered directly into the brain of animals, it stimulates social behaviours, including maternal behaviour; decreases anxiety and aggression; decreases pain; and stimulates growth and healing.[11] Administration of synthetic oxytocin to humans via nasal spray (which appears to bypass the blood-brain barrier in some way[12]) appears to induce some of these effects, in particular social behaviours.

When oxytocin systems are activated in physiological situations such as labour and birth, breastfeeding and skin-to-skin contact, some of these effects are observed. At these times, stimulation of sensory nerves (e.g. in the reproductive tract, nipples, and skin) triggers oxytocin activity in the brain.[2]

Cortisol, the hypothalamic-pituitary-adrenal axis, and hormonal stress adaptations in childbearing

Cortisol is a steroid hormone derived from cholesterol. It is produced in the adrenal glands, which are situated above each kidney. Steroid hormones also include the sex hormones (oestrogen, testosterone etc.) and, unlike polypeptides, can easily pass biological membranes including the blood-brain barrier and placenta.

Cortisol is part of the hypothalamic-pituitary-adrenal axis. The hypothalamic-pituitary-adrenal axis is a hormonal pathway, ultimately controlled by corticotrophin releasing factor (CRF), which is released from the paraventricular nucleus and triggers the release of adrenocorticotrophic hormone (ACTH) from the pituitary into the circulation. Subsequently, ACTH stimulates cortisol release from the adrenal glands. In the brain, CRF release also activates the sympathetic nervous system and physiological fight-or-flight responses.

Cortisol is vital for life and necessary for most biological processes. When cortisol levels are too high, negative feedback processes inhibit activity in the entire hypothalamic-pituitary-adrenal axis, restoring activity to normal levels (homeostasis). Excessive, sustained cortisol levels, reflecting unhealthy stress and an overactive hypothalamic-pituitary-adrenal axis, can cause long-term harms, including in conditions such as hypertension, anxiety and depression.[2]

Oxytocin and cortisol in physiological labour and birth

The physiological (spontaneous) onset of labour is regulated by biological cues from both the baby and the mother. The uterotonic (uterine-contracting) properties of oxytocin play an important role.

Maternal oxytocin levels rise during pregnancy in response to increasing oestrogen levels, which also increase (upregulate) oxytocin receptor numbers in the uterus. This upregulation increases uterine sensitivity to oxytocin, so that relatively low oxytocin levels will effectively stimulate uterine contractions at physiological labour onset. Close to term, transient pulses of oxytocin occur, increasing in amplitude and frequency through labour to reach around three short pulses per ten minutes in late labour.[13, 14]

In the final stages of labour, pressure of the foetal head against the birthing woman's cervix and lower vagina activates sensory nerves that send signals via the spinal cord to her supraoptic nucleus and paraventricular nucleus to release oxytocin into both the circulation and brain. This positive feedback ('Ferguson reflex'[15]) induces more uterine contractions, more pressure on the cervix and vagina, and therefore more oxytocin release. At birth, maternal oxytocin levels, as measured in the blood, are three to four times higher than during late labour.[14, 16, 17] Elevated oxytocin levels in the brain may persist even longer.[18]

The autonomic nervous system also influences uterine contractions. Excessive labour stress, for example due to high levels of fear and pain, leads to increased sympathetic nervous system activity. Elevated noradrenaline, via the sympathetic nerves, causes more prolonged and painful uterine contractions, and at the same time reduces blood supply to the uterus and baby.[19, 20] More intense fear and stress can trigger even stronger labour-inhibiting processes such as adrenaline release from the adrenal gland, which reflects greater recruitment of the sympathetic nervous system.[5] Some types of milder stress, such as unfamiliar surroundings and people, may only inhibit oxytocin release and thereby uterine contractions.[2]

In contrast, activation of the uterine parasympathetic nerves via the sacral plexus increases contraction efficiency as well as uterine blood flow. Touch, warmth and friendly, supportive behaviour are good activators of the parasympathetic nervous system, and may therefore optimise labour efficacy as well as blood supply to the uterus and baby.[5]

The hypothalamic-pituitary-adrenal axis and cortisol also contribute to labour. Physiological cortisol elevations assist with inevitable but biologically adaptive levels of stress ('eustress'[21]), including by mobilising the necessary nutrients for the work of labour.[22] High cortisol levels increase the function of oxytocin receptors in some areas, including the brain,[23] likely to benefit the new mother through to early postpartum.

Skin-to-skin contact and oxytocin after birth

In the immediate postpartum period, when the baby is in skin-to-skin contact, newborn breast massage and suckling stimulate oxytocin release in the mother.[24] Oxytocin release at this time is less pulsatile than during labour, with longer-lasting elevations.[16] Elevated oxytocin levels in the brain, together with increased oxytocin receptor sensitivity at this time due to high cortisol and oestrogen activity, promote interaction and bonding between mother and newborn.[25]

Postpartum oxytocin elevations in the circulation contract the new mother's uterus to prevent bleeding, and dilate blood vessels on her chest wall (vasodilation), providing warmth for her newborn baby.[26]

For the newborn, skin-to-skin contact also stimulates sensory nerves and oxytocin release, optimising readiness for interactions such as breastfeeding and bonding, and promoting resilience to stress.[5, 27]

Postpartum skin-to-skin contact and oxytocin powerfully inhibit stress responses for both mother and baby. Reductions in sympathetic nervous system activity lead to decreases in newborn heart rate and increased circulation in maternal and newborn skin. Decreases in hypothalamic-pituitary-adrenal activity lead to declining cortisol for both mother and baby.[27, 28, 29] Social interactions are stimulated in both.[5]

These anti-stress and pro-social effects during the 'early sensitive period' may contribute to the longer-term benefits of early skin-to-skin contact.[30] For example, studies have found positive effects of early skin-to-skin contact on mother-baby interactions and bonding from birth up to three years later.[31-34] A contemporary randomised study found more positive interactions and better infant stress resilience at one year for those receiving two hours of skin-to-skin contact, compared to those without this contact.[9]

Very high levels of oxytocin released within the maternal brain from birth to the early postpartum period also contribute to pain relief, via endogenous opioids, and activate pleasure and reward centres via dopamine release. Cortisol, endorphins, and adrenaline may also contribute to the euphoric effects for mother and baby following physiological birth.[1] Rewiring of maternal reward centres[35] ensures that the baby is a source of pleasure for the new mother, and is an important motivator of maternal behaviours for all mammals.[1, 36, 37]

The adaptive long-term changes in personality that women have been found to experience following physiological birth, including reduced anxiety and increased sociability,[2, 38] are also likely to be due to perinatal oxytocin released within the so-called 'social brain', especially the amygdala.[2] These personality changes are strongly correlated with maternal oxytocin levels during breastfeeding.[38]

Foetal/newborn hormones in the perinatal period

Foetal/newborn safety during labour and birth is enhanced by parallel hormonal processes, which also promote longer-term offspring wellbeing.

Foetal pre-labour cortisol elevations help to mature foetal organs, including the lungs. Foetal cortisol elevations are coordinated with the maternal oestrogen elevations that prepare the mother's body for labour and birth. This occurs via placental biochemical processes, along with other pre-labour physiological preparations.[1]

The foetal to newborn transition is further facilitated by the late-labour 'foetal catecholamine surge', an enormous outpouring of adrenaline and noradrenaline that is triggered by low oxygen levels (hypoxia) in combination with pressure on the descending head.[39] At this time, catecholamines increase cerebral blood supply, reduce cerebral and metabolic vulnerability to hypoxia, and begin preparations for life outside the womb. These preparations include: reducing lung fluid; dilating the airways; and increasing surfactant (the lung lubricant) to support a successful respiratory transition. Newborn temperature and blood glucose regulation are also enhanced.[39,40] Noradrenaline elevations in the newborn brain support alertness and learning, and facilitate learning the mother's odours.[41]

The baby's oxytocin system is well developed before birth. Foetal oxytocin elevations from labour to postpartum assist with stress and pain reduction[42, 43] and counteract hypoxia and hypoxic cellular damage from labour to the newborn period,[43] likely working in concert with the catecholamines. As described above, postpartum skin-to-skin contact stimulates newborn oxytocin release and promotes readiness for breastfeeding and bonding.[1, 5, 27]

Hormonal impacts of perinatal interventions

Every medical procedure has benefits and risks. Interventions such as caesarean surgery, epidural analgesia, and/or infusions of synthetic oxytocin (Syntocinon, Pitocin) can be clearly beneficial in some situations. However, knowledge about basic biological systems, and the limited research that specifically targets this area, both suggest that many common procedures can disrupt the neuro-hormonal cascades of physiological birth. Possible short- and long-term effects of such disruptions include impacts on breastfeeding and maternal-infant attachment, and even maternal mental health.[1, 2] This section summarises some of this evidence to date.

Caesareans

Caesarean surgery, especially pre-labour (elective) caesarean, is the most impactful intervention because of the absence of the hormonal and neurohormonal orchestration for mother and baby.[1, 2, 39] With pre-labour caesarean, both mother and baby will miss the full pre-labour preparations, as well as in-labour hormonal and neurohormonal processes, including oxytocin pulses and peaks.[1, 2]

In one pre-labour caesarean study, new mothers had no oxytocin release in response to immediate newborn skin-to-skin contact and suckling. These mothers also had reductions in the personality changes that usually follow physiological birth, as discussed above, including reduced anxiety and increased sociability. For those mothers who had received postpartum infusions of synthetic oxytocin for medical reasons, both the release of oxytocin in response to skin-to-skin contact and the personality changes were restored.[44] While the mechanism is unclear, postpartum infusion of synthetic oxytocin may have increased the sensitivity of the skin, facilitating oxytocin release in response to skin-to-skin postpartum. This supports the importance of perinatal oxytocin elevations to sensitise the maternal skin.

In another study, women who experienced either a pre-labour or in-labour (emergency) caesarean were found to have significantly fewer peaks of oxytocin during breastfeeding two days after birth, along with reduced milk ejection and lower levels of prolactin (which is partly triggered by oxytocin), compared to women experiencing vaginal birth.[45, 46] These deficits, likely to be due to a lack of perinatal oxytocin peaks, may contribute to lower breastfeeding success following caesarean.[47, 48]

For pre-labour caesarean newborns, problems that are commonly observed, including difficulties with respiratory transition, thermoregulation, low blood glucose and drowsiness, are predictable effects of the lack of labour-related peaks of catecholamines and cortisol,[39] along with low oxytocin activity.[2]

Together, these findings suggest that women and babies experiencing caesarean, especially pre-labour caesarean, may need extra support with attachment and early breastfeeding. Liberal mother-baby contact, especially skin-to-skin, and long-term breastfeeding may help to fill these hormonal gaps.[1, 27, 28]

Epidural analgesia

Epidurals offer the most effective analgesia for labour and birth, but can have significant impacts on hormonal and neurohormonal processes. This is due to the effectiveness of epidural analgesia, which literally blocks the sensory information from the labouring mother's uterus from reaching her brain. This loss disrupts the positive feedback to her brain, as discussed above, and reduces oxytocin release, as measured in the blood.[20, 49, 50] Infusions of synthetic oxytocin are frequently required to restore contractions and labour progress.[51] Cortisol release is also disrupted by epidural analgesia.[20, 50]

Based on animal studies, epidurals also reduce oxytocin in the maternal brain, which disrupts bonding and maternal behaviours.[18, 52-54] Consistent with this lower oxytocin release, one human study found lower suckling-related prolactin levels two days after birth among women who had used a labour epidural, compared to women who did not use an epidural.[55] Researchers have also found reductions in the adaptive long-term personality changes that follow physiological birth among women using epidurals.[56]

Other studies have also found overall deficits in breastfeeding initiation and continuation, although research in this area is concerningly limited.[57]

In relation to newborn effects, one study looked at epidural-exposed infants two days after birth and found an absence of the usual skin-temperature rise with skin-to-skin/breastfeeding.[58] This suggests some disruption to the warming effects of oxytocin for mother and/or newborn.[26]

Another study found that epidurals, or other analgesics containing local anaesthetic drugs, disturb the immediate behaviours of newborns, including reduced breast-seeking and hand massage.[59] These drugs may also reduce the new mother's skin sensitivity to, and release of, oxytocin in response to breast massage by her newborn.[60] This could be due to numbing of the sensory nerves for mother and/or baby.

Infusions of synthetic oxytocin

Intravenous infusions of synthetic oxytocin are commonly used to initiate or augment labour, and may also be given routinely postpartum, including intravenously, to prevent or stop bleeding.

While synthetic oxytocin is chemically identical to endogenous oxytocin, as discussed, there are major differences from a functional point of view. When endogenous oxytocin is released during physiological labour, it is released into the circulation as short pulses, and is also released into the brain, where it activates the parasympathetic nervous system and reduces pain, among other beneficial effects. When synthetic oxytocin is administered as a constant infusion, flat blood levels are obtained, compared to the short, high oxytocin pulses of physiological labour.[14] Also, due to the blood-brain barrier, synthetic oxytocin doesn't reach the brain, and therefore doesn't directly influence brain function and these beneficial effects.[2]

Synthetic oxytocin administered by infusion at low levels, up to 10 milliunits/minute, gives similar oxytocin levels, as measured in the blood, to physiologic birth.[14, 61] This low dose can effectively trigger contractions when uterine oxytocin receptor numbers and sensitivity are optimal, close to physiological labour onset.[13] Administering synthetic oxytocin via a pulsatile, rather than constant, infusion reduces the total amount of oxytocin required. (For review, see[14])

Some studies have found lower anxiety and increased social interactions in women two days postpartum who had received perinatal synthetic oxytocin, when compared to unexposed women.[44, 56] This may reflect stronger synthetic oxytocin-driven contractions, which increase brain oxytocin release during birth, via an enhanced Ferguson reflex.

However, infusions of synthetic oxytocin during labour, especially in high doses, can have detrimental effects on uterine activity. This is most likely due to the abnormal, flat oxytocin curve that lacks the nadirs seen during physiological labour.[14] Uterine contractions generally become longer, stronger, closer together and more painful, which may alter feedback through nervous mechanisms to the brain.[2] Stress and pain cause increased activity in the hypothalamic-pituitary-adrenal axis and the sympathetic nervous system, leading to elevated noradrenaline and adrenaline, and even more intense and painful uterine contractions. This excessive stress and over-activation of the sympathetic nervous system will disrupt sympathetic-parasympathetic balance in labour, reducing beneficial parasympathetic activity, even when pain is inhibited by epidural.

Some negative postpartum effects of infusions of synthetic oxytocin in labour have been documented. One study found lower breastfeeding-related release of endogenous oxytocin, two days after birth, among women who had been exposed to such infusions in labour, compared to those who were not exposed. In this study, higher synthetic oxytocin exposure, especially in combination with epidural analgesia, correlated with lower oxytocin levels.[62]

These researchers also found higher baseline cortisol levels in new mothers exposed to infusions of synthetic oxytocin in labour, compared to controls, with a delayed and reduced fall during breastfeeding, compared to the larger fall in unexposed women. This difference may reflect a disruption to the normal anti-stress effect of breastfeeding.[63] These findings suggest ongoing increased activity in the mother's stress system following exposure to infusions of synthetic oxytocin in labour, which could have future implications for maternal physical and mental wellbeing.

For the foetus, the longer, stronger, closer-together contractions will reduce uterine blood flow to some extent, which can cause or exacerbate hypoxia.[64, 65] Researchers have also found an exaggerated newborn skin-temperature response to skin-to-skin/breastfeeding following synthetic oxytocin exposure in labour.[58] Such impacts could arise from increased maternal chest-wall vasodilation causing reduced newborn sympathetic nervous system activity, and consequently increased skin temperature in the newborn.

Co-administration of intrapartum interventions

It is very common for interventions to be co-administered, with additive or even multiplied effects for mother and baby. Women receiving infusions of synthetic oxytocin most often receive an epidural because of pain, and those receiving an epidural most often receive infusions of synthetic oxytocin because of a decrease in endogenous oxytocin, leading to ineffective contractions.

In the study mentioned above, women who received both epidurals and infusions of synthetic oxytocin had lower oxytocin levels and higher cortisol when breastfeeding on day two, compared to women who received only synthetic oxytocin, with a dose-dependent effect for both synthetic oxytocin and epidurals.[63] This interaction between epidurals and infusions of synthetic oxytocin seems to cause an imbalance between the stress system (hypothalamic-pituitary-adrenal) and the anti-stress effects of oxytocin. This imbalance was seen two days after birth, but could have longer-lasting effects.

Recent studies have suggested that synthetic oxytocin exposure in labour might increase the risks of maternal anxiety and depression.[66, 67] These findings could reflect a long-term effect of the stress–anti-stress imbalance found in mothers who received both infusions of synthetic oxytocin and epidurals in labour, as described above. The long-term mental health and wellbeing of new mothers is obviously of critical importance. High-quality research is urgently needed, including studies that assess the possible impacts of epidurals and infusions of synthetic oxytocin, including their co-administration.

Discussion and conclusion

During physiological labour and birth, neurohormonal systems induce a multitude of adaptations that promote the processes of labour and birth, and optimise physiology for mother and baby. During labour, oxytocin elevations relieve maternal anxiety and stimulate social interactions, and the oxytocin peaks of late labour activate brain reward centres, creating positive, pleasurable feelings. Pain is relieved for both mother and baby throughout labour.

These neurohormonal processes continue to support mothers and babies after birth. Postpartum skin-to-skin contact releases oxytocin, counteracting the enormous stresses of birth and facilitating the positive interactions that promote bonding. Experiences during this early sensitive period may have long-term consequences for mother and/or baby.

Perinatal interventions can disrupt these delicate neurohormonal systems and critically impact physiological adaptations for mother and baby. For example, with a pre-labour caesarean, lack of the foetal catecholamine surge in labour contributes to increased newborn respiratory morbidity, and the beneficial effects of cortisol and oxytocin elevations will be absent for mother and baby. In addition, the stress relief that is usually facilitated by early skin-to-skin contact can be disrupted by post-operative separation, impacting mother-baby bonding during this sensitive period.

Epidural analgesia has also been found to disrupt these adaptive hormonal processes. Epidurals reduce sensory information from the uterus to the mother. This blocks not only pain, but also the important Ferguson reflex, which drives labour progress via a positive feedback cycle. Maternal oxytocin is reduced in the circulation and also in the brain, where its calming effects are diminished, potentially also impacting postpartum pleasure and bonding, as well as adaptive personality changes.

Infusions of synthetic oxytocin do not reach the brain in biologically significant amounts, but have been shown to negatively impact hormonal processes. In labour, synthetic oxytocin increases activity in the hypothalamic-pituitary-adrenal axis and sympathetic nervous system, probably due to abnormally strong uterine contractions. These effects may be caused by abnormal oxytocin patterns, with high and flat levels and no peaks.

In conclusion, current biological understandings and research, as presented in this chapter, are consistent with the premise that physiological childbirth optimises the transition for mother and baby and enhances wellbeing. These effects can be observed in the short term and might have ongoing, sustained benefits. Common maternity-care interventions may disrupt these adaptive processes.

While studies are urgently needed to confirm and extend these findings, we believe that there is already sufficient evidence to promote a shift in maternity care services towards protecting, supporting and promoting physiological childbirth, and safeguarding healthy mothers and babies from unnecessary interventions.

Key points for consideration

- More research is urgently needed on the short and longer-term hormonal and physiological impacts of common birth interventions for mothers and offspring, including longer-term follow up of breastfeeding, mother-infant attachment, and mental and physical wellbeing.

- In the absence of evidence that obstetric interventions are safe and beneficial in the longer term, these should only be used when a strong indication exists for mother and/or baby.

- In order to facilitate informed decision-making in labour and birth, maternity care providers should give women and families the full information, including the benefits of physiological birth for mothers and babies, and the likely impacts of interventions in the short and longer-terms, as discussed above.

- Increased access to models of care that support physiological birth and have been shown to improve outcomes for mothers and babies, including midwifery care, birth centres, midwife-run maternity units and supportive birth companions (doulas).

- Increased awareness and support for maternity care providers to give friendly, supportive care in labour. This will reduce sympathetic activity and increase parasympathetic activity for the labouring woman and trigger the hormonal and neurohormonal conditions that enable an efficient and safe labour and birth.

- Provide practical and policy support for mother and newborn through immediate postpartum skin-to-skin contact, which promotes oxytocin and parasympathetic nervous system 'rest and digest', and fosters mutual calm and connection. Immediate skin-to-skin also supports newborn-initiated breastfeeding and long-term lactation, with longer-term benefits for both.

References

1   Buckley SJ. Hormonal Physiology of Childbearing: Evidence and Implications for Women, Babies, and Maternity Care. Washington, DC: National Partnership for Women & Families; 2015.
2   Uvnäs Moberg K. Oxytocin: The Biological Guide to Motherhood. Plano, Texas: Hale Publishing; 2015.
3   Kenkel WM, Yee JR, Carter CS. Is oxytocin a maternal-foetal signalling molecule at birth? Implications for development. Journal of neuroendocrinology. 2014;26(10):739-49.
4   Olza-Fernandez I, Marin Gabriel MA, Gil-Sanchez A, Garcia-Segura LM, Arevalo MA. Neuroendocrinology of childbirth and mother-child attachment: the basis of an etiopathogenic model of perinatal neurobiological disorders. Frontiers in neuroendocrinology. 2014;35(4):459-72.
5   Uvnäs Moberg K. How kindness, warmth, empathy and support promote the progress of labour: a physiological perspective. In: Byrom S, Downe S, editors. The Roar Behind the Silence: Why kindness, warmth, compassion and respect matter in maternity care London UK: Pinter and Martin; 2015.
6   Miller SE, Abalos M, Chamillard A, Ciapponi D, Colaci D, Comande V, et al. Beyond too little, too late and too much, too soon: a pathway towards evidence-based, respectful maternity care worldwide. Lancet. 2016;388(10056): 2176-2192.
7   Dahlen HG, Downe S, Wright ML, Kennedy HP, Taylor JY. Childbirth and consequent atopic disease: emerging evidence on epigenetic effects based on the hygiene and EPIIC hypotheses. BMC pregnancy and childbirth. 2016;16:4.
8   Dahlen HG, Kennedy HP, Anderson CM, Bell AF, Clark A, Foureur M, et al. The EPIIC hypothesis: intrapartum

effects on the neonatal epigenome and consequent health outcomes. Medical hypotheses. 2013;80(5):656-62.

9   Bystrova K, Ivanova V, Edhborg M, Matthiesen AS, Ransjo-Arvidson AB, Mukhamedrakhimov R, et al. Early contact versus separation: effects on mother-infant interaction one year later. Birth (Berkeley, Calif). 2009;36(2):97-109.

10 Jones PM, Robinson IC. Differential clearance of neurophysin and neurohypophysial peptides from the cerebrospinal fluid in conscious guinea pigs. Neuroendocrinology. 1982;34(4):297-302.

11 Uvnäs Moberg K. The Oxytocin Factor. Cambridge MA: Da Capo Press; 2003.

12 Neumann ID, Maloumby R, Beiderbeck DI, Lukas M, Landgraf R. Increased brain and plasma oxytocin after nasal and peripheral administration in rats and mice. Psychoneuroendocrinology. 2013;38(10):1985-93.

13 Fuchs AR, Romero R, Keefe D, Parra M, Oyarzun E, Behnke E. Oxytocin secretion and human parturition: pulse frequency and duration increase during spontaneous labor in women. American journal of obstetrics and gynecology. 1991;165(5 Pt 1):1515-23.

14 Uvnäs Moberg K, Ekstrom A, Berg M, Buckley, S, Pajalic, Z, Hadjigeorgiou E, et al. Plasma levels of oxytocin during physiological childbirth- a systematic review with implications for uterine contractions and central actions of oxytocin. 2019; In press.

15 Ferguson J. A study of the motility of the intact uterus at term. Surg Gynaecol Obstet. 1941;73:359-66.

16 Nissen E, Lilja G, Widstrom AM, Uvnäs Moberg K. Elevation of oxytocin levels early post partumin women. Acta obstetricia et gynecologica Scandinavica. 1995;74(7):530-3.

17 Goodfellow CF, Hull MG, Swaab DF, Dogterom J, Buijs RM. Oxytocin deficiency at delivery with epidural analgesia. British journal of obstetrics and gynaecology. 1983;90(3):214-9.

18 Keverne EB, Kendrick KM. Oxytocin facilitation of maternal behavior in sheep. Annals of the New York Academy of Sciences. 1992;652:83-101.

19 Sato Y, Hotta H, Nakayama H, Suzuki H. Sympathetic and parasympathetic regulation of the uterine blood flow and contraction in the rat. Journal of the autonomic nervous system. 1996;59(3):151-8.

20 Alehagen S, Wijma B, Lundberg U, Wijma K. Fear, pain and stress hormones during childbirth. Journal of psychosomatic obstetrics and gynaecology. 2005;26(3):153-65.

21 Selye H. Stress and distress. Compr Ther. 1975;1(8):9-13.

22 Risberg A, Sjoquist M, Wedenberg K, Larsson A. Elevated glucose levels in early puerperium, and association with high cortisol levels during parturition. Scand J Clin Lab Invest. 2016;76(4):309-12.

23 Liberzon I, Chalmers DT, Mansour A, Lopez JF, Watson SJ, Young EA. Glucocorticoid regulation of hippocampal oxytocin receptor binding. Brain research. 1994;650(2):317-22.

24 Matthiesen AS, Ransjo-Arvidson AB, Nissen E, Uvnäs Moberg K. Postpartum maternal oxytocin release by newborns: effects of infant hand massage and sucking. Birth (Berkeley, Calif). 2001;28(1):13-9.

25. Velandia M. Parent-infant Skin-to-Skin Contact Studies. Stockholm, Sweden: Karolinska Institutet; 2012.

26 Bystrova K, Matthiesen AS, Vorontsov I, Widstrom AM, Ransjo-Arvidson AB, Uvnäs Moberg K. Maternal axillar and breast temperature after giving birth: effects of delivery ward practices and relation to infant temperature. Birth (Berkeley, Calif). 2007;34(4):291-300.

27 Bystrova K, Widstrom AM, Matthiesen AS, Ransjo-Arvidson AB, Welles-Nystrom B, Wassberg C, et al. Skin-to-skin contact may reduce negative consequences of "the stress of being born": a study on temperature in newborn infants, subjected to different ward routines in St. Petersburg. Acta paediatrica (Oslo, Norway : 1992). 2003;92(3):320-6.

28 Chi Luong N, Long Nguyen T, Huynh Thi DH, Carrara HP, Bergman NJ. Newly born low birthweight infants stabilise better in skin-to-skin contact than when separated from their mothers: a randomised controlled trial. Acta paediatrica (Oslo, Norway : 1992). 2016;105(4):381-90.

29 Takahashi Y, Tamakoshi K, Matsushima M, Kawabe T. Comparison of salivary cortisol, heart rate, and oxygen saturation between early skin-to-skin contact with different initiation and duration times in healthy, full-term infants. Early human development. 2011;87(3):151-7.

30 Moore ER, Bergman N, Anderson GC, Medley N. Early skin-to-skin contact for mothers and their healthy newborn infants. Cochrane database of systematic reviews (Online). 2016;11:CD003519.

31 Klaus MH, Jerauld R, Kreger NC, McAlpine W, Steffa M, Kennel JH. Maternal attachment. Importance of the first post-partum days. The New England journal of medicine. 1972;286(9):460-3.

32 de Chateau P, Wiberg B. Long-term effect on mother-infant behaviour of extra contact during the first hour post partum. I. First observations at 36 hours. Acta paediatrica Scandinavica. 1977;66(2):137-43.

33 de Chateau P, Wiberg B. Long-term effect on mother-infant behaviour of extra contact during the first hour post partum. III. Follow-up at one year. Scand J Soc Med. 1984;12(2):91-103.

34 Wiberg B, Humble K, de Chateau P. Long-term effect on mother-infant behaviour of extra contact during the first hour post partum. V. Follow-up at three years. Scand J Soc Med. 1989;17(2):181-91.

35 Swain JE, Tasgin E, Mayes LC, Feldman R, Constable RT, Leckman JF. Maternal brain response to own baby-cry is affected by cesarean section delivery. Journal of child psychology and psychiatry, and allied disciplines. 2008;49(10):1042-52.

36 Kristal MB. The biopsychology of maternal behavior in nonhuman mammals. ILAR journal / National Research Council, Institute of Laboratory Animal Resources. 2009;50(1):51-63.

37 Nelson EE, Panksepp J. Brain substrates of infant-mother attachment: contributions of opioids, oxytocin, and norepinephrine. Neuroscience and biobehavioral reviews. 1998;22(3):437-52.

38 Uvnäs Moberg K, Widsröm AM, Nissen E, Björvell H. Personality traits in women 4 days postpartum and their correlation with plasma levels of oxytocin and prolactin. Journal of psychosomatic obstetrics and gynaecology. 1990;11:261-73.

39 Lagercrantz H, Slotkin TA. The "stress" of being born. Scientific American. 1986;254(4):100-7.

40 Hillman NH, Kallapur SG, Jobe AH. Physiology of transition from intrauterine to extrauterine life. Clinics in perinatology. 2012;39(4):769-83.

41 Varendi H, Porter RH, Winberg J. The effect of labor on olfactory exposure learning within the first postnatal hour. Behavioral neuroscience. 2002;116(2):206-11, p 10.

42 Mazzuca M, Minlebaev M, Shakirzyanova A, Tyzio R, Taccola G, Janackova S, et al. Newborn Analgesia Mediated by Oxytocin during Delivery. Frontiers in cellular neuroscience. 2011;5:3.

43 Ceanga M, Spataru A, Zagrean AM. Oxytocin is neuroprotective against oxygen-glucose deprivation and reoxygenation in immature hippocampal cultures. Neuroscience letters. 2010;477(1):15-8.

44 Velandia M, Uvnäs Moberg K, Nissen E. Maternal KSP profile 2 days after elective caesarean: influence of skin-to-skin contact and exogenous oxytocin. Department of Women's and Children's Health2014.

45 Nissen E, Uvnäs Moberg K, Svensson K, Stock S, Widstrom AM, Winberg J. Different patterns of oxytocin, prolactin but not cortisol release during breastfeeding in women delivered by caesarean section or by the vaginal route. Early human development. 1996;45(1-2):103-18.

46 Nissen E, Gustavsson P, Widstrom AM, Uvnäs Moberg K. Oxytocin, prolactin, milk production and their relationship with personality traits in women after vaginal delivery or Cesarean section. Journal of psychosomatic obstetrics and gynaecology. 1998;19(1):49-58.

47 Hobbs AJ, Mannion CA, McDonald SW, Brockway M, Tough SC. The impact of caesarean section on breastfeeding initiation, duration and difficulties in the first four months postpartum. BMC pregnancy and childbirth. 2016;16:90.

48 Prior E, Santhakumaran S, Gale C, Philipps LH, Modi N, Hyde MJ. Breastfeeding after cesarean delivery: a systematic review and meta-analysis of world literature. The American journal of clinical nutrition. 2012;95(5):1113-35.

49 Rahm VA, Hallgren A, Hogberg H, Hurtig I, Odlind V. Plasma oxytocin levels in women during labor with or without epidural analgesia: a prospective study. Acta obstetricia et gynecologica Scandinavica. 2002;81(11):1033-9.

50 Stocche RM, Klamt JG, Antunes-Rodrigues J, Garcia LV, Moreira AC. Effects of intrathecal sufentanil on plasma oxytocin and cortisol concentrations in women during the first stage of labor. Regional anesthesia and pain medicine. 2001;26(6):545-50.

51 Anim-Somuah M, Smyth RM, Jones L. Epidural versus non-epidural or no analgesia in labour. Cochrane database of systematic reviews (Online). 2011(12):CD000331.

52 Krehbiel D, Poindron P, Levy F, Prud'Homme MJ. Peridural anesthesia disturbs maternal behavior in primiparous and multiparous parturient ewes. Physiology & behavior. 1987;40(4):463-72.

53 Levy F, Kendrick KM, Keverne EB, Piketty V, Poindron P. Intracerebral oxytocin is important for the onset of maternal behavior in inexperienced ewes delivered under peridural anesthesia. Behavioral neuroscience. 1992;106(2):427-32.

54 Williams GL, Gazal OS, Leshin LS, Stanko RL, Anderson LL. Physiological regulation of maternal behavior in heifers: roles of genital stimulation, intracerebral oxytocin release, and ovarian steroids. Biology of reproduction. 2001;65(1):295-300.

55 Jonas K, Johansson LM, Nissen E, Ejdeback M, Ransjo-Arvidson AB, Uvnäs Moberg K. Effects of intrapartum oxytocin administration and epidural analgesia on the concentration of plasma oxytocin and prolactin, in response to suckling during the second day postpartum. Breastfeeding medicine : the official journal of the Academy of Breastfeeding Medicine. 2009;4(2):71-82.

56 Jonas W, Nissen E, Ransjo-Arvidson AB, Matthiesen AS, Uvnäs Moberg K. Influence of oxytocin or epidural analgesia on personality profile in breastfeeding women: a comparative study. Archives of women's mental health. 2008;11(5-6):335-45.

57 French CA, Cong X, Chung KS. Labor Epidural Analgesia and Breastfeeding: A Systematic Review. Journal of human lactation : official journal of International Lactation Consultant Association. 2016;32(3):507-20.

58 Jonas W, Wiklund I, Nissen E, Ransjo-Arvidson AB, Uvnäs Moberg K. Newborn skin temperature two days postpartum during breastfeeding related to different labour ward practices. Early human development. 2007;83(1):55-62.

59 Ransjo-Arvidson AB, Matthiesen AS, Lilja G, Nissen E, Widstrom AM, Uvnäs Moberg K. Maternal analgesia during labor disturbs newborn behavior: effects on breastfeeding, temperature, and crying. Birth (Berkeley, Calif). 2001;28(1):5-12.

60 Matthiesen AS, Ransjo-Arvidson AB, Nissen E, Uvnäs Moberg K. Maternal analgesia reduces maternal sensitivity to infant breast massage. 2001.(Unpublished data, see (2).

61 Fuchs AR, Goeschen K, Husslein P, Rasmussen AB, Fuchs F. Oxytocin and initiation of human parturition. III. Plasma concentrations of oxytocin and 13,14-dihydro-15-keto-prostaglandin F2 alpha in spontaneous and oxytocin-induced labor at term. American journal of obstetrics and gynecology. 1983;147(5):497-502.

62 Jonas W, Johansson LM, Nissen E, Ejdeback M, Ransjo-Arvidson AB, Uvnäs Moberg K. Effects of Intrapartum Oxytocin Administration and Epidural Analgesia on the Concentration of Plasma Oxytocin and Prolactin, in Response to Suckling During the Second Day Postpartum. Breastfeeding medicine : the official journal of the Academy of Breastfeeding Medicine. 2009.

63 Handlin L, Jonas W, Petersson M, Ejdeback M, Ransjo-Arvidson AB, Nissen E, et al. Effects of sucking and skin-to-skin contact on maternal ACTH and cortisol levels during the second day postpartum-influence of epidural analgesia and oxytocin in the perinatal period. Breastfeeding medicine : the official journal of the Academy of Breastfeeding Medicine. 2009;4(4):207-20.

64 Clark SL, Simpson KR, Knox GE, Garite TJ. Oxytocin: new perspectives on an old drug. American journal of obstetrics and gynecology. 2008.

65 Sicor Pharmaceuticals. Oxytocin injection (package insert) 2006 [Available from: https://www.accessdata.fda.gov/drugsatfda_docs/label/2008/077453s000lbl.pdf.

66 Gu V, Feeley N, Gold I, Hayton B, Robins S, Mackinnon A, et al. Intrapartum Synthetic Oxytocin and Its Effects on Maternal Well-Being at 2 Months Postpartum. Birth (Berkeley, Calif). 2016;43(1):28-35.

67 Kroll-Desrosiers AR, Nephew BC, Babb JA, Guilarte-Walker Y, Moore Simas TA, Deligiannidis KM. Association of peripartum synthetic oxytocin administration and depressive and anxiety disorders within the first postpartum year. Depress Anxiety. 2017;34(2):137-46.

CHAPTER 3

Anatomy and physiology of labour and associated behavioural clues

Helen Cheyne and Margaret Duff

Introduction

When labour will start, what triggers onset, and at what rate it will progress are superficially simple questions about the physiology of pregnancy and birth, yet in practice they address highly complex processes that are not yet fully understood. This means that while labour and birth are likely to be the most regulated and controlled aspects of a woman's maternity journey, many important judgements and decisions are made in a context of uncertainty, with imperfect information, and outcomes may only become clear retrospectively. Recent research on the anatomy and physiology of labour has challenged many firmly held beliefs about the ways in which women will labour and give birth. These beliefs have underpinned systems of labour care for many decades, and have categorised and constrained the normal birth processes and women's innate behavioural responses. This chapter discusses some of the current research on the physiology of labour and associated behavioural cues, acknowledging that many uncertainties remain. Together with the other chapters in this book, it aims to stimulate and inform new thinking about the ways in which normal birth may flourish in a world that is increasingly interpreted through the lens of technology.

Categorising the labour continuum

While labour is, physiologically, a continuous process, it is typically described in the professional literature as having three distinct stages: latent and active first stage, second stage and third stage. Physiological characteristics and time boundaries are generally attributed to each stage. However, categorising labour in this way is largely pragmatic, and relatively recent. McCourt and Dykes (2010) suggest that the 'industrialisation of birth' through the latter half of the 20th century created an ethos of the production model that required definition of birth stages, so they could be counted, measured and controlled. In a study of historical sources, McIntosh (2013) found that early labour was not viewed as a discrete period until the second half of the 20th century and noted that diagnosis of labour only became important in industrialised models of childbirth, where the central organisation of care providers' workload became critical. Thus, notions of stages and normal or abnormal progress in labour largely arose as a result of the move to hospital birth. In contrast, Dixon et al (2013) found that, from a woman's perspective, labour is a continuous linear experience. They described this as an emotional journey moving through phases, including anticipation and excitement; calm and confidence; increasing intensity and being 'in the zone'; an overwhelming and uncontrollable sense of tiredness and feeling sleepy; and feeling the urge to push. This is reinforced by a recent review (Olza et al, 2018).

Anticipating the start of labour

Making the initial judgement that labour has started is a trigger and benchmark for subsequent assessments of labour progress and decisions about clinical interventions, thus a cascade of subsequent interventions may originate from this first key judgement. Yet it is an inherently uncertain judgement that has been described as one of the most important yet difficult in maternity care (Hanley et al, 2016). This is because the timing of physiological labour onset within the five-week period of normal term pregnancy cannot be accurately predicted, the trigger mechanisms are complex and not yet fully understood, there are no observable biological markers and there is no universal agreement on terminology or definition to guide and inform maternity care providers' prospective judgements and decisions about whether labour has started.

Hormonal trigger mechanisms for labour

As Uvnäs Moberg (2014) and Buckley (2015) have noted in Chapter 2 of this volume, hormonal and physiological processes for labour onset begin in the weeks before birth, long before the outward signs of labour become apparent. In brief, current thinking suggests that the process of normal term labour is triggered by the foetus (Buckley, 2015). A rise in corticotropin releasing hormone (CRH) produced by the placenta contributes to maturation of the foetal adrenal glands (the so-called 'placental clock'). The maturing foetal adrenal glands produce cortisol necessary for maturation of the lungs and other organs, and dehydroepiandrosterone-sulfate DHEAS (an oestrogen precursor) is converted to oestrogen in the placenta, leading to an increase in oxytocin receptors that in turn prepares myometrial cells for coordinated contractions of labour and supports cervical ripening. Rising levels of prostaglandins and relaxin promote loss of collagen in the cervix leading to softening and increased elasticity. Labour onset occurs at the point of peak sensitivity to oxytocin with an increase in the number of gap junctions, intercellular channels that allow direct diffusion of ions and small molecules between cells (Goodenough and Paul, 2009; Hanley et al, 2016). An increase in gap junctions propagates electrical conductivity in the myometrium, supporting the coordinated high-intensity uterine contractions of labour.

Recognising the start of labour

Research indicates that women and maternity care staff view the start of labour very differently. Women describe labour as starting with the earliest signs and report experiencing these in a variety of ways (Gross et al, 2003) including regular or irregular contractions, watery fluid loss, gastrointestinal disorders, sleeping difficulties, emotional disturbance, cramps, pain similar to menstrual pain with or without a mucoid vaginal 'show' and/or rupture of the membranes (Beebe and Humphreys, 2006; Dixon et al, 2013; Gross et al, 2003). In contrast, maternity care providers (and the professional literature) generally focus on the distinction between latent and active first stage, with much less attention given to recognising and defining when labour starts. A systematic review of 62 studies found that four different terms (and a wide range of definitions) were used (Hanley et al, 2016). These were latent, active, first stage, and non-specific 'labour'. The studies that defined the latent phase all included the presence of regular painful contractions, and 79% included cervical dilatation (ranging between >2 cm and <4 cm). Only three included cervical effacement or other symptoms, such as a bloody mucoid 'show' or gastrointestinal disturbance. The majority of studies that described the start of labour as either 'active labour' or non-specific 'labour' generally included cervical dilatation ranging between ≥2 cm to ≥4, or in terms of increasing cervical dilatation and regular painful uterine contractions with a range of definitions of what constituted 'regular'. A minority referred to cervical effacement. Seven studies included admission to hospital in their definition of labour onset, suggesting that current distinctions may be related to operational rather than physiological parameters (Hanley et al, 2016).

Abalos et al (2018) reviewed observational studies that reported on the definitions and duration of stages of normal pregnancy and labour. Of 37 included studies only six defined latent first stage. Three studies defined the end of this phase as, variously, cervical dilatation of 2.5, 3 and 4 centimetres dilatation, while the others described it as the time before admission or from reported onset of regular contractions until the onset of active labour. Similarly, the review found widely varying definitions of the start of active first stage including almost every degree of dilatation of the cervix.

The 2018 WHO intrapartum recommendations (2018) draw on evidence from these two reviews to describe the latent first stage as '*a period of time characterised by painful uterine contractions and variable changes of the cervix, including some degree of effacement and slower progression of dilatation*', thus acknowledging the continuing uncertainty in defining the earliest stage of labour. The WHO recommendations do, however, provide a definition of the start of the active first stage as the presence of '*regular painful uterine contractions, a substantial degree of cervical effacement and more rapid cervical dilatation from 5 cm*' (p35). The Consortium on Safe Labour (Zhang et al, 2010a) similarly does not define the onset of the latent first stage, but defines the onset of active labour as occurring when the woman's cervical os is between 5 and 6 centimetres dilated.

For professionals, the focus on the start of active first stage as a diagnostic point may be in an attempt to reduce uncertainty (Gross et al, 2009). However, when translated into practice this mismatch between the ways in which women and professionals think about and define the start of labour can be confusing and distressing for women, who may experience the dual anxieties of feeling that their labour has started, and of 'getting it wrong' when they try to gain admission to a hospital labour ward (Eri et al, 2015). Research on midwives' decision-making about early labour supports the notion that organisational factors as well as clinical factors influence the judgement that labour has started, with midwives acting as gatekeepers, both to manage labour ward workloads, and in responding to previous research evidence identifying that hospital admission in early labour was associated with increased rates of labour interventions (Cheyne et al, 2006).

Gross et al (2009) compared women's self-diagnosis and midwives' diagnosis of labour onset and the relationship between these and duration of first stage of labour. The study found that there was considerable variation between women's and midwives' judgements about when labour started, with women perceiving that labour was significantly longer than midwives' diagnostic judgements would suggest. However, the authors concluded that although they differed, both were valid and that women's self-report should be regarded and respected by clinicians in making judgements about labour onset and resultant care decisions. This principle has become even more important as emergent evidence has resulted in recommendations to define active first stage of labour as starting from cervical dilatation of six centimetres instead of three or four centimetres as previously indicated. This may be helpful in avoiding premature diagnosis of slow progress of labour (as discussed below). However, it also means that women may experience a sense of being in labour for a considerable length of time, and be considerably 'advanced' in the continuum of labour, at the point when care providers judge that labour has 'started'. It is imperative for maternity care staff to recognise and acknowledge this issue and that women's need for skilled maternity care and support during the whole time they experience labour should not be ignored until a professional makes a formal diagnosis of 'active labour'.

Physiological progress of labour

Until recently, received knowledge about the length and progress of labour had largely been based on work undertaken over 60 years ago (Friedman, 1954; Friedman, 1955). By plotting the degree of cervical dilatation against time in hours, Friedman produced a graphical representation of the 'ideal labour', and described latent, active, deceleration or transition phases. The latent phase was described as from labour onset to the start of the acceleration phase at around 4cm dilatation. Active labour was further subdivided into acceleration, maximal slope and deceleration (transition) phases. Cervical dilatation in the active phase was expected to be greater than 1.2cm per hour in a primiparous woman and greater than 1.5cm per hour in multiparous women. As Friedman's work became widely accepted and used, slower rates of dilatation came to be diagnosed as dysfunctional. Friedman's curve has dominated labour care throughout the last 60 years, forming the accepted parameters of normal and therefore abnormal patterns of labour progress. However, there is a growing body of research indicating that normal labour is likely to last considerably longer than suggested by Friedman. In a study of 1,473 women in 1996, Albers et al found that, based on Friedman's norms, 20% had a 'prolonged' active phase of labour, without increased morbidity. Hildingsson et al (2015) studied the duration of labour in 1,612 women who had planned home birth and spontaneous labour onset supported by midwives in four Nordic countries, finding that the median length of labour (from onset to birth) was 14 hours for primiparous women and 7.25 for multiparous women. The Consortium on Safe Labour (Zhang et al, 2010a) studied over 60,000 singleton, term spontaneous births. They found that cervical dilatation from 4 to 6 centimetres could take up to 9 hours in both primigravid and parous women. In this study, after 6 centimetres of cervical dilatation parous women experienced more rapid progress than primiparous women, and the second stage of labour was as long as 2.8 hours in primiparous women if they did not have an epidural in situ. Oladapou et al (2018) examined labour progression in a cohort of women in Uganda and Nigeria who had experienced spontaneous labour onset and vaginal birth. Findings indicated that for some women (primiparous and multiparous) the rate of cervical dilatation up to 5 centimetres was less than one centimetre per hour and that, within the parameters of normal, some primiparous women could take more than three hours to progress from five to six centimetres dilation.

These studies all indicate that physiological labour is more variable, and can progress at a far slower rate, than previously thought, and that a substantial number of women do not have a consistent pattern of cervical dilatation during the active phase of labour. Zhang et al, 2010a recommend a revision of definitions of the parameters of normal labour accounting for the acceleration phase of cervical dilatation starting at 6 centimetres (Zhang et al, 2010b; Zhang et al, 2010a). The American Congress of Obstetricians and Gynecologists (ACOG) now recommend adopting these findings (2017). The National Institute of Health Care Excellence (NICE) guidance (2017) also currently acknowledges the wide variation and non-linearity of normal active first-stage labour progress of up to 18 hours for primiparous women, and up to 12 hours for multiparous women, without the need for intervention to speed labour up. The 2018 WHO intrapartum care recommendations (2018) concur with this position. It appears that there is now no justification to implement rigid standardised timelines for physiological labour progress. Care should instead be individualised to the needs of each woman and her baby.

The impact of birth environment on women's experiences

Although childbirth is a biological process, it is also a psychosocial event. McCourt (2010) has observed that the way in which women respond to labour and birth may vary due to culturally enforced rules and rituals. The place of birth is both a physical and a spiritual space, which may affect the biophysical and hormonal changes that occur throughout labour, and as a result the woman's behavioural responses.

In a study to explore how different designs and birthing spaces affect women's labours and births the researchers compared childbirth in seven women: five who birthed in hospitals; one who birthed in a free-standing birthing centre and one who had a home birth. Through filming, the researchers observed that the women behaved differently depending on the birth space they occupied. Four of the five women who birthed in hospital became patients, responding passively to events and care providers, while women who birthed in the birth centre and at home took control of the space, moving about freely, doing as they wished. The researchers suggest that when women are in an environment they feel they can control, they behave differently and have more positive experiences (Mondy et al, 2016). This may include the shower. In a study which investigated the effects of showering for 30 minutes in 24 labouring women with no complications, Stark (2013) found that women moved around more freely in the shower than out of it, changing positions frequently, from sitting to standing, and support people were more likely to respect their privacy.

Psychological separation from the physical space was a theme that emerged from a study by Reed et al (2015). They explored women's stories of their physiological labour and birth and interpreted the women's stories into three phases: separating from the external world, being in their own world, and reintegration with the external world. In common with the findings of Mondy and colleagues (2016) and of Stark (2013), women talked about isolating themselves from supporters in the separation phase, and minimising external noise by moving away from the centre of a room, or to a smaller space, or creating a physical and aural barrier, for example, by using the shower.

Maternal physiological response to labour

As Uvnäs Moberg (2014) and Buckley (2015) have observed in Chapter 2 of this volume, unlike synthetic oxytocin which does not cross the blood–brain barrier, maternal oxytocin is released within the hypothalamus, flooding the brain and other systems with oxytocin levels up to 10 times higher than those found in maternal blood. At this time, high levels of oxytocin in the brain, fuelled by the sensations of uterine contractions, help the labouring woman by reducing fear, pain and stress, and increasing calm and connection, including through activation of her pleasure and reward centres in preparation for motherhood. It also assists in reducing blood pressure, heart rate, and digestion, and promotes rest, creating a calming effect. Oxytocin also stimulates beta-endorphins which aid in pain relief. These maternal oxytocin-based systems trigger reduction in stress, pain and fear during physiological labour (Buckley, 2015).

Oxytocin produced during labour also causes vasodilation of superficial blood vessels (Buckley, 2015) which can be observed as facial flushing (Johnstone, 1974). In a study that examined women's responses to labour when birthing in hospital, flushing of the women's faces was frequently recorded, but there were observed differences between spontaneous (n=63) and induced (n=31) labours (Duff, 2005). The study found that as labour progressed more nulliparous women labouring spontaneously developed flushed faces. Within three hours of full dilation of the cervix, 60% (n=38) had flushed faces. By the time the cervix was fully dilated, most women (90% or n=57) had flushing recorded. However, in the induced group, flushing increased dramatically from five hours before full cervical dilation. Within three hours of full cervical dilation 84% (n=26) of the women who had induced labours were flushed but in 7 women, flushing reduced or disappeared an hour before full cervical dilation. While the mechanism is not clear, this interesting finding could possibly be linked to disruption to the oxytocin system from synthetic oxytocin exposure.

Oxytocin has also been linked to relaxation and sleep (Uvnäs Moberg et al, 2014). Walmsley (2003) and Davis (1992) described women's eyes in active labour as being '*drowsy*', nulliparous women were recorded as having '*glazed eyes*' four hours prior to full cervical dilation in Duff's study. Women themselves described feeling tired and sleepy in the period prior to active pushing (Dixon et al, 2014). This is possibly the result of the oxytocin surge in late labour.

During periods of excessive stress, such as changes in the birthing environment, or the appearance of new carers, extremely high levels of epinephrine-norepinephrine and beta-endorphins are produced. Buckley (2015) asserts that these changes can disrupt or slow labour by reducing oxytocin production. In Duff's (2005) study, 35% of primiparous women in spontaneous labour had a lull in contractions, or the contractions became less frequent, at various times. Unfortunately, why this occurred is not known as changes in the environment and/or carers were not documented. In support of Buckley's theory, midwives who were interviewed by Winter about changes in contractions during labour considered that this may be caused by changes in emotional or environmental situations (Winter and Duff, 2009).

Assessing labour progress

Vaginal examinations

Digital vaginal examination is currently the principal intervention to assess labour progress. The assessment is based on the degree of cervical dilatation and effacement, and the descent and position of the foetal head. The UK National Institute for Health and Care Excellence (NICE) recommends that vaginal examination is undertaken, with the woman's permission, on admission and at four-hourly intervals throughout labour (NICE, 2017). However, despite its long standing and routine use there is little evidence of the reliability or effectiveness of vaginal examination (Downe et al, 2013). Studies using simulation models have found digital assessment of cervical dilatation to be correct in only between 19% and 56% of cases (Phelps et al, 1995; Tuffnell et al, 1989) with high levels of discrepancy between judgements of experienced clinicians (Tuffnell et al, 1989).

Other physical signs that may indicate labour progress

A line of purple or red skin discolouration has been observed, arising from the anal margin in some women in early labour and extending between the buttocks as labour progresses. This has been proposed as a non-invasive indicator of labour progress. A study of 48 women found it was present in 89% of participants, and that it was significantly correlated with cervical dilatation and station of the foetal head (Byrne and Edmonds, 1990). In a prospective study, Shepherd et al (2010) observed 144 women through labour and found that the purple line was present at some point during labour for 109 (76%) women, and that there was a moderate correlation between the length of the line, cervical dilatation and station of the foetal head. The line was more likely to be present in spontaneous than induced labours, but it did not vary by parity. What causes this line is not known. It is thought to result from increasing intra-pelvic pressure due to descent of the foetal head causing vaso-congestion in the basivertebral and intervertebral veins at the sacrum (Byrne and Edmonds, 1990). These two small studies were undertaken largely with Caucasian women and it is not known to what extent the line may be readily visible in other ethnic populations.

During labour women sometimes have the urge to push when the cervix has not been confirmed as being fully dilated (Downe et al, 2008). This has been termed the 'early pushing urge'. It has been explored by a number of researchers (Borrelli et al, 2013; Downe et al, 2008), and the incidence appears to range between 20 and 40%, although 60% of women in Duff's study, who were in spontaneous labour, reported rectal pressure and pain up to three hours prior to full dilation (2005). It has been traditional practice to help women to stop pushing in these circumstances, to avoid damage to the remaining cervix. However, there is increasing awareness that the early pushing urge might be physiological for some women, especially if the foetal head is in the anterior position, and midwives are increasingly taking a 'wait and see' approach in this situation.

Women's behaviour as a sign of progress

Winter and Duff (2009) found that women's behaviours changed with time during labour, and few behaviours were correlated with Friedman's phases of labour. Burvill (2002) interviewed eight experienced midwives who described using reactions of the women to assess their labour progress. This included observation of their breathing, conversation, mood, movements and posture, as well as external signs (such as contractions, red line, vaginal loss), and clinical assessment through vaginal examinations. Cues were mapped onto five phases, termed: late pregnancy; latent/pre labour; early labour; early active labour; and active labour with distinct behavioural changes in cues identified between early compared to later phases.

Nolan et al (2009) found that in early labour women were described as being happy and excited, while, in Duff's (2005) study, the descriptors *normal movements; appears comfortable and relaxed; normal skin; eyes bright; talkative and social*, and *a normal tone of voice* were all descriptors that were only associated with the early portion of labour *between* contractions. Duff also found that 90% (n=32) of nulliparous women in spontaneous labour displayed *'rhythmic movements'* (such as rocking) during contractions while 50% or more also used gripping behaviours. Both actions occurred early in the labours but decreased dramatically one hour before full cervical dilation was recorded. Why this occurred is unknown, but a rocking or swaying action may ease pain during labour and assist the foetal head to navigate the architecture of the pelvis. During late labour, as the foetal head descends further into the pelvis, *'rhythmic movements'* may become more uncomfortable, causing the women to stop.

Mobilisation during labour

Throughout history, upright positions for labour and birth have been the norm in almost all cultures. The practice of requiring women to remain mobile and semi-recumbent or supine during labour is relatively recent, and is associated with the move into hospital birth settings, and increased technical surveillance and intervention during labour and birth (Priddis et al, 2012). There is good evidence from a Cochrane systematic review (Gupta et al, 2017) that encouraging women to adopt upright positions and to remain mobile during labour is beneficial when compared to recumbent positions. These findings were echoed in a review of the impact of labour and birth positions and of facilitators and inhibitors for mothers adopting various positions (Priddis et al, 2012). This review also found that in different birth settings women were more or less likely to adopt upright positions for labour and birth (discussed below). In a narrative review, including 22 studies, using a broad range of methods to assess the effect of maternal physical activity on the length of the first stage of labour, the researchers found 11 studies that reported no difference in the length of first stage of labour when women adopted various labour positions. However, seven studies indicated that first stage was shorter if the women remained mobile, and none indicated that mobilisation lengthened first stage of labour (Hollins Martin and Martin, 2013).

There are good physiological reasons to support upright and mobile postures during the first stage of labour. In upright positions gravity assists the descent of the foetal head. This in turn increases direct pressure on the cervix, resulting in hormonal feedback which, in turn, generates more intense and regular contractions (Buckley, 2015; Gupta et al, 2012). A study using Magnetic Resonance pelvimetry to compare dimensions of the pelvis in non-pregnant women adopting hand to knee, squatting and supine positions found significant increases in pelvic dimensions in hand to knee and squatting positions compared to supine (Michel et al, 2002). In contrast, adopting supine positions during labour may result in supine hypotension and reduced foetal oxygen saturation (Carbonne et al, 1996).

In contrast to the generally positive evidence about upright and mobile positions in labour, the evidence on upright positions for birth is less clear. A Cochrane review of benefits and risks of different birth positions during second stage of labour (Gupta et al, 2012) included 32 trials whic found that women who gave birth in upright positions had a reduction in mean length of the second stage. However, the authors describe this finding as based on low-quality evidence. The review found that women adopting upright birth positions were significantly less likely to have an assisted birth and an episiotomy. They also found a possible increase in second degree tears and an increase in estimated blood loss above 500ml. The authors speculate that ease of blood collection in births using a birth stool when compared with women using a bed may account for this finding.

Subsequent studies have also demonstrated inconsistent findings. A study that compared 102 women allocated to give birth in either a squatting or supine position found that women allocated to a squatting position had a shorter second stage with no increased blood loss (Moraloglu et al, 2017). Another study compared birth in the hands and knees position to the supine position for 886 women, and found lower rates of episiotomy and higher rates of intact perineum in the hands and knees group, with no difference in blood loss (Zhang et al, 2016). However, a large cohort study of 7,832 vaginal births found that squatting (2.9%) and kneeling (2.1%) positions for birth were associated with a significant increase in anal sphincter tears compared to birth positions on a bed (1%) (Haslinger et al, 2015). Overall the evidence for upright birth positions remains inconclusive. There is, however, sufficient evidence to recommend that women should be encouraged to adopt positions for birth, including upright positions, in which they feel most comfortable.

Techniques to support physiological labour and birth

Antenatal education and training

A range of techniques have been introduced in the antenatal period with the aim of providing women with the tools to support physiological labour and birth. These include antenatal education and exercise; various complementary therapies; use of water; breathing and relaxation techniques; acupressure and hypnosis. This section examines some of these techniques that can be taught during pregnancy.

Levett et al (2016) examined nulliparous women's labour and birth outcomes associated with multi-component antenatal education. The RCT compared outcomes for women randomised to standard antenatal classes or to sessions where specific education included training in complementary therapies consisting of acupressure, breathing, massage, visualisation and relaxation, yoga techniques and facilitated partner support. Results indicated significantly less epidurals in the intervention group (absolute reduction of 45% and a relative reduction of 63% (RR=0.37, p<0.001), and a reduction in augmentation, caesarean sections, length of second stage and perineal trauma.

Hypnosis is another technique that can be taught during the antenatal period. A Cochrane review (Madden et al, 2016) of nine trials with 2,954 participants investigated the effect of hypnosis on managing labour pain. They found women who used hypnosis required less pharmacological pain relief or analgesia. There were no other clear differences in the trials, although the qualitative evidence supports its acceptability for women and their birth partners. For example, Finlayson et al (2015) explored women's experiences and views of using self-hypnosis as part of the SHIP trial, in which groups of women and their partners were taught hypnosis techniques for labour in the third trimester of pregnancy (Downe et al, 2015). The participants found the hypnosis education and training beneficial in building their confidence, and that they, and their partners, used the technique both for labour and birth and in other situations.

Water, acupuncture, relaxation, and massage

Water is frequently used to assist in relaxation, and to reduce anxiety during labour, either through showering or through baths. Two studies have found showering to be therapeutic (Stark, 2013; Stark, 2017). In addition, a systematic review to establish if labouring and birthing in water was appropriate for use in hospitals found that women relaxed more and required less analgesia during labour (Poder and Larivière, 2014). Furthermore, a Cochrane review (Jones et al, 2012) supports immersion in water and also suggests that use of acupuncture and relaxation techniques may improve satisfaction and decrease labour pain. In addition, massage may also assist in decreasing pain sensation.

Manual techniques to reduce pain in labour have been reviewed in a Cochrane review (Smith et al, 2018b) which included 10 trials involving 1,055 women. Massage, warm packs and thermal manual procedures were found to be effective in reducing pain. Another Cochrane review (Smith et al, 2018a) included 19 studies of which 15 (1,731 women) met selection criteria. The review aimed to examine the effect of mind-body relaxation techniques on labour compared to usual care. They found that relaxation, yoga and music may play a role in reducing pain.

Continuous support during labour

There is good evidence from a Cochrane review (Bohren et al, 2017) of 27 trials, that women having a continuous support person during labour and birth are more likely to have a vaginal birth and a shorter labour, and less likely to be dissatisfied with their care, require analgesia or have a caesarean section. The trials in the review included continuous support from a range of people including midwives, doulas and birth partners. A study of continuous support provided by midwives during labour described the elements of supportive midwifery care. In 49 labours and more than 100 hours of observations, the authors found that midwives provided almost continuous emotional support, while simultaneously giving physical support, including aspects such as massage, helping the woman move into comfortable positions, providing fluids and nutrition, advising, informing and listening.[52]

Discussion

Over the last century the trend in increased technical surveillance has included attempts to delineate, describe and manage labour and birth through rigid patterns and graphs that have been accepted over time as being 'true'. This has meant that women's experiences and responses to normal labour have been largely deprioritised and dismissed. However, as this chapter has highlighted, many important aspects of labour onset and progress are not yet completely understood. There is little consensus about definition or description of labour onset. Long-accepted patterns defining labour progress are now recognised as being flawed. At the same time evidence suggests that the predominant method of assessing labour progress, the vaginal examination, is also a poor predictor of labour progress and of outcome.

Where does this 'erosion of certainty' leave healthcare providers who are charged with providing safe and effective care to each woman and baby every time? Everyone responsible for planning and providing intrapartum care should acknowledge current uncertainties, and the impact these have on the interactions between mothers and maternity care providers. For example, there is no justification for rigid gatekeeping of access to healthcare facilities or for routine, time-constrained assessment of progress independent of maternal and foetal wellbeing, and maternal experiences, values and behaviours. At the same time labour and birth is a time of increased risk for some women and babies, and skilled vigilance is essential. All women should be given the opportunity to build trusting, respectful, supportive relationships with their maternity care providers and have access to a safe birth environment that supports and encourages rather than constrains the normal hormonal, emotional and physiological processes of labour and birth.

Conclusion

Many aspects of physiological labour are not yet fully understood. There are no biological markers that define the start of labour. The triggers for labour onset, and the mechanisms of birth itself are a complex continuum, and this is how women experience labour. Yet, in practice, maternity care providers artificially create standard boundaries and definitions in the belief that this is the best way to organise safe care. Recognition of the uncertain and sometimes arbitrary nature of these boundaries, prioritising women's understanding and observing their behaviours during physiological labour, may enable midwives and other maternity healthcare providers to provide the supportive care that women need through labour and birth.

Key points for consideration

Women and their families should be made aware of the uncertainties surrounding timing of onset and recognition of physiologic labour.

- Decisions about admission to maternity care facilities or provision of skilled maternity care should be based on women's individual care needs and not on cervical dilatation alone.
- There is no justification to implement rigid standardised timelines for physiological labour progress: care should be individualised to the needs of each woman and baby.
- Continuous support during labour by midwives, birth partners and doulas encourages shorter labours, vaginal births and women's satisfaction with their care.
- Encouraging women to feel comfortable during labour, including support to adopt upright positions and to be mobile, is beneficial.
- Women should be offered a variety of techniques for reducing discomfort in labour and promoting relaxation, including: immersion in water; acupuncture; massage; warm packs; yoga and music. Observing the purple line is a non-invasive method that can indicate labour progress for women in spontaneous labours. Observing women's changing reactions to labour, by the same midwife, may provide cues to the woman's progress. Women should be supported to choose a position for birth in which they are most comfortable, this should include upright positions.

Points for consideration for research

- Not enough is known about environmental stress and its impact on normal labour and birth.
- There is a significant gap in the evidence base on non-invasive or alternative means of assessing labour progress.
- Further research is needed on the amount of blood lost during different birth positions and how this is accurately measured, and what the physiological consequences are for the mother into the postnatal period.
- Larger-scale studies are needed into techniques to aid pain relief to support physiological labour. Research should detail when in pregnancy the intervention commences, how many sessions are included, and the experience and education of the educators /therapists would be of value.
- In all cases, pre-determined sub-group analysis should include whether women are in spontaneous labour, or if they have experienced induced or augmented labour.

References

Abalos E, Oladapo OT, Chamillard M, Díaz V, Pasquale J, Bonet M, Souza JP, Gülmezoglu AM. 2018 Duration of spontaneous labour in 'low-risk' women with 'normal' perinatal outcomes: A systematic review. Eur J Obstet Gynecol Reprod Biol. 2018 Apr;223:123-132. doi: 10.1016/j.ejogrb.2018.02.026. Epub 2018 Feb 27.

Albers, L., Schiff, M. & Gorwoda, J. 1996. The length of active labor in normal pregnancies. *Obstetrics and Gynecology*, 87, 355-9.

Beebe, K. R. & Humphreys, J. 2006. Expectations, perceptions, and management of labor in nulliparas prior to hospitalization. *J Midwifery Womens Health*, 51, 347-53.

Bohren, M. A., Hofmeyr, G. J., Sakala, C., Fukuzawa, R. K. & Cuthbert, A. 2017. Continuous support for women during childbirth. *Cochrane Database of Systematic Reviews*.

Borrelli, S. E., Locatelli, A. & Nespoli, A. 2013. Early pushing urge in labour and midwifery practice: A prospective observational study at an Italian maternity hospital. *Midwifery*, 29, 871-875.

Buckley, S. J. 2015. Hormonal Physiology of Childbearing: Evidence and Implications for Women, Babies, and Maternity Care. Washington, D.C.: Childbirth Connection Programs, National Partnership for Women & Families.

Burvill, S. 2002. Midwifery diagnosis of labour-onset. *British Journal of Midwifery*, 10, 600-605.

Byrne, D. & Edmonds, D. K. 1990. Clinical method for evaluating progress in first stage of labour. *The Lancet*, 335, 122.

Carbonne, B., Benachi, A., Leveque, M., Cabrol, D. & Papiernik, E. 1996. Maternal position during labor: effects on fetal oxygen saturation measured by pulse oximetry. *Obstet Gynecol* 88, 797-800.

Cheyne, H., Dowling, D. W. & Hundley, V. 2006. Making the diagnosis of labour: midwives' diagnostic judgement and management decisions. *J Adv Nurs*, 53.

Davis, E. 1992. *Heart and hands,* Berkeley, Celestial Arts.

Dixon, L., Skinner, J. & Foureur, M. 2013. Women's perspectives of the stages and phases of labour. *Midwifery*, 29, 10-17.

Dixon, L., Skinner, J. & Foureur, M. 2014. The emotional journey of labour—Women's perspectives of the experience of labour moving towards birth. *Midwifery*, 30, 371-377.

Downe, S., Finlayson, K., Melvin, C., Spiby, H., Ali, S., Diggle, P., Gyte, G., Hinder, S., Miller, V., Slade, P., Trepel, D., Weeks, A., Whorwell, P. & Williamson, M. 2015. Self-hypnosis for intrapartum pain management in pregnant nulliparous women: a randomised controlled trial of clinical effectiveness. *BJOG: An International Journal of Obstetrics & Gynaecology*, 122, 1226-1234.

Downe, S., Gyte, G. M. L., Dahlen, H. G. & Singata, M. 2013. Routine vaginal examinations for assessing progress of labour to improve outcomes for women and babies at term. *Cochrane Database of Systematic Reviews*.

Downe, S., Young, C. & Moran, V. H. 2008. The early pushing urge: practice and discourse. *In:* DOWNE, S. (ed.) *Normal Childbirth: Evidence and Debate.* 2nd ed.

Duff, M. 2005. *A study of labour.* PhD, University of Technology.

E., A., Oladapo O.T, Chamillard M, Díaz V, Pasquale J, Bonet M, Souza J.P & A.M., G. 2018. Duration of spontaneous labour in 'low-risk' women with 'normal' perinatal outcomes: A systematic review. *European Journal of Obstetrics and Gynecology and Reproductive Biology*, 1, 123-32.

Eri, T. S., Bondas, T., Gross, M. M., Janssen, P. & Green, J. M. 2015. A balancing act in an unknown territory: A metasynthesis of first-time mothers' experiences in early labour. *Midwifery*, 31, e58-e67.

Finlayson, K., Downe, S., Hinder, S., Carr, H., Spiby, H. & Whorwell, P. 2015. Unexpected consequences: women's experiences of a self-hypnosis intervention to help with pain relief during labour. *BMC Pregnancy and Childbirth*, 15, 229.

Friedman, E. A. 1954. The graphic analysis of labor. *The American Journal of Obstetrics and Gynecology*, 68, 1568-1575.

Friedman, E. A. 1955. Primigravid labor: A graphicostaticial analysis. *American Journal of Obstetrics and Gynecology*, 6, 567-589.

Goodenough, D. A. & Paul, D. L. 2009. Gap Junctions. *Cold Spring Harbor Perspectives in Biology*, 1, a002576.

Gross, M. M., Burian, R. A., Fromke, C., Hecker, H., Schippert, C. & Hillemanns, P. 2009. Onset of labour: women's experiences and midwives' assessments in relation to first stage duration. *Arch Gynecol Obstet*, 280.

Gross, M. M., Haunschild, T., Stoexen, T., Methner, V. & Guenter, H. H. 2003. Women's recognition of the spontaneous onset of labor. *Birth*, 30.

Gupta, J., Hofmeyr, G. & Shehmar, M. 2012. Position in the second stage of labour for women without epidural anaesthesia. . *Cochrane Database of Systematic Reviews 2012, Issue 5. Art. No.: CD002006. DOI: 10.1002/14651858. CD002006.pub3.*

Gupta, J. K., Sood, A., Hofmeyr, G. J. & Vogel, J. P. 2017. Position in the second stage of labour for women without epidural anaesthesia. *Cochrane Database of Systematic Reviews*.

Hanley, G. E., Munro, S., Greyson, D., Gross, M. M., Hundley, V., Spiby, H. & Janssen, P. A. 2016. Diagnosing onset of labor: a systematic review of definitions in the research literature. *BMC Pregnancy and Childbirth*, 16, 71.

Haslinger, C., Burkhardt, T., Stoiber, B., Zimmermann, R. & Schäffer, L. 2015. Position at birth as an important factor for the occurrence of anal sphincter tears: a retrospective cohort study. *Journal of Perinatal Medicine. ,* 43, 715-20.

Hildingsson, I., Blix, E., Hegaard, H., Huitfeldt, A., Ingversen, K., Ólafsdóttir, Ó. Á. & Lindgren, H. 2015. How Long Is a Normal Labor? Contemporary Patterns of Labor and Birth in a Low Risk Sample of 1,612 Women from Four

Nordic Countries. . *Birth: Issues In Perinatal Care,* 42, 346-353.

Hollins Martin, C. J. & Martin, C. R. 2013. A narrative review of maternal physical activity during labour and its effects upon length of first stage. *Complementary Therapies in Clinical Practice,* 19, 44-49.

Johnstone, M. 1974. Facial vasomotor behaviour. *Br J Anaesth,* 46, 765-9.

Jones, L., Othman, M., Dowswell, T., Alfirevic, Z., Gates, S., Newburn, M., Jordan, S., Lavender, T. & Neilson, J. P. 2012. Pain management for women in labour: An overview of systematic reviews. *The Cochrane Library.*

Levett, K. M., Smith, C. A., Bensoussan, A. & Dahlen, H. G. 2016. Complementary therapies for labour and birth study: a randomised controlled trial of antenatal integrative medicine for pain management in labour. *BMJ Open,* 6.

Madden, K., Middleton, P., Cyna, A. M., Matthewson, M. & Jones, L. 2016. Hypnosis for pain management during labour and childbirth. *Cochrane Database of Systematic Reviews.*

Maharana, S., Nagarathna, R., Padmalatha, V., Nagendra, H. R. & Hankey, A. 2013. The effect of integrated yoga on labor outcome: A randomized controlled study. *International Journal of Childbirth,* 3, 165-177.

Mccourt, C. 2010. Cosmologies, concepts and theories: Time and childbirth in cross-cultural perspectives. *In:* MCCOURT, C. (ed.) *Childbirth, Midwifery and Concepts of Time.* Oxford: Berghahn Books.

Mccourt, C. & Dykes, F. 2010. From tradition to Modernity: Time and childbirth in historical perspective. *In:* MCCOURT, C. (ed.) *Childbirth, Midwifery and Concepts of Time.* New York: Berghahn Books.

Mcintosh, T. 2013. The concept of early labour in the experience of maternity in twentieth century Britain. *Midwifery,* 29, 3-9.

Michel, S., Rake, A. T., K., Seifert, B., Chaoui, R., Huch, R., Marincek, B. & Kubik-Huch, R. 2002. MR obstetric pelvimetry: Effect of birthing position on pelvic bony dimensions. *American Journal of Roentgenology,* 179, 1063-7.

Mondy, T., Fenwick, J., Leap, N. & Foureur, M. 2016. How domesticity dictates behaviour in the birth space: Lessons for designing birth environments in institutions wanting to promote a positive experience of birth. *Midwifery,* 43, 37-47.

Moraloglu, O., Kansu-Celik, H., Tasci, Y., Karakaya, B., Yilmaz, Y., Cakir, E. & Yakut, H. 2017. The influence of different maternal pushing positions on birth outcomes at the second stage of labor in nulliparous women. *The Journal of Maternal-Fetal & Neonatal Medicine. ,* 30, 245-9.

National Institute for Health and Care Excellence 2017. Intrapartum care for healthy women and babies (CG190). London: NICE.

Nolan, M., Smith, J. & Catling, J. 2009. Experiences of early labour (1) Contact with health professionals. *The Practising Midwife,* 12, 21-24.

Oladapo OT, Souza JP, Fawole B, Mugerwa K, Perdoná G, Alves D, Souza H, Reis R, Oliveira-Ciabati L, Maiorano A, Akintan A, Alu FE, Oyeneyin L, Adebayo A, Byamugisha J, Nakalembe M, Idris HA, Okike O, Althabe F, Hundley V, Donnay F, Pattinson R, Sanghvi HC, Jardine JE, Tunçalp Ö, Vogel JP, Stanton ME, Bohren M, Zhang J, Lavender T, Liljestrand J, Ten Hoope-Bender P, Mathai M, Bahl R, Gülmezoglu AM. 2018 Progression of the first stage of spontaneous labour: A prospective cohort study in two sub-Saharan African countries. PLoS Med. 2018 Jan 16;15(1):e1002492. doi: 10.1371/journal.pmed.1002492. eCollection 2018 Jan.

Olza, I., Leahy-Warren, P., Benyamini, Y., Kazmierczak, M., Karlsdottir, S. I., Spyridou, A., Crespo-Mirasol, E., Takács, L., Hall, P. J., Murphy, M., Jonsdottir, S. S., Downe, S. & Nieuwenhuijze, M. J. 2018. Women's psychological experiences of physiological childbirth: a meta-synthesis. *BMJ Open,* 8, e020347.

Phelps, J. Y., Higby, K., Smyth, M. H., Ward, J. A., Arredondo, F. & Mayer, A. R. 1995. Accuracy and intraobserver variability of simulated cervical dilatation measurements. *American Journal of Obstetrics and Gynecology,* 173, 942-945.

Poder, T. & Larivière, M. 2014. Advantages and disadvantages of water birth. A systematic review of the literature. *Gynecol Obstet Fertil. ,* 42, 706-13.

Priddis, H., Dahlen, H. & Schmied, V. 2012. What are the facilitators, inhibitors, and implications of birth positioning? A review of the literature. *Women and Birth,* 25, 100-106.

Reed, R., Barnes, M. & Rowe, J. 2015. Women's experience of birth: Childbirth as a rite of passage. *International Journal of Childbirth,* 5, 46-56.

Shepherd, A., Cheyne, H., Kennedy, S., Mcintosh, C., Styles, M. & Niven, C. 2010. The purple line as a measure of labourprogress: a longitudinal study. *BMC Pregnancy and Childbirth,* 10, 54.

Smith, C. A., Levett, K. M., Collins, C. T., Armour, M., Dahlen, H. G. & Suganuma, M. 2018a. Relaxation techniques for pain management in labour. *Cochrane Database of Systematic Reviews.*

Smith, C. A., Levett, K. M., Collins, C. T., Dahlen, H. G., Ee, C. C. & Suganuma, M. 2018b. Massage, reflexology and other manual methods for pain management in labour. *Cochrane Database of Systematic Reviews.*

Stark, M. 2013. Therapeutic showering in labor. *Clinical Nursing Research,* 22, 359-374.

Stark, M. 2017. Testing the effectiveness of therapeutic showering in labor. *J Perinat Neonatal Nurs,* 31, 109-117.

The American College of Obstetricians and Gynecologists 2017. Approaches to Limit Intervention During Labor and Birth - Committee Opinion 687. *Obstet Gynecol,* 1-9.

Tuffnell, D. J., Johnson, N., Bryce, F. & Lilford, R. J. 1989. Simulation of cervical changes in labour: Reproducibility of expert assessment. *The Lancet,* 334, 1089-1090.

Uvnäs Moberg, K., Handlin, L. & Petersson, M. 2014. Self-soothing behaviors with particular reference to oxytocin release induced by non-noxious sensory stimulation. *Frontiers in Psychology,* 5, 1529.

Walmsley, K. 2003. Caring for women during the latent phase of labour. *In:* WICKHAM, S. (ed.) *Midwifery: Best practice.*. London: Elsevier.

Winter, C. & Duff, M. 2009. The progress of labour: orderly chaos? . *In:* MCCOURT, C. (ed.) *Childbirth, Midwifery and Concepts of Time.* London: Berghaun Books.

World Health Organization 2018. WHO recommendations: intrapartum care for a positive childbirth experience. Geneva: World Health Organization.

Zhang, H.-Y., Shu, R., Zhao, N.-N., Lu, Y.-J., Chen, M., Li, Y.-X., Wu, J.-Q., Huang, L.-H., Guo, X.-L., Yang, Y.-H., Zhang, X.-L., Zhou, X.-Y., Guo, R.-F., Li, J. & Cai, W.-Z. 2016. Comparing maternal and neonatal outcomes between hands-and-knees delivery position and supine position. *International Journal of Nursing Sciences,* 3, 178-184.

Zhang, J., Landy, H. J., Branch, D. W., Burkman, R., Haberman, S., Gregory, K. D., Hatjis, C. G., Ramirez, M. M., Bailit, J. L., Gonzalez-Quintero, V. H., Hibbard, J. U., Hoffman, M. K., Kominiarek, M., Learman, L. A., Van Veldhuisen, P., Troendle, J. & Reddy, U. M. 2010a. Contemporary Patterns of Spontaneous Labor With Normal Neonatal Outcomes. *Obstetrics and gynecology,* 116, 1281-1287.

Zhang, J., Troendle, J., Mikolajczyk, R., Sundaram, R., Beaver, J. & Fraser, W. 2010b. The natural history of the normal first stage of labor. *Obstet Gynecol,* 115.

CHAPTER 4

The 'trusting communion' of a positive birth: an existential perspective

Gillian Thomson and *Claire Feeley*

Introduction

Childbirth is a liminal life experience; a transcendental journey through which a mother and baby are born. However, as with other significant life transitions, childbirth can be experienced on a spectrum from an inherently positive and empowering event to one that is deeply distressing, with short and long-term implications for maternal wellbeing, family functioning and infant/child development. Positive and distressing accounts of birth have tended to be associated with a specific mode of birth, i.e. normal/ vaginal=good and medical/instrumental or surgical=bad. However, such dichotomies are unhelpful, and do not necessarily reflect women's realities. It is not what, or where childbirth happens that makes a difference for women's birth appraisals. A positive birth is an embodied experience of 'being one's body' irrespective of how the baby is born (Thomson, 2007). In this chapter, we draw upon lifeworld existentials (van Manen, 1997) and use our own research and that of others to illustrate how interconnected interpersonal, corporal, temporal and spatial features of intrapartum care influence women's experiences and psychological responses. We highlight how a 'trusting communion' in the birth space enables a state of wholeness, as women, irrespective of how their baby is born, become 'one' to achieve a positive birth.

Through a lifeworld lens

Lifeworld, a concept introduced by Edmund Husserl, relates to how our realities are influenced by the dynamic world in which we live. Van Manen (1997) went on to describe interconnected facets of the lifeworld that are always present and influence any life experience ('existentials'), namely lived time, lived body, lived space and lived relations. We now describe these four features and, together with real-life accounts, illuminate the impact of connection or disruption of these characteristics on women's experiences and psychological wellbeing.

Being with

Lived human relations concerns our relationships; the communications and connections we share with others during life events (van Manen, 1997). While all existentials are ever-present in our lifeworld, childbirth is a potentially isolating, vulnerable experience in which relationships with others in the social space are crucial. Women have evolutionary needs to seek companionship during labour – needs based on heightened emotional states and desires for physical safety (Rosenberg & Tervathan, 2002). The key mechanism through which these inherent needs can be met is through 'trust'. Women need to trust the expertise of those in attendance, and to trust the individual(s) providing the care. A trust-based woman-caregiver relationship requires sensitive communication and meaningful connections to enable women to feel safe and protected, and to know they are cared for. Positive relationships are more easily achievable if the woman experiences continuity of carer. However, it is possible to forge a shared communion without the woman and caregiver having met before, if both parties maintain an aligned and open attunement to each other. As a woman said in an interview undertaken by one of us: *'you* [self and midwife] *just click'* (Thomson, 2007, p274).

Underpinning meaningful relationships is the extent to which caregivers offer 'presence', which is the sense of 'being with' a woman during labour. 'Being with' concerns the emotional, physical, spiritual and psychological attunement of the caregiver (Osterman & Schwartz-Barcott, 1996). The subtle cues of presence, as reflected by Diane in the following quote, reinforce an inner belief that a positive outcome could be achieved:

> *'I just felt like, because I had so much trust in her [midwife] I knew that whatever happened it would be OK.'* (Diane, Thomson, 2009, p196)

'Presence' relates to responsive care, where women feel themselves to *'be seen and heard'* (Karlström et al, 2015, p3). Presence can be subtle, visceral and difficult to describe. For Sonia, in the following interview account, the midwife's presence was a 'sublime' facilitation:

> *'It was facilitation that was almost sublime, it wasn't really there, it was definitely there, but it wasn't really felt.'* (Sonia, Thomson, 2007, p278)

Conversely, when trust-based relationships are absent (due to care provided by multiple care providers and/or when care does not align with the woman's needs), this can erode women's feelings of safety during labour and birth, and augment negative emotions. As reflected by Cat below, a lack of care could be experienced as dehumanising:

'It's not because of what happened to me that made it traumatic, it would have been a bad birth anyway, but the fact that nobody wanted to listen to me, nobody treated me like a human being, that's the part that really really hurt me... It was all so just barbaric [crying].' (Cat, Feeley, 2015).

The importance of time

Lived time is time as we experience it rather than objective 'factual' linear time (van Manen, 1997). It relates to how our past, present and future are fundamentally intertwined, thereby emphasising the importance of women's childbirth expectations. Pregnant multigravida women who have had a previous traumatic birth may require additional and/or specialist support. However, temporality also concerns how our emotions impact on our experience of time, and how constraints or the imposition of time can affect how we feel. Childbirth is often governed by linear clock time in which women's bodily rhythms are monitored through regular clinical checks, vaginal examinations and expectations of 'timely' progress. While arguably such events are important to assess for maternal and infant wellbeing, there are marked differences in how time-based procedures are performed and experienced.

During births that women recall as being 'positive', maternity professionals tend to adopt a *'watchful waiting'* approach (Carlson & Lowe, 2014). Observation and expert intuition are used to assess women's progress, with clinical assessments used intermittently, only if necessary, and as unobtrusively as possible (Carlson & Lowe, 2014). This approach instils trust and can enable women to feel free to labour at their own pace. Linear time fades as they enter a private, inner world: as one woman recounted, *'time didn't really exist anymore, and the rest of the world kind of disappeared'* (Reed, 2013, p109).

However, during a birth that is experienced as traumatic and/or stressful, women often report regulated invasive procedures that they feel they have to endure, irrespective of their wishes. As reflected by Lesley below, these clock-based procedures served to reinforce a sense of her 'failing' body:

'It was a case of every three hours somebody coming in the room with a rubber glove on and shove their hand up and say you're still 4cms.' (Lesley, Thomson 2011, p142)

In contrast to the cyclical, embodied basis of a positive birth, women in a number of studies report that time was not their own during a traumatic birth. A woman from Reed et al's (2016) study reported:

'...I was basically told that if I didn't have a c-section on their timetable I would kill my baby, even though they couldn't tell me what exactly was "wrong" as to why I was not delivering vaginally... They broke me down gradually until they declared my baby was "in distress" (she wasn't... I could see the screens)' (Participant 559, p5)

For some women, the unsafe and precarious nature of their situation led to panic and fear. As recounted by Diane, this situation can lead to women becoming suspended in a distorted sense of 'now' time:

'Forty, forty-five, fifty minutes at the most, that was it, the whole thing. But to me it felt like forty-five hours – it was like I was suspended in time.' (Clare, Thomson, 2007, p279).

Being the body

The concept of the lived body relates to our physical body and our psyche (van Manen, 1997); *'It is through our lived body that we communicate, feel, interact, and experience the world'* (Rich, Graham, Tacket & Shelley, 2012, p501). It concerns how our bodies can be experienced subjectively and/or objectively.

A sense of (not being out of) control is a key attribute of a positive, empowering birth. This is a paradoxical concept where women need to feel in control over what is happening in order to 'let go' to give birth. Through trust-based care, women are able to focus inwards and achieve a unifying experience where cognitive and emotional responses are relinquished in order to submit to the physiological forces of childbirth (Anderson, 2000):

'I was just able to get on with what my body was doing and I didn't think about anything' (Janet, Thomson 2009, p200)

'Letting go' is frequently associated with a normal/vaginal birth. However, this phenomenon is also evident among women who experience labour interventions. As reflected by Clare below, when women felt that they had enough information and enough choice, this could enable them to feel 'at one' with the birth:

'He [doctor] asked me, and it was amazing really, so it was my choice and even though she [daughter] was breech and needed forceps with the head and stuff it was me, it was still me, I was in control' (Clare, Thomson 2009, p198)

Conversely, many accounts of negative birth experiences are associated with women having a sense of limited or no control. Women can feel that their bodies are restrained by restrictive procedures (such as foetal monitoring), and they lose a sense of selfhood if they are marginalised, minimised, ostracised and objectified by clinical providers. In one study, women used terms like *'faceless', 'invisible', 'lump of meat'* on a *'conveyor belt'* to express their feelings (Thomson, 2007). In a more recent study, some participants felt that their bodies had become an objectified *'spectacle'* for staff who wanted a *'learning opportunity'* due to their unusual birth (Reed et al, 2017):

'... and the amount of people that filled the room to watch a vaginal breech delivery, when I failed at this, everyone left.' (pn-662, Reed et al, 2017, p4)

Such negative and negating experiences can lead to a psychic disturbance called dissociation, which is a psychological experience of physical and emotional detachment:

'it felt like an absolutely, out of body unreal experience, it was like I was like in a corner watching everything' (Kate, Thomson & Downe 2008, p271).

Women's entry into *'labour land'* (Reed, 2013, p109) can be blocked when their bodies are governed by external control, creating a heightened sense of vulnerability, and bodily and emotional conflict:

'I was absolutely desperate and just heartbroken, absolutely heartbroken because I didn't have any control over it [...] I felt like they'd just ripped her out of my body and I had no choice no option but to go with what was happening'
(Diane, Thomson 2007, p190).

Within the space

Lived space is the felt subjective space in which sentient being exists; it concerns how the self and the environment interact to influence our emotions (van Manen, 1997). Within a childbirth context, it relates to the dynamic interaction of the external environment upon the birthing woman and vice versa. Feeling at ease in her birth environment fosters a woman's sense of wellbeing, enhancing feelings of trust and safety (Jenkinson et al, 2014). Birth settings comprise a range of physical features such as home comforts or technical machinery, or, more usually, a mixture of such artefacts. It is how this space is mediated by maternity caregivers that can make the difference to women. During a positive birth, maternity professionals skilfully *'hold the space'* for women (Siebold et al, 2010). They operate as a loving guardian to protect the women's birthing zones, free from distractions or interferences (Fahy and Parratt, 2006). A midwife in Reed et al's study (2017) explains:

'Just try and keep the room nice and calm, dark, try and you know make the ins and outs of the room to a minimum. Don't have too many people knocking on the door.'
(Gina, midwife/mother, p11)

Subtle actions by maternity professionals can mitigate clinical environments to create a calm, ambient birth space. Kathy, who gave birth in an operating theatre, explained:

'It was dead peaceful, you read about books in natural birth having candles and soft music and this environment was great, it was like that even though I was in an operating theatre, it was calm and happy' (Kathy, Thomson, 2009, p199)

In contrast, negative birth stories are depicted by a lack of 'ownership' of the birth environment; situations in which neither caregivers nor women 'hold the space'. A lack of privacy, intrusions, chaos, noise and panic all feature in women's accounts of a traumatic birth (Thomson, 2007). These disruptions force women to concentrate on the external environment as they try to ensure they are safe, thereby preventing them from engaging with their unconscious brain, which, as is noted in earlier chapters in this section, is essential for effective labour progress. In this hyper-aware emotional state, features of the event become fixed in recurring unconsciously mediated recollections:

'That's the thing with flashbacks that something you don't think is in your head and next minute you're living it, you're reliving it, you're in theatre with a mask on, being operated on, and yet seconds before you can't even recall it'
(Jules, Thomson 2007, p241)

Discussion

Through drawing on existing qualitative research and van Manen's (1997) lifeworld existentials, we have highlighted how interpersonal, corporal, temporal and spatial features of intrapartum care can influence women's experiences and psychological responses. A traumatic and/or stressful birth is characterised by a lack of trust with care providers. Poor and fragmented care, intrusive time-based procedures, and the active management of women's objectified bodies in a stressful, chaotic birth environment can lead to women feeling unsafe, dehumanised and can experience a loss of selfhood. During a positive birth, women describe a trust-based relationship with health providers – a relationship underpinned by sensitive needs-led care and a positive woman-provider attunement. Women are encouraged and enabled, within a peaceful birth environment, to succumb and feel connected to the birthing process.

Currently, there is a predominance of research into women's experiences and the implications of a traumatic (Fenech & Thomson, 2014), rather than a positive (Hill & Firth, 2018) birth event. This focus arguably reflects the current 'risk society' (Beck, 1992) that pervades modern maternity care. While there is limited prospective research into the impact of divergent birth experiences, available evidence suggests that a woman's birth can have a long-term influence on maternal, child and family outcomes (McKenzie-Harg et al, 2015; Reisz et al, 2015). The intrapartum guidelines from the World Health Organization (2018) highlight the need for maternity services to promote a positive pregnancy and birth to enable a successful transition into parenthood (WHO, 2016). The *Better Birth* maternity review (NHS England, 2016) recognises the need for individualised care, with home-type birth environments and continuity of care models perceived necessary to optimise the birthing experience. However, while physical aesthetics and opportunities for women and professionals to build relationships over time are important, what our work has highlighted is the primacy of the social space of birth. What matters most is that a trust-based caregiver-woman union is forged – for women to feel safe, cared for, listened to and valued, and to facilitate an embodied connection to the birth irrespective of where or how it occurs.

Conclusion: What matters most

Based on the accounts provided in this chapter, van Manen's existentials provide a powerful lens through which to consider how both birth environment and caregiver behaviour serve to facilitate or impede a positive birth. While none of the lifeworld features have primacy in lifeworld theory, in a childbirth context the qualitative evidence used as the basis for analysis in this chapter suggests that trust-based 'being with' is the central force which permeates and influences all others. A 'trusting communion' is reported when women feel taken care of, and are able to preserve their selfhood through connections with intuitive caregivers who protect women's bodies within the birth space. This enables women to 'become their bodies', to succumb to physiological impulses, and to retain an embodied connection to the birth should intervention be required. We advocate that this type of care is not ascribed to a particular model of practice (i.e. caseload/continuity models), or a place of birth, but rather takes place in a caregiver-mother union, where a trust-imbued space, place and bodily responses facilitate a state of wholeness as women are 'one' with the process of birth.

Key points for consideration

- Forging a trusting relationship, regardless of care model, requires the health professional to be attentive, responsive and mentally, emotionally and physically 'present'.
- Maternity workers should minimise interruptions and disturbances in the birth space to help facilitate an ambient and calm environment.
- Maternity care should be provided in an unobtrusive manner that respects the woman's rhythm of labour.

References

Anderson, T., (2000). Feeling safe enough to let go: The relationship between a woman and her midwife during the second stage of labour. *In* M Kirkham, ed. *The Midwife-Mother Relationship*. MacMillan Press Limited, 92-118.

Bauer, A. Parsonage, M. Knapp, M. Lemmi, V. & Adelaja, B. (2014). The costs of perinatal mental health problems. Centre for Mental Health and London School of Economics, London.

Beck, U. (1992). Risk Society: Towards a New Modernity. Sage Publications: London.

Carlson, N.S. & Lowe, N.K. (2014). A concept analysis of watchful waiting among providers caring for women in labour. Journal of Advanced Nursing, 70(3), 511-522.

Fahy, K., & Parratt, J. (2006). Birth territory: a theory for midwifery practice. *Women and Birth,* 19 (2) 45-50.

Feeley, C. (2015). *Making sense of childbirth choices; exploring the decision to freebirth in the UK.* Master's Thesis, University of Central Lancashire, Preston.

Fenech, G. & Thomson, G. (2014). 'Tormented by Ghosts of their Past': A meta-synthesis to explore the psychosocial implications of a traumatic birth on maternal wellbeing. *Midwifery*, 30,185–193.

Hill, E. & Firth, A. (2018) Positive birth experiences: a systematic review of the lived experience from a birthing person's perspective. MIDIRS Midwifery Digest. 28(1): 71-78.

Jenkinson, B., Josey, N., & Kruske, S. (2014). Birth- Space: An evidence-based guide to birth environ- ment design (Research Report of the Queensland Centre for Mothers & Babies, The University of Queensland). Retrieved from https://espace. library.uq.edu.au

McKenzie-McHarg, K., Ayers, S., Ford, E., Horsch, A., Jomeen, J., Sawyer, A., Stramrood, C., Thomson, G. & Slade, P. (2015). Post-traumatic stress disorder following childbirth: an update of current issues and recommendations for future research. *Journal of Reproductive and Infant Psychology (Special Edition),* 33, 219-237.

NHS England (2016). Better Births. Improving outcomes of maternity services in England. A Five Year Forward view for maternity care. London: NHS England.

Osterman, P., Schwartz-Barcott, D., (1996). Presence: Four ways of being there. *Nursing Forum*, 31, 23-30.

Reed, R. (2013). *Midwifery Practice During Birth: Rites of Passage and Rites of Protection.* PhD Thesis. University of the Sunshine Coast, Queensland.

Reed, R., Sharman, R., & Inglis, C. (2017). Women's descriptions of childbirth trauma relating to care provider actions and interactions. *BMC Pregnancy and Childbirth,* 17:21.

Reisz S, Jacobvitz D, George C (2015). Birth and motherhood: childbirth experiences and mothers' perceptions of themselves and their babies. Infant Mental Health Journal 36(2):16778

Rich, S., Graham, M., Taket, A. & Shelley, J. (2013). Navigating the Terrain of Lived Experience: The Value of Lifeworld Existentials for Reflective Analysis. *International Journal of Qualitative Methods, 12,* 498-510.

Siebold, C., Licqurish, S., Rolls, C., & Hopkins, F. (2010). 'Lending the space': Midwives perceptions of birth space and clinical risk management. *Midwifery*, (26), 526-531.

Thomson, G. (2007). A Hero's Tale of Childbirth: An Interpretive Phenomenological Study of Traumatic and Positive Childbirth. Unpublished PhD Dissertation.

Thomson , G. (2009). Birth as a Peak Experience. In Walsh, D. and Downe, S. (Eds) *Intrapartum Care (Essential Midwifery Practice)*, Wiley Blackwell Publishers: Oxford, pp. 191-122.

Thomson, G. (2011). Abandonment of Being in Childbirth. In: Thomson, G., Dykes, F., Downe, S. (eds). Qualitative Research in Midwifery and Childbirth: Phenomenological Approaches. Routledge: London.

Thomson, G. & Downe, S. (2008). Widening the trauma discourse: the link between childbirth and experiences of abuse. *Journal of Psychosomatic Obstetrics & Gynaecology*, 29(4), 268-273.

World Health Organization (2018). *Intrapartum care for a positive childbirth experience.* WHO: Geneva.

CHAPTER 5

What works to promote physiological labour and birth for healthy women and babies?

Practical responses to new evidence on birth physiology, and consequent outcomes

Mercedes Perez-Botella, Logan van Lessen, Sandra Morano and Ank de Jonge

Introduction

While it is important to understand how interventions can reduce the negative effects of pathological conditions during childbearing, much can be learnt from understanding the normal physiology of labour and birth, and how this can be facilitated (WHO, 2013; McDougall, Campbell, and Graham, 2016). These principles can then be more widely applied, even when the pregnancy is not considered strictly 'normal'. If women are provided with the appropriate support, respect and expertise, most women are able to give birth physiologically.

This chapter summarises the evidence available on what works in facilitating physiological labour and birth for women who have more or less uncomplicated pregnancies and the potential impact this can have on outcomes such as maternal and neonatal wellbeing, breastfeeding, parental capacity and self-efficacy. It will highlight the physiological factors that aid birth and it will explore the multiple external factors that influence and affect outcomes of physiological births, including the carer(s), models of care, and environments in maternity care.

An overview of the normal physiology of labour and birth

Having a sound understanding of normal physiology of labour and birth provides mothers and caregivers with enhanced opportunities to achieve positive outcomes. Even though it is widely accepted that labour is divided into three stages, current debates question whether the boundaries between the different parts of labour may actually be more dynamic (Walsh, 2012; Neil, Ryan and Hunter, 2015).

Traditionally, labour is said to occur when regular uterine contractions are accompanied by cervical dilatation and descent of the foetus (NICE, 2014; Neal, Ryan and Hunter, 2015). However, how frequent or strong the contractions should be and at what pace dilatation should occur are still contentious issues and, as of yet, there is no agreement in the literature as to what constitutes 'prolonged labour' (Nysdedt and Hildingsson, 2014). Even though it is believed that 0.5cm to 1cm dilatation of the cervical os per hour is adequate for both multiparous and nulliparous women (WHO, 2014), recent research has shown that labour patterns and duration have changed over the last decades (Laughton, Branch, Beaver & Zhang, 2012) and an extensive study on the progress of labour confirms that the cervical os does not dilate at the same speed for all women, nor does it follow a standard progression in velocity (Oladapo et al, 2018; WHO, 2018a). In fact, in response to the pulsatile production of oxytocin intrapartum, spontaneous labour progression is more like a stepped process, with periods of more intense activity, and then subsequent periods of more stable or restful periods throughout labour. This includes the 'labour plateau' or 'rest and be thankful' periods that often occur after the intensity of the 'transition' period that happens towards the end of labour (Oladapo, 2018). This has important implications for the optimal support of physiological labour, as misjudging labour as 'slow' or 'failing to progress' may initiate a cascade of unnecessary and potentially harmful interventions (Nysdedt and Hildingsson, 2014). It is therefore important for caregivers to take into account other factors that indicate progress of labour, such as cervical changes (not necessarily dilatation), maternal indicators (such as change in position, breathing pattern or involuntary noises) and descent and rotation of the foetus (Walsh, 2012, and see Chapter 3 in this volume). This can be facilitated by low levels of noise and lighting, and by the mother's instinctive adoption of the most suitable position at each point in their labour (Neal, Ryan & Hunter, 2015). Crucially, the Curve of Carus that characterises the pelvic axis maps directly to the upright forward leaning positions that women adopt spontaneously. This suggests that such positions are ideal, as they allow foetal rotation into the most optimal position (Romano & Lothian, 2008).

The neurohormonal adaptations the foetus makes, including the adoption of a more restful pattern of movement at certain points in labour, mirrors neurohormonal changes in the mother. These include surges of oxytocin, followed by release of endorphins, allowing adjustment to the change of pace in each case (Romano & Lothian, 2008). Such delicate, simple and complex orchestration of hormones indicates the importance of undisturbed birth if all is well with mother and baby (Odent, 1992).

The use of forced pushing (the Valsalva technique – Lemos et al, 2017) and fundal pressure (the Kristeller manoeuvre – Hofmeyr, Vogel, Cuthbert, Sygnata, 2017) may contribute to foetal descent in a malposition, or in an attitude of relative deflexion, both of which increase the risk of vaginal and perineal trauma. This is theoretically exacerbated when the woman is in the supine or semi-supine position, as the force of the descending head is exerted on the perineum, against the Curve of Carus, which is angled upwards when women are in this position. There is evidence that none of these factors (forced pushing, the Kristeller manoeuvre, and the supine position) should be used routinely in labour (Lemos et al, 2017; Hofmeyr, Vogel, Cuthbert, Sygnata, 2017).

Practical responses to normal birth physiology

It is widely acknowledged that technology and interventions should be reserved for those who really need them based on clinical need rather than on service or practitioner preference (*BMJ*, 2016; McDougall, Campbell and Graham, 2016). *The Lancet* series on midwifery (Renfrew et al, 2014) has identified aspects of care provision which capitalise on birth physiology, minimising the need for technical intervention. The next section provides approaches that may help maternity care providers to do this.

The midwifery philosophy of care

Significant evidence is emerging about the pivotal role that midwifery care provision plays in supporting physiological birth (Renfrew et al, 2014; Vedam et al, 2018; Escuriet, 2016). Provision of care that is aligned with a midwifery philosophy of care represents the single most effective strategy in the achievement of positive birth outcomes and improved health status in the long term (Renfrew et al, 2014, and see Chapter 23 in this volume). This philosophy of care is articulated in the framework for Quality Maternal and Newborn Care (QMNC) which places emphasis on delivering care that is socially and culturally sensitive, respectful, woman-centred and which optimises biological and psychological processes, reserving interventions for when they are indicated only. It also calls for practitioners who are knowledgeable and interpersonally and culturally competent (Renfrew et al, 2014).The qualities the framework calls for embrace the essence of ethical healthcare provision (beneficence and non-maleficence) and are applicable to all professionals providing maternity care.

Models of maternity care to support continuity of care and caregiver

A recent review of what matters to women in pregnancy around the world indicates that their fundamental concern is for a positive childbirth experience (Downe, Finlayson, Tuncalp and Gulmezoglu, 2016).

As explored in Chapter 11 in this volume, evidence suggests that midwife-led care which is delivered by a known midwife or small group of midwives, in effective collaboration with medical colleagues where this is needed, is associated with numerous benefits, including a positive childbirth experience. In particular, midwife-led continuity of care models, (continuity of care and carer) are associated with better clinical and psychological outcomes and fewer medical interventions compared to other models of care (Sandall et al, 2016; Homer, Brodie and Leap, 2008).

Midwife-led care is based on the same midwife, two midwives or a group of midwives providing care throughout pregnancy and birth (de Jonge, Stuijt, Westerman, 2014; Sandall et al, 2016). This care is based on the premise that birth is a normal physiological process and promotes a holistic approach to individualised care (Sandall, 2014). Primary care providers in midwife-led care models collaborate with obstetricians and paediatricians when clinical advice and treatment are required (Homer et al, 2001).

A systematic review of 15 studies by Sandall, Soltani, Gates, Shennan and Devane (2016) on midwife-led continuity models of care versus other models of care showed, among other outcomes, fewer preterm births, fewer foetal and neonatal deaths, more spontaneous vaginal births, fewer instrumental vaginal births and less use of regional analgesia. There was no statistically significant difference for caesarean sections or intact perinea. Most of the studies in this review reported increased satisfaction among women in midwife-led continuity of care.

Similarly, a Cochrane review (Bohren, Hofmeyr, Sakala, Fukuzawa and Cuthbert, 2017) of 26 studies found that continuous support in labour from hospital staff or from persons either known or unknown to the women was more likely to result in 'spontaneous' births, less need for analgesia, fewer caesarean sections, shorter labours, and more satisfaction. In this case, supporters who were not professional caregivers (for example, doulas) were more likely to be associated with better outcomes.

Continuity of care models are varied and influenced by local priorities and geographical, demographic and financial pressures in maternity services across the UK. The scope of midwifery practice in providing continuity of care is growing in countries such as Canada (Stoll and Gallagher, 2018), while in the Netherlands, UK and Ireland a combination of midwife-led care, medical care and shared care options are available for women (Sandall et al, 2016). In New Zealand (as in the UK), publicly funded midwives can be chosen as the maternity care provider directly by women (Grigg and Tracy, 2012), although this model has been under pressure recently due to competing professionals and budget reforms (Guililland 1999, Midwifery Council New Zealand, 2018).

Place of birth

An important concern for women when deciding where to give birth is that of safety (National Maternity Review, 2016). This refers not only to physical care, but also to its psychosocial aspects such as being respected by healthcare providers and feeling at ease with the birth environment (Downe, Finlayson, Oladapo, Bonet and Gulmezoglu, 2018; WHO 2018a). International literature seems to offer diverging conclusions about the safety of birth in different settings, especially between countries with different arrangements of service provision (Scarf et al, 2018). In many countries, birth has progressively moved to hospital, amid claims of increased safety when compared to out-of-hospital birth (Olsen & Clausen, 2012). However, there is mounting evidence of the benefits of out-of-hospital birth for women without complications in health systems which have adequate provision to ensure good collaboration and communication channels between professionals in and out of hospital, and good transport networks (Olsen and Clausen, 2012; Brockelhurst et al, 2011).

The Birthplace in England study (Brockelhurst et al, 2011), included 64,000 'low-risk' women and compared outcomes for mothers and neonates for births planned at home, in free-standing midwife units, alongside midwife units, and hospital labour wards. The study found that, among planned out-of-hospital births there were more spontaneous vaginal births and fewer interventions, such as epidural anaesthesia, instrumental deliveries and caesarean sections, than among planned births in an obstetric unit (OU). For multiparous women, there were no significant differences in adverse perinatal outcomes between the different birth settings. For nulliparous women birthing in a birth centre was found to be the safest option. The only situation in which adverse perinatal outcomes were higher out of hospital was for primiparous women giving birth at home (9/1,000 versus 5/1,000).

These findings are not unique to the UK, as seen in a case-control study involving more than 1,000 women in France, which demonstrated more spontaneous vaginal births and fewer perineal tears in a homelike birth centre than in a standard labour ward, with no statistically significant difference in adverse neonatal outcomes (Gaudineau, 2013). A large Dutch nationwide study of low-risk women has shown no significant differences for intrapartum and neonatal deaths for those having a planned home birth versus a planned midwife-led hospital birth, and babies among multiparous women born at home were less likely to have Apgar scores below seven, and less likely to be admitted to a neonatal intensive care unit (de Jonge et al, 2015). Another study found more spontaneous births, fewer episiotomies and less use of oxytocin for augmentation and in the third stage of labour, with no significant difference in caesarean sections, instrumental deliveries and postpartum haemorrhage (Bolten et al, 2016). In Canada, a meta-analysis of two matched cohort studies found that the rate of intrapartum intervention was lower in planned home births and found no significant difference in stillbirths and neonatal deaths between the two groups (Hutton et al, 2015).

In contrast to the above, a meta-analysis on place of birth concluded that neonatal mortality was increased (Wax et al, 2010) in home versus hospital births. However, this study has been criticised for the inclusion of unplanned as well as planned home births, and for the inclusion of births with varying levels of risk (Michal, Janssen, Vedam, Hutton and de Jonge, 2011; Gyte, Dodwell and McFarlane, 2011; Kirby and Fost, 2011).

Overall, for women with limited or no complications in pregnancy who are giving birth in countries with well-trained midwives with good links and relations to local hospitals and medical support, choosing an out-of-hospital care setting for birth seems to be safe, and to promote physiological birth and reduce interventions, as well as being associated with a range of other positive outcomes (including higher maternal satisfaction – Hodnett, Downe and Walsh, 2012) and very few adverse effects (Scarf et al, 2018).

The provision of midwife-led care settings (MLUs), alongside midwife-led units (AMU) and freestanding midwifery units (FMUs) in any specific country is influenced by geographical, service, organisational and cultural factors (McCourt, Rance, Rayment and Sandall, 2011), which affect women's choice in place of birth. Therefore, when out-of-hospital birth provision does not exist in such well-resourced contexts, there are good grounds for political lobbying to ensure that such provision is expanded. In those contexts where conditions are not optimal for out-of-hospital birth, the drive should be to improve conditions so that this can be a safe, viable and desirable option for women.

It is likely that the beneficial effects of out-of-hospital settings are associated with the social and relational philosophy of care that often features in these kinds of birthplace, and that are also seen in midwifery-led care (discussed in the next section). This results in the use of pain-relief methods that interfere minimally in labour progress, as well as the opportunity for women to adopt more upright and mobile positions, and for them to have more time before intervention is considered. These factors are considered in the next sections of this chapter. Although they are more usually associated with out-of-hospital birth and midwife-led care (Bohren et al, 2017; Sandall et al, 2016), there is no logical reason why they could not also be applied in hospital settings and with the full range of maternity care providers.

Care practices during labour to support physiological labour and birth

Physiological labour is characterised by spontaneous onset and hormonal surges of oxytocin, which help sustain uterine contractions while the foetus adapts to labour stresses such as hypoxia with catecholamine rises which are triggered by epinephrine-norepinephrine receptor changes (see Chapter 2). There is reduced likelihood of foetal compromise when labour remains physiological and any interventions, such as use of epidural for pain relief, can reduce the effectiveness of oxytocin on uterine contractions thus increasing the risk of further interventions (Buckley 2005; Buckley, 2015).

A birth environment which facilitates free movement (RCM, 2012) provides dignity, privacy and comfort, respects women's choices (Prochaska, 2013), encourages eating and drinking in labour (Singata, Tranmer and Gyte, 2013), offers non-pharmacological pain relief (Jones et al 2012), including freedom of movement, and uses intermittent monitoring strategies (NICE 2014) that enhance the physiological birth process (Bohren, Hofmeyr, Sakal, Fujuzawaand and Cuthbert, 2017).

Supportive strategies for working with pain

Among the available pain-relief techniques and strategies, pharmacological methods have traditionally been favoured due to their effectiveness. As Leap et al discuss (see Chapter 16), resorting to the 'pain menu' of pharmacological pain relief has a number of adverse consequences, particularly for healthy women without complications.

Other pain-relief methods are more conducive to facilitating birth physiology. These include complementary therapies such as relaxation, acupuncture, massage, yoga, hypnosis, aromatherapy, reflexology, homeopathy and breathing techniques. Their efficacy is yet to be tested in large randomised controlled trials, but these non-pharmacological pain-relief methods have been found to offer some benefits with the likelihood of minimal side effects (Smith et al, 2018; Cluett, Burns and Cuthbert, 2018).

Given the potential for improved outcomes, and the unlikely detrimental effects, non-pharmacological pain relief methods, coupled with other strategies discussed below, should be considered as important facilitators of birth physiology.

Dynamic movement and maternal position

Most of the evidence on the outcomes of labour and birth is based on births in which women are in the supine or semi-recumbent position, or in lithotomy. It is known that there are physiological advantages to being upright in labour. Being upright reduces aorto-caval compression, increases efficiency of uterine contractions, supports optimal foetal alignment and (especially in terms of squatting and kneeling) increases the pelvic outlet dimension.

The advantages for women who labour in more upright positions both during the first and the second stage of labour have been reported in two Cochrane reviews (Lawrence, Lewis, Hofmeyr and Styles, 2013; Gupta, Hofmeyr and Shehmar, 2012) and by Pridis, Dahlen and Schmied (2012), and they include shorter labours, less use of epidural analgesia, fewer abnormal foetal heart rate patterns and a lower incidence of instrumental births, caesarean sections and episiotomy, but a higher incidence of second-degree tears and estimated blood loss above 500ml. A cohort study showed that upright positions were only associated with an increase in blood loss greater than 500ml among women with perineal damage, which suggests the origin is not uterine (de Jonge A et al, 2007).

When women are free to follow their feelings and needs, they adopt a range of positions as labour progresses, thought to be instinctively aimed at helping the foetus adopt an optimal position of flexion and descent (Romano and Lothian, 2008). Importantly, when women move freely during labour, they report an increased sense of control (Albers et al, 1997) and satisfaction (Pridis, Dahlen and Schmied, 2012).

Intermittent auscultation of the foetal heart

Continuous electronic foetal heart rate monitoring (EFHM) is a widely used tool to check the foetus' health during labour in developed countries. It was devised with the intention of identifying foetal hypoxia in labour, but introduced without evidence of effectiveness (Devane, 2005). Indeed, some limitations were evident from its inception, including its low specificity and the difficulty in accurately interpreting the traces (Nelson et al, 1996; Ayres-de-Campos, Bernardes, Costa-Pereira and Pereira-Leite, 1999). A Cochrane review comparing continuous vs intermittent cardiotocography (CTG) and intermittent auscultation (Alfirevic, Devane, Gyte and Cuthbert, 2017) concluded that continuous cardiotocography during labour is associated with a reduction in neonatal seizures, but no significant differences in cerebral palsy, infant mortality or other standard measures of neonatal wellbeing. It was also associated with increased caesarean section and instrumental vaginal birth rates. In addition, conducting an admission CTG when the woman is considered to have a low-risk pregnancy increases by 20% her risk of having a caesarean section (Devane et al, 2017).

Importantly, continuous EFHM tends to interfere with a woman's ability to mobilise during labour, which, as discussed above, is one of the most important factors in supporting its physiology.

In the absence of reliable methods to interpret electronic continuous foetal monitoring in labour, intermittent auscultation for the low-risk mother remains the most effective method to promote labour physiology and is a safe method to assess foetal wellbeing (NICE, 2014).

Observations of labour progress

Assessment of progress in labour is a central element in modern maternity care and it is usually determined through vaginal examination. However, this is an uncomfortable procedure which can also disturb the woman's mental 'space' and consequently the interplay of labour hormones and potentially the progress of labour. In addition, no good evidence to support or reject the routine use of vaginal examination has been found (Downe, Gyte, Dahlen and Singata, 2013). Downe et al (2013) recommend that other ways of assessing labour progress should be investigated, especially in view of the invasiveness of the procedure and its lack of accuracy. These observational cues are discussed in more detail in Chapter 3.

Some evidence indicates that an abdominal examination can reveal descent of the foetus, and that this is a sign of effective labour progress (Higgins and Farine, 2013). During the second stage of labour the occurrence of a so-called 'purple line' can be seen in about 90% of labouring women, running from the upper part of the anus up and between the buttocks. This has a 76% correlation with cervical dilatation (Sheperd, Cheyne and Kennedy, 2010).

Dixon, Skinner and Fourer (2013) found that labouring women display a certain pattern of distinct behaviours as they progress through their labour (findings which correlate with other studies). The authors postulate that these may in fact represent normal labour physiology and progress. Indeed, these results probably resonate with clinicians who may be aware of women changing their demeanour and behaviour as labour progresses.

These findings suggest that a thorough assessment of factors other than vaginal examination is needed before intervention is considered for so-called 'slow progress', since, in fact, labour may be 'slow but normal'. These factors include asking if the woman is free to adopt any position that works for her as labour progresses, the degree to which the environment is conducive to her doing labour work, and if all other parameters of maternal and foetal wellbeing are reassuring.

Effects of physiological birth on positive maternal and neonatal outcomes

Birth is a defining moment for later life health. It is recognised that a straightforward vaginal birth is associated with multiple health benefits for most mothers and their babies (New Zealand College of Midwives, 2006). Mothers recover quicker when compared to other modes of birth (Fenwick, Gamble and Hauck, 2007; McGovern et al, 2006) and there is less blood loss (Lumbiganon et al. 2010; Shamsa, Bai, Raviraj and Gyaneshwar, 2013).

The normal stress response of labour has been associated with benefits such as improved neonatal respiratory response (Herrera-Gomez et al, 2015). As discussed in Chapter 13, there are other potential benefits to neonates, in the short and longer term (and see Simon-Areces et al, 2012; Peters et al, 2018).

Physiological birth is associated with an increased likelihood that a woman will commence and continue breastfeeding (Buckley, 2015; Smith and Kroger, 2010). As a consequence, the Standards for Improving Quality of Maternal and Newborn Care in Health Facilities (WHO, 2016) recommend that in order to improve breastfeeding women should be encouraged to adopt the position of their choice during labour. The Implementation Guidance for Protecting, Promoting and Supporting Breastfeeding

(WHO, 2018b) advocates for respect and maintenance of dignity and privacy for women and newborns. These are all essential elements for the promotion and protection of physiological births.

Psychosocial outcomes – positive maternal health, self-efficacy and parenting capacity

Given concerns about maternal mental health in the UK (MBRRACE, 2017) and beyond, it is important to consider the psychology of childbirth. The birth experience represents a milestone that deeply impacts on the woman's emotional and social life (Kwee and McBride, 2016; Salmela-Aro et al, 2012). Most women, in most cultures, would prefer to experience a safe, physiological labour, resulting in the birth of a healthy baby (Downe et al, 2018; WHO 2018a). For these women, such an experience optimises a positive transition to parenthood (Leap, Sandall, Buckland & Huber, 2010; Salmela-Aro et al, 2012) which has been linked to improved parental skills, parental efficacy and an increased sense of achievement (Loto, et al, 2010), leading to a reduction in maternal mental health problems, and in infant behavioural problems (WHO and UNFPA, 2008; Stewart, Robertson, Dennis, Grace and Wallington, 2003).

Those who are supported through physiological births are more likely to enjoy increased self-esteem (Loto et al, 2010). This helps them overcome some of the challenges that new motherhood entails and this will further reinforce their self-esteem, thought to be essential when developing parenting capacity (Loto et al, 2010). In addition, the woman's satisfaction with the birth experience is related to the development of a sense of maternal identity which has positive effects beyond herself: it positively affects the family's psychosocial wellbeing (Howarth, Swain and Treharne, 2011).

Longer-term outcomes

As Chapters 13 and 14 demonstrate, there may be a protective effect of physiological labour and birth on medium and longer-term outcomes for the baby. This includes a reduced risk of chronic auto-immune disease, linked to the positive effects of the maternal vaginal microbiome on the neonatal gut flora, and of epigenetic factors. There is also recent evidence emerging that links postnatal depression to the use of synthetic oxytocin in labour (Kroll-Desroisers, 2017) which, again, would suggest a protective effect of maternal oxytocin produced in spontaneous labour and birth. Some of the possible pathways for this effect are explored in Chapter 2.

Conclusion

The importance of supporting normal birth physiology cannot be overestimated. The available evidence shows that this is best capitalised on when intrapartum care is provided in an environment where maternal hormones can work optimally, through the strategies discussed in this chapter and by limiting the use of routine interventions. This should be viable, possible and easily achievable for the vast majority of mothers and babies worldwide.

Because of the positive effects for mother and baby in both the short and longer term, caregivers from all disciplinary backgrounds have a duty to facilitate safe physiological birth for healthy women with uncomplicated pregnancies when this is what they want to achieve, regardless of the care setting, and to be skilled and confident in their abilities to do so.

This can be achieved through adopting an underpinning shared philosophy of care which considers birth a normal, physiological process. Such a philosophy has been described as the midwifery philosophy of care in the latest *Lancet* series on midwifery (Renfrew et al, 2014). Since at the core of that philosophy lie the principles of beneficence and non-maleficence, such a philosophy should be the default position for all professionals providing maternity care.

Key points for consideration

- Whenever you're with a labouring woman, listen to her needs, respect her feelings, look into her eyes and not at your watch.
- Remember the importance of 'watchful waiting'.
- Create a sensitive and caring environment.
- Be mindful of the language you use.
- Respect the physiology of labour.

References

Albers LL, Anderson D, Cragin L, Daniels SM, Hunter C, Sedler KD, et al. The relationship of ambulation in labor to operative delivery. Journal of Nurse Midwifery. 1997; 42 (1):4-8

Alfirevic Z,Devane D, Gyte GML, Cuthbert A. Continuous cardiotocography (CTG) asa form of electronic fetal monitoring (EFM) for fetal assessment during labour. CochraneDatabaseof SystematicReviews 2017, Issue 2. Art. No.: CD006066. DOI: 10.1002/14651858.CD006066.pub3.

Anim-Somuah M, Smyth RMD, Cyna AM, Cuthbert A. Epidural versus non-epidural or no analgesiafor pain management in labour. CochraneDatabaseof SystematicReviews 2018, Issue 5. Art. No.: CD000331. DOI: 10.1002/14651858.CD000331.pub4.

Ayres-de-Campos D., Bernardes J., Costa-Pereira A. & Pereira-Leite L. (1999) Inconsistencies in classification by experts of cardiotocograms and subsequent clinical decisions. British Journal of Obstetrics and Gynaecology 106, 1307–1310.

Bohren MA, Hofmeyr GJ, SakalaC, Fukuzawa RK, Cuthbert A. Continuous support for women during childbirth. Cochrane Database of Systematic Reviews 2017, Issue 7. Art. No.: CD003766. DOI: 10.1002/14651858.CD003766.pub6.

Bolten N, De Jonge A, Zwagerman E, Klomp T, Zart JJ, Geerts CC (2016) Effect Of Planned Place Of Birth On Obstetric Interventions And Maternal Outcomes Among Low-Risk Women: A Cohort Study In The Netherlands. BMC Pregnancy and Childbirth. 16:329.

British Medical Journal (2016). Too much medicine. BMJ. Available at www.bmj.com/too-much-medicine [Accessed 3rd February 2016].

Brocklehurst P, et al (2011). Perinatal and maternal outcomes by planned place of birth for healthy women with low risk pregnancies: the Birthplace in England national prospective cohort study. Birthplace in England Collaborative Group. BMJ; 343 doi: https://doi.org/10.1136/bmj.d7400 BMJ 2011;343:d7400

Buckley SJ. (2005) Gentle birth, gentle mothering: the wisdom and science of gentle choices in pregnancy, birth and parenting. Brisbane, Australia: One Moon Press

Buckley, SJ. (2015) Hormonal Physiology of Childbearing: Evidence and Implications for Women, Babies, and Maternity Care. Washington, D.C.: Childbirth Connection Programs, National Partnership for Women & Families.

Cheng YW, Shaffer BL, Nicholson JM, Caughey AB. (2014). Second Stage of Labor and Epidural Use: A Larger Effect Than Previously Suggested. Obstetrics & Gynecology: 123 - Issue 3 - p 527–535 doi: 10.1097/

AOG.0000000000000134

Cluett ER, Burns E, Cuthbert A. Immersion in water during labour and birth. Cochrane Database of Systematic Reviews 2018, Issue 5. Art. No.: CD000111. DOI: 10.1002/14651858.CD000111.pub4

de Jonge, A. et al., 2015. Perinatal mortality and morbidity up to 28 days after birth among 743 070 low-risk planned home and hospital births: a cohort study based on three merged national perinatal databases. BJOG : an international journal of obstetrics and gynaecology, 122(5), pp.720–728

de Jonge A, Stuijt R, Eijke I, Westerman MJ ; Continuity of care: what matters to women when they are transferred from primary to secondary care during labour? A qualitative interview study in the NETHERLANDS, BMC PREGNANCY AND CHILDBIRTH 2014, 14:103 DOI:10.1186/1471-2393-14-103

De Jonge A, Van Diem M Th, Scheepers PLH, Van der Pal-de Bruin KM, Lagro-Janssen ALM (2007). Increased blood loss in upright birthing positions originates from perineal damage. BJOG, 114: 349-55.

Devane D, Lalor JG, Daly S, McGuire W, Cuthbert A, Smith V. Cardiotocography versus intermittent auscultation of fetal hearton admission to labour ward for assessment of fetal wellbeing. CochraneDatabaseof SystematicReviews 2017, Issue 1. Art. No.: CD005122. DOI: 10.1002/14651858.CD005122.pub5.

Dixon L, Skinner J and Foureur M (2013). The emotional and hormonal pathways of labour and birth: integrating mind, body and behaviour. New Zealand College of Midwives. 48 15-23

Downe S, Gyte GML, Dahlen HG, Singata M. Routine vaginal examinations for assessing progress of labour to improve outcomes for women and babies at term. CochraneDatabaseof SystematicReviews 2013, Issue 7. Art. No.: CD010088. DOI: 10.1002/14651858.CD010088.pub2.

Downe S, Finlayson K. Oladapo Ot, Bonet M, Gulmezoglu AM: What matters to women during childbirth: a systematic qualitative review (Plos One (2018) 13:4 (E0194906) DOI 10.1371/journal.pone.0194906). PLOS ONE. 2018;13(5):1–17.

Downe S, Finlayson K, Tunçalp Ö, Metin Gülmezoglu A. (2016). What matters to women: a systematic scoping review to identify the processes and outcomes of antenatal care provision that are important to healthy pregnant women. BJOG. 2016 Mar;123(4):529-39.

Escuriet, R. (2016) Midwives' contribution to normal childbirth care. Cross-sectional study in public health settings ISRCTN17833269 https://doi.org/10.1186/ISRCTN17833269

Fenwich J, Gamble J, Hauck Y. (2007). Believing in birth – choosing VBAC: the childbirth expecttions of a self-selected cohort of Australian women. Journal of Clinical Nursing 16 (8) https://doi.org/10.1111/j.1365-2702.2006.01747.x

Gamble LA, Hesson A, Burns T (2015). Sticking to the Plan: Patient Preferences for Epidural Use During Labor. Medical Student Research Journal 4 issue Winter

Gaudineau A, Sauleau EA, Nisand I, Langer B. Obstetric and Neonatal Oucomes in a home-like birth centre: a case control study. Arch Gynecol Obstet. 2013 Feb;287(2):211-6.

Grigg CP, Tracy SK (2013), New Zealand's unique maternity system, Women and birth : Journal of the Australian College of Midwives, ISSN: 1878-1799, Vol: 26, Issue: 1, Page: e59-64 https://doi.org/10.1016/j.wombi.2012.09.006

Guililland K: Midwifery In New Zealand (1999), Birth International, Posted Feb 11, 2016 By Abby Sutcliffe. Available From Https://Birthinternational.Com/Article/Midwifery/Midwifery-In-New-Zealand/

Gupta JK, Hofmeyr GJ, Shehmar M. Position in the second stage of labour for women without epidural anaesthesia. Cochrane Database of Systematic Reviews 2012, Issue 5. Art. No.: CD002006. DOI: 10.1002/14651858.CD002006.pub3

Gyte G, Dodwell M, Macfarlane A (2011). Home birth metaanalysis: does it meet AJOG's reporting requirements? Am J Obstet Gynecol. 204(4):e15; author reply e18-20, discussion e20. doi: 10.1016/j.ajog.2011.01.035. Epub 2011

Herrera-Gomez A, Garcia-Martinez O, Ramos-Torrecillas J, Luna-Bertos E, Ruiz C, Ocana-Peinado FM. (2015). Retrospective study of the association between epidural analgesia during labour and complications for the newborn. Midwifery 31 613-616

Higgins M and Farine D (2013) Assessment of labor progress. Expert Rev Obstet Gynecol. 8 (1) 1-13

Hodnett ED, Downe S, Walsh D. Alternative Versus Conventional Institutional Settings For Birth. Cochrane Database Of Systematic Reviews 2012, Issue 8. Art. No.: Cd000012. Doi: 10.1002/14651858.Cd000012.Pub4

Hofmeyr GJ, Vogel JP, Cuthbert A, Singata M. (2017) Fundal pressure during the second stage of labour. Cochrane Database of Systematic Reviews 2017, Issue 3 DOI: 10.1002/14651858.CD006067.pub3.

Homer CS, Davis GK, Brodie PM, Sheehan A, Barclay LM, Wills J, Chapman MG: Collaboration in maternity care: a randomised controlled trial comparing community-based continuity care with standard hospital care, BJOG 2001 Jan:108(1):16-22

Homer C, Brodie P, Leap N. (2008). Midwifery Continuity Of Care: A Practical Guide. Elsevier Australia

Howarth AM, Swain N and Treharne GJ (2011). Taking personal responsibility for well-being increases birth satisfaction of first time mothers. Journal of Health Psychology. DOI: 10.1177/1359105311403521

Hutton EK, Cappelletti A, Reitsma AH, Simioni J, Horne J, Mcgregor C, Ahmed RJ: Outcomes Associated With Planned Place Of Birth Among Women With Low Risk Pregnancies Cmaj 2015. Doi:10.1503/ Cmaj.150564

Jones I, Othman M, Dowswell T, Alfirevic Z, Gates S, Newburn M, Jordan S, Lavender T, Neilson J. Pain management for women in labour: An overview of systematic reviews. Cochrane Database of Systematic Reviews 2012, issue 3. Art. No.: cd009234. Doi: 10.1002/14651858.cd009234.pub2

Kirby RS, Frost J (2011) Maternal and newborn outcomes in planned home birth vs planned hospital births; a meta-analysis – letter to the editor. AJOG e16

Kroll-Desrosiers AR, Nephew BC, Babb JA, Guilarte-Walker Y, Moore Simas TA, Deligiannidis KM (2017). Association of peripartum synthetic oxytocin administration and depressive and anxiety disorders within the first postpartum year. Depress Anxiety. 34(2):137-146. doi: 10.1002/da.22599.

Kwee JH, McBride HL. Working together for women's empowerment: Strategies for interdisciplinary collaboration in perinatal care. J Health Psychol. 2016;21(11):2742-2752.

Laughton SK, Branch DW, Beaver J and Zhang J (2012). Changes in labour patterns over the last 50 years. American Journal of Obstetrics and Gynecology. 206(5):419.e1-9. doi: 10.1016/j.ajog.2012.03.003. Epub 2012 Mar 10.

Lawrence A, Lewis L, Hofmeyr G, Styles C. Maternal positions and mobility during first stage labour. Cochrane Database of Systematic Reviews 2013, Issue 10. Art. No.: CD003934. DOI: 10.1002/14651858.CD003934.pub4

Leap N, Sandall J, Buckland S, Huber U. Journey to confidence: women's experiences of pain in labour and relational continuity of care. J Midwifery Womens Health 2010;55:234–42.

Lemos A, Amorim MMR, Dornelas de Andrade A, de Souza AI, Cabral Filho JE, Correia JB (2017) Pushing/bearing downmethods for the second stage of labour.Cochrane Database of Systematic Reviews. Issue 3. DOI: 10.1002/14651858.CD009124.pub3.

Loto OM, Adewuya AO, Ajenifuja OK, Orji EO, Ayandiran EO, Owolabi ET & Ade-Oj IP (2010) Cesarean section in relation to self-esteem and parenting among new mothers in southwestern Nigeria. Acta Obstetricia et Gynecologica. 2010; 89: 35–38

Lumbiganon, P., Laopaiboon, M., Gülmezoglu, A.M., Souza, J.P., et al. (2010) Method of delivery and pregnancy outcomes in Asia: The WHO global survey on maternal and perinatal health 2007-08. The Lancet, 375, 490-500

MBRRACE (2017). Lessons learned to inform maternity care from the UK and Ireland Confidential Enquiries into Maternal Deaths and Morbidity 2013–15. Maternal, Newborn and Infant Clinical Outcome Review Programme; MBRRACE.

Mccourt, C., Rance, S., Rayment, J. Sandall, J. Birthplace Qualitative Organisational Case Studies: How Maternity Care Systems May Affect The Provision Of Care In Different Birth Settings Birthplace In England Research Programme 2011, Final Report Part 6. Hmso.

McDougall M, Campbell OMR and Graham W (2016). Maternal Health Series; Executive Summary. The Lancet

McGovern P, Dowd B, Gjerdingen D, Gross CR, Kenney S, Ukestad L,McCaffrey D and Lundberg U (2006). Postpartum Health of Employed Mothers 5 Weeks After Childbirth. Ann Fam Med 2006;4:159-167. DOI: 10.1370/afm.519.

Michal CA, Janssen PA, Vedam S, Hutton EK And De Jonge A (2011) Planned Home Vs Hospital Birth: A Meta-Analysis Gone Wrong. Medscape

Midwifery Council New Zealand Newsletter (Mcnz). Midpoint (2018),

National Maternity Review: Better Births, Improving Outcomes Of Maternity Services In England, A Five Year Forward View Of Maternity Care, 2016

National Institute for Health and Care Excellence (NICE) (2014). Intrapartum care for healthy women and babies. Clinical guideline 190. 2014. http://nice.org.uk/guidance/cg190

Neal JL, Ryan SL and Hunter LA. (2015) The first stage of labour. In: King TL, Brucker MC, Kriebs JM, Fahey JO, Gregor CL, Varney H (eds) Varney's Midwifery. 5th ed. Jones and Bartlett Learning: Burlington.

Nelson K.B., Dambrosia J.M., Ting T.Y. & Grether J.K. (1996) Uncertain value of electronic fetal monitoring in predicting cerebral palsy. New England Journal of Medicine 334, 613–618.

New Zealand College of Midwives (2006). Consensus statement normal birth.

Nystedt A, Hildingsson I. (2014) Diverse definitions of prolonged labour and its consequences with sometimes subsequent inappropriate treatment. BMC Pregnancy and Childbirth 14:233 https://doi.org/10.1186/1471-2393-14-233

Odent, M (1992). The fetus ejection reflex. In: The nature of birth and breastfeeding. Westport, CT: Bergin and Garvey. 29-43.

Oladapo OT, Souza JP, Fawole B, Mugerwa K, Perdona AG, Alves D, et al (2018) Progression of the first stage of spontaneous labour: A prospective cohort study in two sub-Saharan African countries. PLoS Med 15(1):e1002492. https://doi.org/10.1371/journal.pmed1002492

Olsen O, Clausen JA. Planned hospital birth versus planned home birth. Cochrane Database of Systematic Reviews 2012, Issue 9. Art. No.: CD000352. DOI: 10.1002/14651858.CD000352.pub2

Peters, L.L, Thornton C, de Jonge A, Khashan A, Tracy M, Downe S, Feijen-de Jong E.I, and Dahlen HG (2018). The effect of medical and operative birth interventions on child health outcomes in the first 28 days and up to 5 years of age: A linked data population-based cohort study. Birth, 00, pp.1–11.

Priddis H, Dahlen H, Schmied V. What are the facilitators, inhibitors and implications of birth positioning? A review of the literature. Women and Birth (2012) 25, 100-106

Prochaska E. (2013). The importance of dignity in childbirth, British Journal of Midwifery Vol. 21 (11).

RCM: Evidence Based gGidelines for Midwifery-led Care in Labour; Positions for labour and birth (2012)

Renfrew MJ, McFadden A, Bastos MH et al. (2014) Midwifery and quality care: findings from a new evidence-informed framework for maternal and newborn care. The Lancet. Published online June 23 http://dx.doi.org/10.1016/SO140-6736(14)60789-3

Romano AM and Lothian JA, (2008). Promoting, protecting and supporting normal birth: A look at the evidence.

JOGNN, 37 , 94-105; 2008. DOI: 10.1111/J.1552-6909.2007.00210.x

Salmela-Aro K, Read S, Rouhe H, Halmesmäki E, Toivanen RM, Tokola MI et al. Promoting positive motherhood among nulliparous pregnant women with an intense fear of childbirth: RCT intervention. J Health Psychol. 2012;17(4):520-534.

Sandall J (2014). The Contribution Of Continuity Of Midwifery Care To High Quality Maternity Care, A Report By Professor Jane Sandall For The Royal College Of Midwives.

Sandall J, Soltani H, Gates S, Shennan A, Devane D. Midwife-Led Versus Other Models Of Care For Childbearing Women. Cochrane Database Of Systematic Reviews 2016, Issue 4. Art. No.: Cd004667. Doi: 10.1002/14651858. Cd004667.Pub5

Scarf VL, Rossiter C, Vedam Saraswathi V, Dahlen HG, Ellwood D, Forster D, Foureur M, McLachlan H, Oats J, Sibbritt D, Thornton C and Homer C (2018).Maternal and perinatal outcomes by planned placed of birth among women with low-risk pregnancies in high-income countries: A systematic review and meta-analysis. Midwifery 62. 240-255.

Schytt E, Waldenstrom U. (2010). Epidural analgesia for labor pain: whose choice? Acta Obstetricia et Gynecologica. 89: 238–242

Shamsa A, Bai J, Raviraj P, Gyaneshwar R (2013). Mode of delivery and its associated maternal and neonatal outcomes. Open Journal of Obstetrics and Gynecology. Vol. 3 No. 3 DOI:10.4236/ojog.2013.33057

Shepherd A, Cheyne H and Kennedy S (2010) The purple line as a measure of labour progress: a longitudinal study. BMC Pregnancy and Childbirth, 10:54

Simon-Areces J, Dietrich MO, Hermes G, Garcia-Segura LM, Arevalo MA, Horvath TL (2012). Ucp2 Induced by Natural Birth Regulates Neuronal Differentiation of the Hippocampus and Related Adult Behavior. Plos One. https://doi.org/10.1371/journal.pone.0042911

Singata M, TranmerJ, Gyte GML: Restricting oral fluid and food intake during labour. Cochrane Database of Systematic Reviews 2013, issue 8. Art. No.: cd003930. Doi: 10.1002/14651858.cd003930.pub3.

Smith LJ, Kroger M. Impact of birthing practices on breastfeeding, 2nd ed.Sudbury: Jones and Bartlett; 2010

Smith, V., Daly, D., Lundgren, I., Eri, T., Benstoem, C. and Devane, D. (2014). Salutogenically focused outcomes in systematic reviews of intrapartum interventions: A systematic review of systematic reviews. Midwifery 30 e151-e156. Available at http://dx.doi.org/10.1016/j.midw.2013.11.002

Smith CA, Levett KM, Collins CT, Armour M, Dahlen HG, Suganuma M. Relaxation techniques for pain management in labour. Cochrane database of systematic reviews 2018, issue 3. Art. No.: cd009514. Doi: 10.1002/14651858.cd009514.pub2

Stewart DE, Robertson E, Dennis C-L, Grace SL and Wallington T (2003). POSTPARTUM DEPRESSION: LITERATURE REVIEW OF RISK FACTORS AND INTERVENTIONS. University Health Network Women's Health Program. Toronto Public Health

Stoll K, J. Gallagher, A Survey Of Burnout And Intentions To Leave The Profession Among Western Canadian Midwives, Women Birth (2018), Https://Doi.Org/10.1016/J.Wombi.2018.10.002

Vedam S, Stoll K, MacDorman M, Declercq E, Cramer R, Cheyney M, Fisher T , Butt E, Yang YT, Powell Kennedy H. (2018) Mapping integration of midwives across the United States: Impact on access, equity, and outcomes. PLoS ONE 13(2) e0192523. https://doi.org/10.1371/journal.pone.0192523

Walsh D. (2012) Evidence and Skills for Normal Labour and Birth; A Guide for Midwives. 2nd ed. Routledge: London

Wax Jr, Pinette Mg, Cartin A, Et Al. Maternal And Newborn Morbidity By Birth Facility Among Selected United States 2006 Low-Risk Births. Am J Obstet Gynecol 2010;202:152.E1-5.

World Health Organization. The world health report 2013: research for universal health coverage. Geneva: WHO; 2013.

World Health Organization (2014). WHO recommendations for augmentation of labour. WHO: Geneva ISBN 978 92 4 150736 3

World Health Organization (2016). Standards for improving quality of maternal and newborn care in health facilities. Geneva; ISBN: 978 92 4 151121 6

World Health Organization (2018a). WHO recommendations Intrapartum care for a positive experience. WHO: Geneva; ISBN 978-92-4-155021-5

World Health Organization (2018b).Implementation Guidance; Protecting, promoting and supporting Breastfeeding in facilities providing maternity and newborn services. The revised baby-friendly hospital initiative. Unicef;.WHO

World Health Organization and United Nations Population Fund (2008). Maternal mental health and child health and development in low and middle income countries. Report of the meeting held in Geneva, Switzerland.

PART II

Philosophies and theories

CHAPTER 6

From being to becoming: reconstructing childbirth knowledge

Soo Downe and Christine McCourt

This chapter was first published in 2004, and updated in 2008. The 2008 version is included here. It is seen as relevant because it was the first time that discussions of complexity and salutogenesis were introduced into the maternity discourse, and the arguments are still current for maternity research, policy, and practice.*

As a reprint, the references and internal chapter links appear as they were then, without updates (though some footnotes have been added, for clarity). Of particular note: the current volume does not include a separate chapter on the definition of 'normality', because this chapter addresses the issue of 'unique normality', which is at the heart of Squaring the Circle. *Footnotes direct the reader to more recent texts that address this issue of definitions.*

Introduction

The impetus for the work set out in this chapter was frustration with the near invisibility of normal physiological processes in Western approaches to childbirth. This included the apparent inability even to define 'normal birth', except as an absence of technical intervention. Thinking through the factors which have led to this point has given us the opportunity to share some of the insights and observations we have previously reported separately.[1-4] In the process, the synergy between our separate but connected areas of knowledge has become apparent to us. We hope that we have been able to make this clear in the account we give in this chapter.

In order to explain the conclusions at the end of the chapter, it is necessary to

* Downe S and McCourt C 2008 From Being to Becoming: Reconstructing childbirth knowledge In: Downe S (ed) *Normal Birth, evidence and debate* (2nd ed). Elsevier, Oxford. Reprinted by kind permission from Elsevier.

describe the recent history of some of the philosophies and theories that we feel have influenced current perspectives in the context of health. We also briefly describe the theories that are the basis of our proposal for new 'ways of seeing'.[5] We are aware that, in places, some of these accounts may seem to be very far from clinical practice, or from personal experiences of birth. Where we can, we have drawn theory–practice connections through reference to research based in practice.

In 1972, Archie Cochrane, then director of the Medical Research Council Epidemiology Unit, published a seminal book entitled *Effectiveness and Efficiency*.[6] He put forward the apparently simple view that 'all effective treatment must be free'. Its implication was revolutionary in that, by default, it proposed that ineffective treatment should not be free. This agenda has become central to political developments in healthcare in many countries worldwide since the early 1990s.

A problem arises, however, when we try to define and measure effectiveness. This is not merely a matter of asking 'does it work?' but, fundamentally, of deciding what should be evaluated, and how, and how the results should be interpreted. Who decides the nature of accepted knowledge? Even within so-called 'hard' numerical, controlled studies, findings depend on a series of assumptions about what is to be studied, how the study is framed, what is seen as bias or 'noise' and how the findings are interpreted. All evidence is culturally bound and all is framed by the nature of the questions that are asked. As Ann Oakley pointed out: 'Science and knowledge are socially produced: that is, they are subject to the very influence of social processes and practicalities that their common-sense representations would dismiss as quite beyond their frames of reference' (p335).[7] This has an impact on what is termed the 'authoritative knowledge' of health.[8,9] Such knowledge is characterised through its dominance and authority. This can be expressed at any level of a social system, usually through a combination of structural and explanatory power. It is generally so well established that it is difficult to question and tends to be taken for granted as right and proper, or even simply part of the natural order. At the extreme, powerful social groups may affirm the superiority of their way of knowing by associating it with established truths, such as with God or with nature. Jordan argues:[8]

> *To legitimise one way of knowing as authoritative devalues, often totally dismisses, all other ways of knowing. Those who espouse alternative knowledge systems tend to be seen as backward, ignorant or naïve troublemakers ... The constitution of authoritative knowledge is an ongoing social process that both builds and reflects power relationships within a community of practice. It does so in such a way that all participants come to see the current social order as a natural order, i.e. as the way things (obviously) are.* (p152)

With these observations in mind, we intend to examine the nature of childbirth knowledge (the 'epistemology' of childbirth) with particular reference to our understanding of normality. This chapter examines four aspects of current authoritative knowledge in childbirth: certainty, simplicity, linearity and pathology. We propose a new approach, based on uncertainty, complexity and the generation of well-being (salutogenesis). In presenting our case, we also make the claim that we need to see the world and the natural processes within it from a cyclical and complex paradigm, rather than by the simple, linear model that underpins most of the current authoritative knowledge applied in healthcare.

The current childbirth paradigm

Certainty as a given

The kind of science that investigates ever more advanced technical solutions to human problems is arguably the fundamental guiding force in most 21st century societies. Although eco-warriors and anti-globalisation campaigners seek to challenge this hegemony, it is firmly and deeply established. Healthcare is a prime example of the authority of this kind of science in our lives. This kind of authority is generally accepted by most members of a society, as it is taken to be the norm, but the issue of power is especially evident when the norms and certainties of applied health science are enforced legally on those who deviate from accepted practices. This phenomenon has been evident in US and UK cases where women who refuse caesarean section have been ordered by the courts to submit to surgery.[10,11]

The philosophical underpinnings of the approach to science used by the judge in such cases can be located in what has been termed 'enlightenment science'.[12] However, as we will illustrate, enlightenment science, paradoxically, also bore the seeds of scientific uncertainty. The enlightenment movement is identified by historians as having taken place in the 18th century in Europe. Bacon, Newton and Descartes were key thinkers influencing the science that developed in this period.[13] They were interested in understanding how the natural world and the phenomena within it worked. The analogy they used was that of the machine. This reflected their social context of rapid technical and industrial development. This model was characterised by simplicity and elegance. It offered a unified way of analysing all aspects of the natural (and human) world by reducing it to its constituent building blocks. It was believed that complex phenomena could be understood and explained by reducing them to these basic parts, and then by looking for the mechanisms through which they interacted. Newton hoped to use his theories to develop an overall, unifying explanation of the workings of this 'clockwork universe'.[14]

Hampson notes that this new science, which held that all previously believed 'truths' should be questioned, should have undermined the social certainties that had previously rested in traditional and religious ideas.[12] However, in an era of tremendous social and cultural change, societies of the time sought new certainties; as Capra wrote: 'as science seemed to establish itself on an impregnable basis of experimentally verified fact, doubt and confusion eventually gave way to self-confidence and the belief that the unknown was merely the undiscovered' (p35).[14]

In contradiction to this desire by societies to find certainty, the 20th-century philosopher Popper argued that science should proceed according to the principle of falsifiability. In his view, scientific knowledge should proceed incrementally, in an orderly fashion, by systematic testing of theories. Thus, 'truths' cannot be proven but only tested and falsified.[15] Such a philosophy of science does not appear to support the notion of certainty – quite the opposite in fact. However, writers such as Kuhn have shown that, although scientists may claim to operate according to Popperian principles, most scientific enquiry does not in fact follow this course.[16] He noted that research tends to proceed within what he called 'paradigms' of knowledge. These are the current accepted world views. There is considerable investment and security vested in working within the prevailing paradigm, and it is held tenaciously, even in the face of evidence that contradicts it. Kuhn wrote:[16]

> *Normal science, the activity in which most scientists inevitably spend almost all their time, is predicated on the assumption that the scientific community knows what the world is like. Much of the success of the enterprise derives from the community's willingness to defend that assumption, if necessary at considerable cost.* (p5)

This brings us back, then, to the example of legally enforced caesarean sections. The scientific community, almost in spite of its epistemological origins, has been adopted into a societal view of the certainty of science. This apparent certainty marks out the behaviour of individuals as acceptable or deviant, depending on the degree to which the behaviours fit with the scientific norms of the day, which implicitly also reflect moral and social norms.

Having very briefly explored the historical background to the relationships between science and health, it is not surprising to find that critical theorists in this area have claimed that the current paradigm of childbirth has been fundamentally based on the metaphor of the (female) body as a machine.[17] Metaphorically, from this perspective, research and practice rules tend to proceed on the basis that the machine is fundamentally faulty, and these faults can best be contained by setting strict 'quality control' rules within which the machine is known to function optimally. Behaviours and physiological processes outside of these parameters become, by default, pathologies. We discuss the role of pathology in current ways of seeing later in the chapter.

The implications of certainty

The currently held authoritative scientific and practice paradigm in most Westernised countries is based on the belief that the best, most certain evidence is that gained from research based on the study of specific elements of the system, with enough individuals to be fairly sure that the results can be generalised to whole populations. The ideal has been termed 'large trials with simple protocols'.[18] It is believed that this model increases certainty, and that the findings from such trials, if they are carried out well, should be applied wholesale to individuals.

In 1985, Bateson, a biologist, anthropologist and one of the founders of cybernetics, commented on the widespread assumption that generalisability to a population implies generalisability to each of the individuals in that population.[19] He described this tendency as a logical confusion between 'class' and 'individual'. He illustrated this point with the example of Brownian motion: molecules in boiling water. Although the boiling point of water can be reasonably accurately predicted, the point at which 'boiling' begins for a particular molecule cannot. Later in this chapter we will give several examples of ways in which this logical confusion has occurred in the implementation of 'evidence-based' practice in maternity care, where once a probability estimate of risk is established, a new protocol, such as timing of induction of labour for post-maturity, may be applied to all women, regardless of their individual characteristics.

One example of the way that the dominant paradigm of knowledge has come to override alternative views of the world is, then, the current interpretation of the concept of evidence-based medicine. We will set out the original philosophy behind this approach, and some specific clinical examples associated with it. We intend to illustrate the point that, while the concept of evidence has now become the underpinning feature of accepted knowledge in the health services, this only became possible after the original concept of evidence-based medicine as a fluid entity had been subverted by the wider professional demand for certainties.

Evidence-based practice and certainty

The pioneers of evidence-based medicine recognised that 'best practice' was an amalgam of good quality data with practitioners' skills and experience, and the individual service user's beliefs, knowledge and values.[20–22] As Jelinek points out, in arguing for a clinical approach to clinical trials: 'the randomised controlled trial ... has to be balanced with other evidence of a biomedical, psychological and sociological nature: and with previous experience derived from both a core of relevant literature and of a personal or institutional base. It has to be applied to the individual patient as perceived by both patient and doctor' (p86).[20]

This concept of best practice allows for fluidity in the interpretation of research, with individual variables and partnership between practitioner and client built in to the final clinical decision. However, the evidence-based medicine agenda as currently promoted in many countries is firmly rooted in certainty, with very little emphasis on the practitioner and the service user. This is illustrated by the very narrow definition of 'best evidence' that has been promoted within this field.[23]

The inexorable move towards a demand for maximum certainty has led to the creation of practice and clinical protocols in many countries that are written and adhered to as though the evidence were comprehensive, without limitations and equally applicable to all members of the population. Two examples will illustrate the point. The first is that of foetal auscultation policies during labour, and, specifically, the recommended time interval between periods of listening to the foetal heart.

Electronic foetal heart rate monitoring

For many centuries, midwives have listened to the foetal heart during labour intermittently. There does not appear to be any published evidence relating to the range of practice among midwives in terms of the interval between periods of auscultation, or to women's views of the acceptability of different monitoring intervals. However, it is clear from the personal clinical and birth experiences of one of us (SD), and from observation of the practices of midwives by both of us, that, where protocols allow for flexibility, this interval varies from irregular listening in every few hours or so to regular monitoring several times within the hour. Auscultation appears to become more frequent as labour advances, or if the midwife feels from other signs that there may be an impending problem with the labour or the baby. Such flexible practices appear to be more common during home births or in other out-of-hospital settings.[24] In contrast, in the context of the development of protocols for many aspects of labour in UK hospitals during the late 20th century, this flexible time interval was often standardised to every 30 minutes in the first stage of labour, and then after every contraction in the second stage.

Since the early 1990s, professional and governmental bodies across the world have responded to the accumulating evidence that labouring women and their babies, at least at the population level, may benefit from intermittent rather than continuous foetal monitoring in labour.[25-28] However, the main trial on which this evidence is based used an unusually intensive regimen of intermittent auscultation as the control for the intervention of electronic foetal monitoring. This involved listening in to the foetal heart every 15 minutes in the active first stage of labour, and more frequently in the second stage.[29] The guidelines of national professional bodies cited above generally adopt a 15 (or 15–30) minute interval for auscultation in the first stage of labour, in contrast to preceding centuries of custom and practice. In the process, this practice is reified as the only safe way to undertake auscultation, despite the preceding decades of empirical evidence on less frequent regimens of monitoring. The frequency of the new regimen has made it very difficult to implement in many busy labour wards. Indeed, this is the rationale given by some practitioners for continuing with continuous electronic foetal monitoring.[30] This particular regimen is increasingly seen as mandatory and 'certain' because it is based on a trial, even if it is unachievable in actual practice. The issues of an individual practitioner's skills and knowledge, or a specific woman's beliefs and values and particular pattern of labouring, do not appear to feature widely in most formal protocols or guidelines in this area. Two specific points arise from this example. The first is that, even when there is evidence of an authoritative nature, according to the rules of 'normal science', it may not fit with the prevailing socio-cultural paradigm and set of beliefs around childbirth. This leads to non-adoption of the evidence. Secondly, in this case the 'normal science' rules were violated in the process of undertaking the research. The trial design compared continuous electronic foetal monitoring with an intensive pattern of intermittent monitoring which had not been previously evaluated for efficacy, acceptability or utility. Alternative patterns that were in common use at the time the trial was conducted may have generated different results, one way or the other.

Induction of labour for post-maturity

Our second example is induction of labour for post-maturity. Based on the Cochrane review in this area,[31] benefits for populations of women and babies only begin to become clear after 41 weeks of gestation. Indeed, these advantages do not become really apparent until after 42 weeks of gestation. Rather than a clear cut-off point occurring, the balance of risks and benefits of induction shifts in a continuum over time. This shift follows an exponential curve, so the balance changes more rapidly as time goes on. Despite the recommendations that women be offered induction routinely after 41 weeks, anecdotally inductions for post-maturity are now routinely carried out in a number of settings and countries soon after the woman has reached 40 weeks of gestation. The routine nature of these practices is an example of Bateson's argument regarding logical confusion in interpreting probability statistics. This has occurred in parallel with rising rates of induction of labour, which, for example, were over 20% in the UK in 2003/4,[32] from around 17–18% between 1989 and 1993. Again, very little notice appears to be taken of the relationship between the practitioner and the woman, of the woman's skills and knowledge or, indeed, of the complexity of the relevant evidence. This raises serious questions about the application to individuals of population-level protocol or guideline-driven practices.

Rather than valuing certainty as illustrated above, it is possible to see science as a continuous process. Instead of taking a linear approach to evidence, in which we ask the question and we find the answer, such a paradigm sees science as an ongoing dialogue. In this case, evidence is a complex and fluid phenomenon, continually moving between developing and testing ideas. Before we come back to this possibility, however, we will examine the principle of simplicity, which is central to the experimental design of the randomised controlled trial.

Simplicity as a framework

Thinkers such as Descartes, Bacon and Newton aimed to develop theory that had simplicity. Bacon, for example, saw his method of experiment and induction as one that would offer 'an infallible method of distinguishing between truth and error' (p36).[12] Newton built on this approach, aiming to identify simple basic principles that would allow generalisation about the nature of the world: 'The beautiful simplicity of a single law which appeared to explain the operation of every kind of earthly and celestial movement was a triumphant example of the possibilities of the new learning' (p37).[12]

Much research in the area of childbirth is based on this notion of simplicity. It also has resonance for practices that are regulated by protocols and guidelines. The assumption is that there is a straightforward cause–effect relationship in the physiology of birth. This can be found and codified if birth can be reduced to its essential components and then systematically examined. It is inherent in this paradigm that the single summary finding from the whole population of individuals in a trial can be directly and uniformly applied to the complex situations of individuals in practice, as we have discussed above. The promotion of large trials with simple protocols illustrates this simplicity-based approach. Additionally, this vision of knowledge assumes that clinical parameters are of overriding importance, in isolation from almost all other parameters that impinge on birth, such as social interactions and environmental impact, which may act independently and may also interact with clinical parameters in complex ways.

Randomisation is used to get as close as possible to samples that are similar to each other and which represent the relevant population as a whole. This is intended to remove all possible sources of systematic bias, so that what is found in the samples can be said to hold true for that population. Randomisation is used effectively to resolve the problem of achieving simplicity and control in experimental research involving people. In order to design an effective randomised controlled trial, simplicity is needed to achieve the required level of control. Control is crucial to ensure that the findings are not 'contaminated' by potentially confounding variables. This is particularly difficult to achieve with complex interventions, which are the very interventions that are often particularly relevant to maternity care. It requires considerable knowledge to be able to identify the nature of the intervention to be studied as well and to have the capacity to 'unpick' different aspects of an intervention. This is not always possible or desirable in complex systems, such as childbirth, where both input and outcome are influenced by an interacting 'net' of cultural, social, environmental, psychological and physiological factors.

Similarly, meta-analysis relies strongly on the principle of simplicity, as illustrated by attempts to control for heterogeneity in data synthesis. Examination of two particular meta-analyses within the Cochrane library illustrates the difficulties of operating on the principle of simplicity in a complex environment.

An overview of trials of antenatal support interventions with a primary outcome measure of reduction in low birth weight includes interventions as diverse as antenatal classes (of various types), home-based support and peer and professional support, in a wide range of cultural and health service contexts.[33] The studies measured a range of different, although overlapping, outcomes. Few of the trials studied in depth the degree to which women perceived the intervention to be supportive, despite a body of psychological research suggesting that perception of support is a key measure.[34,35] Similarly, the Cochrane meta-analysis of position in labour summarises any position that is not supine as 'upright'.[36] The physiological variability between trials using the lateral position and those using squatting is not explored in the analysis.

The problem of interpretation without attending to potential underlying variables is neatly illustrated by the published accounts of so-called 'active management of labour'.[37,38] This highly prescriptive approach originated at the National Maternity Hospital in Dublin. Active management comprised a range of elements, including monitoring, augmentation of labour and constant midwifery support. A review of published accounts of the system in the mid-1990s suggested that active management could reduce emergency caesarean section rates, but that the most effective ingredient of the package was probably continuous support for labouring women.[39] In practice, however, the findings of the original work were interpreted as suggesting that the surveillance and intervention elements of the package were the most important aspects to implement. It is of interest that more recent data from the home of active management in Ireland, published in 2004, indicate a sharply rising caesarean section rate among nulliparous women.[40] Both the tendency to adopt the technical aspects of the package over the social ones, and the trend to rising caesarean rates are not surprising in the context of what has been termed the 'technocratic' paradigm of childbirth currently prevailing across most of the world.[41] Although evidence from trials of continuing support in labour[42] has been used to challenge the prevailing interpretation of active management of labour, practices in many labour wards continue to favour a simplistic, technocratic implementation.

Bateson argued that seeking the simplest, most elegant explanation that will cover the known data (parsimony) is an obligation of science.[19] However, he also noted that reductionism becomes a problem if the simplest explanation is seen as the only explanation. Although many writers in this field, even those publishing in the medical journals, have begun to question the framing of issues in terms of certainty and predictability,[43] the telling factor which indicates where the beliefs of the current system lie is the allocation of resources. As we have indicated, large, preferably multicentre trials and meta-analyses head the list of 'best evidence' in all the standard lists. Big trials are not funded unless they are powered for a single primary outcome. Subanalysis is written off as 'data trawling' since it is always possible for researchers to find some significant difference, purely by chance, with a large number of measures. Knowledge that is generated by hands-on experience, by messy interactions with people and with events, and by intuitive understandings and decisions[44–46] is dismissed as being biased or unscientific. The term 'noise' is used to describe anything in the environment or context that is not defined as part of the issue of interest.[47] These elements are dismissed as confounding variables.

Linearity of thinking

Linear thinking is particularly characteristic of certain cultural/religious philosophies. Christianity and Judaism, for example, provide views of history and time that have a clear beginning, a line of development and a clear endpoint (such as Judgement Day). Other religious philosophies, such as Buddhism or Hinduism, have more cyclical views. Such basic cultural concepts and philosophies have been shown by historians and anthropologists to have profound effects on the way enquiry and knowledge are framed.[48,49] Reflecting on this, Hampson writes: 'scientific evidence can only answer the questions that scientists think fit to ask' (p21).[12] Examples of linear thinking include the interpretation of Darwin's theory of evolution, which saw the development of *Homo sapiens* as a process of orderly change (despite its basis in random mutation) towards a higher evolutionary point, and 19th-century European liberal economics, which sought continual progress through competition.

It is not surprising then that such concepts of time and of progress also frame Western medical thought. The standard interpretation of Friedman's work on definitions of normal progress of labour is a particularly clear example of this.[50] Although Friedman did not necessarily intend his work to form the authoritative account of 'normal' progress in labour, his findings, and those of subsequent researchers in this area,[51] have become seminal in modern obstetrics. However, we suggest that this classic work has involved unexamined assumptions about the linearity of physical time and physiological processes of birth. Friedman undertook his research with women who laboured in a particular hospital setting in South Africa. Although the findings were then tested in other hospitals, the work has never been undertaken for births out of hospital. Given the emphasis in hospitals on time as the principal delineator of progress,[52–54] studies of physiological processes in such settings run the risk of providing the answer to the wrong question. These findings are about typical progress of labour in a hospital, and in a particular cultural context, rather than the physiology of labour in women labouring spontaneously. Friedman's curve does allow for differential rates of progress at different stages. However, the interpretation of his findings, and the development of action and alert lines for labour, has led to the creation of powerful beliefs about normal progress in labour.

The socially situated nature of these beliefs can be illustrated by the changes in norms of labour duration given in successive obstetric textbooks. While in 1962 Lennon's text described normal labour as lasting up to 24 hours, by 1980 standard texts such as *Obstetrics Illustrated* described labour as lasting up to 12 hours in a primigravida or 6–8 hours in a parous woman.[55,56] In neither case was any supporting evidence given for these firm statements, as was usual until recently in textbooks, but they clearly reflected both the voice of authority and the norms of practice of their time. This phenomenon has also been reported by one of us in a chronological review of midwifery textbooks.[57] Many hospital protocols specify the number of centimetres of cervical dilation per hour a woman's cervix should progress before intervention should be considered, with little allowance for physiological variation or plateaux in progress. The irresistible nature of these beliefs is illustrated in a series of recent studies of the progress of labour, which sought to escape the rigidity of post-Friedman definitions by using the assessments of nurse-midwives in hospitals deemed to be more relaxed in their approach.[58,59] While the interpretation of the data generated allows slightly slower cervical dilation per hour than in the prior standard definitions of progress, the authors still propose that cervical dilation increases regularly hour by hour. This is in contradistinction to the clearly variant progress evident in Friedman's curve itself.

These findings stand in stark contrast to anecdotal accounts of midwives undertaking home births. Such stories report an ebb and flow of labour, which may take days rather than hours and which moves on in increments rather than in a smoothly linear process.[60] These accounts allow for the possibility that 'progress' is influenced by a range of emotional, spiritual, psychological and environmental factors as well as factors such as parity and previous birth history.*

Positivist approaches to knowledge rest on the view that direct, simple cause–effect relationships can be established, in the manner of logical operations, as in the example of support in labour given in Figure 1.

Figure 1.
Logical operations: support in labour

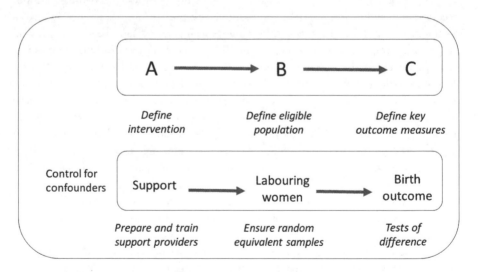

---

*   Recent analyses undertaken by WHO support these observations, and illustrate that asking different questions generates different kinds of answers: see, for example, Souza JP, Oladapo OT, Fawole B, Mugerwa K, Reis R, Barbosa-Junior F, et al, 2018 Cervical dilatation over time is a poor predictor of severe adverse birth outcomes: a diagnostic accuracy study. *BJOG.* 125(8):991-1000.

However, this notion of cause and effect is not very efficient when real-life research encounters complexity. The model where A, operating on B, leads to C begins to break down unless it can cope with the kind of 'noise' mentioned above. This 'noise' may be the individual practitioner's skills and attitudes, the culture of an organisation, the efficiency of administration systems or any number of factors that actually influence the nature of care delivery. The context of practice becomes a problem to be dealt with because it does not conform to the philosophical models inherent in the formal evidence base. Even the issue of complexity in the physiological process of labour is not accommodated well in such a model. We will come back to the issue of linearity later in the chapter when we discuss alternative approaches that may take us closer to an understanding of normality in childbirth.

Pathology as pivotal

The central place of pathology in the current childbirth paradigm is underpinned by assumptions of certainty, and by the primacy of risk, as we have discussed. Concepts of risk are discussed in more detail in another chapter.* From an economic perspective, it is clear that where health is framed by a constant expectation of danger, there is money to be made in providing investigative, preventative or curative products to counteract the risks. The largely hidden, unacknowledged and unaccountable influence of markets such as the pharmacological, biotechnological and 'hi-tech' equipment industries on our everyday construction of health risk is an element in the promotion of a pathological perspective.

As we note above in the context of clinical trials, the evidence for the central place of pathology in mainstream beliefs about childbirth is most clearly indicated in the budget allocated to it. This spending can be seen in clinical risk systems, in insurance premiums and in the widespread application of equipment and treatments that were originally designed to maximise 'safety' for the very few who are truly at high and imminent risk of serious pathology if an intervention does not take place.

This emphasis is also evident in the standard outcome measures used in intervention-based research in childbirth. Most published studies utilise short-term measures of clinical mortality and morbidity, such as rates of caesarean section, depression, anxiety, back pain, tiredness and urinary incontinence in the mother, and perinatal mortality or morbidity in the baby. Aside from breastfeeding uptake or, occasionally, satisfaction or quality-of-life scores, positive experiences are usually not accommodated, except as the absence of morbidity or mortality.

It may be argued that there is no point in assessing wellness, since it does not need to be treated, and therefore it is not of interest to health services. However, this very argument illustrates a pathological paradigm. If health and wellbeing is only defined as what is left over after illness is dealt with, then illness becomes the defining characteristic of healthcare. Such an approach ignores the possibility that understanding wellbeing may be the key to minimising illness. In terms of childbirth, such an approach may

---

* Chapter 6 in Walsh et al, 2008 'Rethinking risk and safety in maternity care', in: Downe, S. (ed) *Normal Birth, evidence and debate*, 2nd ed., Elsevier, Oxford. In the current volume, risk is discussed in Chapter 7.

also render the potential benefits of physiological labour and birth invisible. In fact, even in the context of 'normal' birth, the outcome measures proposed by at least one authoritative UK body included maternal death and incontinence.[61] Subtle, positive longer-term outcomes, such as capacity to parent or maternal and infant wellbeing, are rarely measured in routine assessments of care delivery.

Having expressed our view that many randomised controlled trials operate on the basis of maximising certainty, we also acknowledge that the use of confidence intervals, and of sensitivity analyses in economic studies, indicates that ideas of uncertainty do feature in the authoritative knowledge of mainstream health research. Unfortunately, as we have already discussed, this is not generally translated from the trials to evidence-based medicine as it is applied in maternity unit protocols or to individuals. In the next section of this chapter, we present an alternative way of seeing. We suggest that we cannot begin to understand 'normal childbirth' without reframing some of our basic assumptions about knowledge in general. We also note that some of these alternative ideas are beginning to feature in medical publications, particularly where the focus is general practice and community care.[62]

Alternative ways of seeing

Uncertainty

In the previous section, we discussed the importance of certainty as a goal of modern science. We noted that certainty arose from 'enlightenment' ideas about seeking general explanatory scientific theories, based on mechanical metaphors. As long ago as the 18th century, scepticism regarding the new certainties of enlightenment science was developing, partly influenced by contact with different cultures. Hampson cites the philosopher Kant, who, in his *Critique of Pure Reason* published in 1781, argued that empirical knowledge could convey information to a human observer not about things as they existed (noumena) but only as they were perceived (phenomena).[12] The observer imposes his or her perceptions of the dimensions of space and time onto the object. Anthropologists began to develop the argument that the way in which the world is perceived is a product of mental processes, and of interactions with the environment, which are, at least partly, culturally and socially shaped.[48] This theoretical perspective was echoed a century later in the theories of relativity and thermodynamics. These ideas presented a significant challenge to assumptions of certainty in science.[14] While physics may seem to be very far away from normal birth, the insights gained from these new areas are relevant to human understanding of all phenomena, including biological processes. Capra has explored this area in detail,[14] and we summarise some of his insights next.

Maxwell's laws of thermodynamics represented an important shift in concepts of nature from those that pertained previously. While his first law described the principle of conservation of energy, the second described its dissipation (such as by movement producing heat). This implied a shift from order to disorder and led to the concept of entropy (that all matter breaks down over time). Einstein's relativity and quantum theories built on this work. The new capacity to observe subatomic particles was also of importance. In keeping with a mechanical model of the universe, particles had always been thought of as 'matter' or 'things'; the new theory proposed that particles might be better understood as forms of energy and relationships. Electrons, for example, were understood to be in a continual state of flux, sometimes with the properties of waves, sometimes of particles. This observation led to Heisenberg's 'uncertainty principle' and to Bohr's 'complementarity principle', which argued that the properties of particles are only definable and observable through their interaction with other systems.

The implication of the new subatomic physics was that certainty was replaced by probability, or the notion of tendencies rather than absolutes: 'we can never predict an atomic event with certainty; we can only predict the likelihood of its happening'.[14] Equally, the implication was that the properties and behaviour of things are better thought about in terms of systems and relationships rather than as individual components that can be examined separately. This directly contradicts the mechanistic model we explored above, and it implies that a subject such as normal birth needs to be looked at as a whole rather than by its parts. We discuss this further in the section on complexity.

If this approach is accepted, cause and effect need to be approached in a very different way. In particular, the role of the individual and relationships within the system must be taken into account. As we have noted, cross-cultural theory within anthropology proposed that the world is experienced and understood differently by different individuals according to the environmental, social and cultural shaping of that experience. Similarly, quantum and relativity theory in physics proposed that the consciousness of the observer is a part of and necessary to the whole. To do the experiment is to become part of it. Consciousness influences what is observed and the types of question asked influence the answers that can be obtained. This challenges the basic notion of an objective, certain and value-free science.

When we turn to the implications of this paradigm shift for our understanding of health, it becomes clear that the benefit or harm of an intervention for an individual can only be established with reasonable certainty by identifying and taking into account all the relevant 'noise'. This includes environment, carer attitudes, skills and beliefs and the expectations of the woman and her family. Similarly, the appraisal of research evidence needs to consider the concepts, attitudes and roles of the researchers and how these may have framed or influenced the process of generating evidence. Such an approach may seem to be impossibly open-ended and complex. However, it is exactly the approach set out in the original proposals for evidence-based medicine described at the beginning of this chapter. In this version, best practice is a constructed position, dependent on the interactions between the practitioner, the research evidence and the service user; it will be different for each separate set of circumstances. Interpretation of these variables depends on the weight given to the potential factors involved by the individuals concerned. Since it is likely that all the risks and benefits relative to an intervention will never be established for populations, let alone for individuals, and that research produces probabilistic statistical findings, decisions must be made in a state of relative uncertainty. As David Sackett and his colleagues state: 'Diagnosis is not about finding absolute truth, but about limiting uncertainty ...' (p92).[22]

There are a number of techniques that have been proposed for use in clinical practice to address these issues. These include likelihood ratios for diagnostic tests[22] and Bayesian techniques.[63–65] Both these approaches are based on finding out what the current state of evidence might be before adding in the results of a new trial or test. In the case of the likelihood ratio, the pre-test probability that an individual has a certain disease is estimated, based on their circumstances, the clinician's expertise and the evidence. A clinical test is undertaken, and the findings are put alongside the pre-test probability to estimate the likelihood that the individual does indeed have the condition being considered. In Bayesian theory, so-called 'priors' are established to find out the consensus about an intervention before a further study is undertaken. These priors can be established by groups of stakeholders, including service users. They can then be moderated by data arising from formal investigation, whether the data are generated from a strictly controlled randomised trial of sufficient size or not. This approach depends on recalculations of relative risk and sensitivity analyses after a new study or other piece of evidence is added to the prior probability.

The value of these methods of interpreting data lies in the fact they do not depend on black and white acceptance or rejection of a null hypothesis. They can give far more information to an individual than simply that based on aggregated population-based data. They also explicitly accept the fact that most researchers, and most users of research, have strong views about an intervention, and they bring this to their interpretation of new data.

To examine the issue of interpretation further, we want to explore another phenomenon. This is the issue of the time it takes to implement formal evidence into practice. The first example is of a technique that has been examined over many years and many trials, but which is still not well accepted or established in many hospitals. This is auscultation in labour for well women and babies. We have discussed the evidence in this area earlier in the chapter. However, there are recent examples of single trials that have led to widespread changes on the ground, even before authoritative guidelines from august bodies have been produced. The Term Breech Trial is a case in point.[66] A multicentre audit of practice in the sites where the trial was run, undertaken two years after the results were published, indicated that the vast majority had instituted the findings of the trial wholesale.[66,67] This is despite the findings in the original study that the advantages of caesarean section were less evident in some sites taking part in the study than in others, and also despite the warning of the authors of the current Cochrane review in this area: 'The data from this review cannot be generalised to settings where caesarean section is not readily available, or to methods of breech delivery that differ materially from the clinical delivery protocols used in the trials reviewed ...'.[68] In this case, it seems that the evidence arising from the Term Breech Trial was so convincing, so certain, that changes were made immediately, worldwide, across disparate groups of individuals and without attention to the healthcare setting, practitioners' variable skills and knowledge, and women's beliefs and values or the impact of resource issues on how care is delivered. It is not clear if this change has persisted following publication of the two-year follow-up data which demonstrated that, taking account of deaths and neurodevelopmental delay from the point of randomisation to two years after birth, there were no differences between the two groups: while mortality was higher in the vaginal birth group, neurodevelopmental delay was higher in the caesarean section group.[69]

What is the explanation for the difference in implementation of formal evidence between the two areas of practice? In each case, the studies seem to have been carefully designed and implemented. Why has one approach been so resistant to change and the other so amenable? There are probably a number of possible explanations, from the economic to the technical. However, it seems likely that a good case could be made for suggesting that this response is based on belief systems, which, in turn, can be located in the cultural norms of post-industrial societies. At root, many if not most doctors, midwives, managers and birthing women believe that electronic foetal monitoring must be good for babies, as it provides apparently objective technical data. In addition, many if not most of us do not believe that women can birth breech babies spontaneously and safely, as this is an uncommon, and therefore, we assume, an abnormal/pathological position for the foetus to adopt. Prior beliefs in both the utility of cardiotocography and in the efficacy of caesarean section for breech babies are so strong that they continue to override the accumulating evidence against the belief in the former and rapidly accommodated the evidence for caesarean section in the latter. This may be seen as a case against the use of the creation of prior hypotheses as part of 'evidence', as recommended in Bayesian theory, since they can give credence to what may be unfounded certainties.[70] However, the advantage of using something like Bayes' theorem in interpreting evidence is that it makes researchers and practitioners face up to the role of belief. As Merry and colleagues state: 'Bayes' theorem provides the key to the ways in which beliefs should fit together in the light of changing evidence ... [it allows us] to establish rules and procedures for ... disciplined uncertainty accounting (while maximising utility) ...'.[71]

In the use of such theory, priors could be constructed for population-based evidence, with input from a variety of views and beliefs, including those of lay commentators. They could also be constructed in clinical practice, with the input of both the practitioner(s) concerned and the individual childbearing woman. Such 'disciplined uncertainty accounting', if we were to formalise it, may reveal a number of profound flaws in our current approach to birth. Its use would allow us to acknowledge the relative uncertainties of applying formal research to individuals. While all good-quality evidence is valid in this construction of knowledge, one trial with simple protocols, or even an infinite number of such trials, cannot give us certainty of acting in the context of any single individual. Such trials can only give us more or less support for our beliefs. Very convincing trials may even change our beliefs, as in the case of the Back to Sleep studies.[72,73] As Salsburg states:[74]

> *There is no 'correct' (approach). Scientific reasoning consists of attempts to fit the complexities of reality into models useful for the organisation of observations ... some fit for the time being until we can find one that fits better, or until the lack of fit begins to trouble us. But we must always recognise that we fit our observations to very arbitrary models, and we must be prepared to abandon a model if it leads to nonsense.*

Acknowledging uncertainty leads us to question some current accepted views about the nature of normal birth. As discussed in Chapter 4,[**] the commonly quoted definitions tend to include specific features, such as gestation, position of the foetal head and length of labour, as prerequisites for 'normality'. However, issues of relativity, uncertainty and belief systems begin to suggest that the absolutism of these kinds of approach may be misleading. They may be a factor in the nonsense of our apparently headlong rush to intervene in large numbers of labours that would otherwise progress physiologically if left alone. This leads us to explore alternative ways of approaching the problem, through theories of complexity and chaos.

Complexity and chaos

A solution to the dissonance between the evidence claims of much of the current research in health and healthcare, and its apparent lack of application to individuals, may lie in the very heart of quantitative knowledge, namely quantum physics. This profoundly 'scientific' branch of physics is fundamentally linked to observations that the natural systems of the world are not simple and predictable, but complex and chaotic.

Theories of complexity and chaos arose simultaneously in a number of fields. The terms are often used interchangeably, though some maintain that chaos is a function of the non-linearity, or non-periodic pattern, of complex systems. The meteorologist Edward Lorenz is credited with the crucial first insights into 'deterministic non-periodic flow' in the early 1960s.[75] The rapidly expanding theoretical and mathematical developments in complexity and chaos have influenced fields as diverse as management theory and cardiac regulation.[76, 77] However, a number of authors have cautioned against oversimplistic generalisation of the seductive post-modernist aspects of multiplicity and connectivity that are expressed in these theories. Carol Haigh, writing from a nursing perspective, sees the misuse of chaos theory as being particularly prevalent within nursing research and philosophy.[78] She cautioned that application of the chaos construct is not relevant without a thorough understanding and use of the mathematical underpinning of the theories. While we accept her thesis to some extent, we depart from her apparent rejection of the potential for the insights of complexity and chaos to provide new ways of seeing health at the macro level. We agree, however, that applied research in this area will need to pay attention to the mathematical and statistical tools that have been developed to support research from this perspective.

Carol Haigh alluded to a number of nursing theorists in her critique of the use of chaos theory. As we have noted above, primary care practitioners have also published accounts of complexity in practice.[62,79] However, only very recently have a small number of researchers begun to engage with the potential of this approach for understanding childbirth.[79–81] The rest of this section sets out some of the central tenets of complexity

---

* Beech, Phipps, 2008 'Normal Birth, Women's Stories', in: Downe, S. (Ed) *Normal Birth, evidence and debate*, 2nd ed, Elsevier, Oxford

** For more recent discussions of the nature and range of definitions of 'normal' or 'physiologic(al)' birth, see: birthtools.org/What-Is-Physiologic-Birth; Kennedy et al, 2015 'The development of a consensus statement on normal physiologic birth: a modified Delphi study', *J Midwifery Womens Health*. 60(2):140-5. doi: 10.1111/jmwh.12254; Darra, Murphy, 2016 'Coping and help in birth: An investigation into 'normal' childbirth as described by new mothers and their attending midwives', *Midwifery* 40:18-25. doi: 10.1016/j.midw.2016.05.007. Epub 2016 May 13.

theory and provides some initial insights into how it could be applied in the context of childbirth.

The power of complexity theory lies in the observation that events are profoundly interconnected. The concept of a simple linear process is replaced with the metaphor of a web or network of interconnections. It therefore challenges the assumption that there is a one 'right' way of doing things for everyone, and all we have to do is to find it and then stick to it. Rightness becomes 'problematised', because we are usually basing our judgement on only one part of the story. Take the professional insistence on laying all babies on their face to prevent inhalation of vomit until more recent evidence has persuaded us that this practice is linked to higher rates of cot death for some babies. We still do not know which babies benefit from the new approaches and which may be disadvantaged. Complexity holds that, even if we have good trial data for populations, we cannot know many of the wider long-term consequences of implementing such a policy, or any other such policy (such as auscultation every 15 minutes in labour, widespread implementation of midwife-led units or caesarean section for babies presenting by the breech).

The phenomenon of connectivity is formally termed 'sensitive dependence on initial conditions'. It has been brought to the popular imagination through the concept of the 'butterfly effect': the idea that 'a butterfly flaps its wings in the jungle and there is a hurricane in New York'. This suggests that small changes within systems may achieve large effects while large changes may achieve small effects.[79] While the example may sound overly romantic, the point is that any simple input into a dynamic system, such as the weather, an organisation or a labouring woman, will have consequences that are not linear but which bifurcate – that is, a + b = c & d, b + c = e & f, b + d = g & h and so on ad infinitum. Figure 2 sets this out graphically. The diagram is generated from a computer set to track changes in a chaotic

Figure 2.
Bifurcation diagram

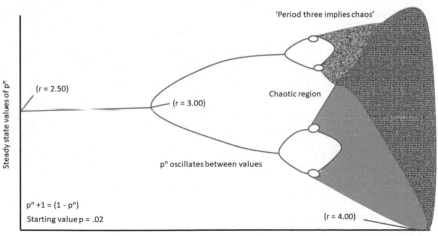

'Period three implies chaos'

(r = 2.50)

(r = 3.00)

Chaotic region

Steady state values of p^n

p^n oscillates between values

$p^n +1 = (1 - p^n)$
Starting value p = .02

(r = 4.00)

Value of r

system (such as the weather or heart rate patterns). It is clear that the way the system progresses is, at first, predictable: it is a straight line. However, at a certain point, the system reaches a moment when it tips from this smoothly linear progression into a so-called 'chaotic region'. It may go one of two ways at this point and then, quickly, the divisions (or bifurcations) happen again and again, until they become so frequent that the system becomes chaotic and unpredictable.

What is apparent is that, although the way the individual paths divide may seem to be random and chaotic, the overall pattern is regular (as in Bateson's example of Brownian motion and the boiling point of water molecules). There is order in the chaos. This is determined by the connections between and the overall connectivity of the wider system. This reverses the notion in positivistic science that the parts determine the behaviour of the whole.

So, to take an extremely simplified example, a woman who is 'overdue' and who is told that this is dangerous for her baby and she should accept induction (or who is fed up and wants induction) has an emotional response to the news, which has neurohormonal consequences. This responsive neurohormonal state provides an unpredictable basis for receiving prostaglandin. The effects of the prostaglandin interact with her emotional state and her feelings of loneliness if her chosen companions are not there, or relaxation if they are. Her unpredictable response to pain interacts with her unknown physiology to create an unpredictable physiological response to the prostin gel ... and so on. While the overall pattern (the labour proceeds and the baby is born) may be predictable, the interacting elements and process that produce this outcome are not simple.

In opposition to this physiological reality, labour and birth are currently managed in a framework that seeks to bind these essentially complex and relatively unpredictable processes into ever tighter constraints to ensure certainty. This clash of realities carries potential dangers on the physiological, emotional, spiritual and psychological level, for both mother and baby. Some of these consequences are explored in other chapters in this book.

Beyond the issue of constraining unpredictable processes, complexity theorists indicate that change as opposed to stasis is an indication of an effective dynamical system, and that: 'complex adaptive systems adapt to, and on, the edge of chaos ... Systems in the complex region ... can adapt most readily ...'.[71] This means that systems that show unpredictable behaviour are those most likely to be healthy, and to innovate. The metaphor often given here is of a heart in persistent sinusoidal rhythm – the pattern is smooth and highly predictable at both the macro and the micro level. It often indicates pathology. In contrast, a healthy heart produces a clear pattern of activity at the macro level, but shows wide variation and unpredictability at the micro level. This indicates its capacity to adapt dynamically to changing situations and stressors within and outside of the body. Applying this thinking to labour seems to imply that it is at the time when labour is at its most complex, its most unpredictable, its least controllable, that the maternal and infant system can most easily make the necessary changes in so-called 'phase space' to move from one aspect of labour to another: to make a 'phase transition'.[79] It may even imply that if systems such as labour are not allowed to progress to the edge of chaos, the body cannot make the dynamic changes necessary to accomplish essential phase transitions. Ilya Prigogine, Nobel Prize winner in the area of quantum physics, talked of this as 'from being to becoming' in the context of quantum mechanics.[82] It is also termed a *far-from-equilibrium state*. This is not necessarily a negative concept. It is in far-from-equilibrium states that the most positive changes to systems can occur. This does not mean states that are fundamentally out of control. It does mean states that do not conform to obvious and predictable patterns. They are subject to the phenomenon called the 'strange attractor'. James Gleick describes the process by which David Ruelle and Floris Taken came to this concept (p132–4),[75] which they saw as a phenomenon that pulls processes and organisms out of the edge of chaos and into a new more stable phase space.

An example of the strange attractor at work in labour may be transition. This is a time when the rhythm of labour changes pace, when many women feel themselves to be in an unfamiliar place, and when their requests and pleas can be interpreted as demanding a 'fix', rather than support for the adjustment needed. If women are supported through transition, it moves from an apparently chaotic state into the calmer more organised space of spontaneous bearing down, or to the so-called 'rest and be thankful' phase. Such states in labour are within the pull of the 'strange attractor', which may be a hormonal cue, a function of the practitioner's technological or physiological outlook or any number of other interconnected factors: '[the state of] ..."far from equilibrium"... allow(s) an alternative attractor to define a new context for the system ...'.[83] The actual attractors in operation remain to be discovered by formal research.

Complex systems have emergent properties. Sweeney and Griffiths understood emergence to be 'the phenomenon by which new properties arise through the complex interactions and connectivity of lower order processes' (p42).[79] This implies that the sum of the functioning of parts considered separately is seldom equal to the functioning of the whole. Ackoff gave the example of constructing a car to illustrate this: 'if you picked the best parts from a range of vehicles to make up a supercar you may well find it doesn't work at all'.[84] This is because the whole is dependent on interactions of parts. As Merry states: '... behaviour can be predicted by studying how elements interact and how the system adapts and changes throughout time ... the complex system cannot be understood by reducing it to its parts' (p58).[71] However, raising the possibility that birth is a complex adaptive process raises the possibility that we can begin to understand it in a different and possibly more meaningful way in the future. This work has still barely begun.

Applying complexity: from linearity to cycles of knowledge development

This complexity theory way of seeing may seem to be seductive but ultimately useless. If labour is seen as being so incredibly complex, how can it ever be understood? Luckily, one of the current theories of complex adaptive systems is that they may be underpinned by simple rules. This may seem to be counterintuitive. The classic example of the flocking behaviour of computer-generated birds (termed 'boids') may make it more understandable. Observed casually, the way birds flock in the sky seems to be completely random or non-predictable and yet it forms a pattern. However, as Sweeney and Griffiths note,[79] three simple rules (derived originally from studies of chemical reactions, and modelled on the computer-generated 'boids') may explain the ability of this apparently chaotic behaviour to produce patterns. These are:

1. Maintain a minimum distance from other boids.
2. Match the velocity of the other boids in the neighbourhood.
3. Try to move towards the perceived centre of the flock.

Running a computer program based on these rules results in apparently random flocking behaviour that, nevertheless, exhibits underlying if complex patterning. It is of interest that the rules describe the dynamic nature of the relationship between each boid and the next. They are not reductive to the parts of the flock, but descriptive of how the parts fit together. This emphasises the importance of connectivity in complex systems.

The observation that simple rules of relationship may help in describing the behaviour of complex systems offers the potential for understanding a phenomenon such as transition in labour without recourse to exhaustive description of every influence upon it. If similar rules of connectivity could be identified that encompass the wide range of normal-but-not-average variation in pregnancy and labour, we may be in a position to begin to move away from rules of practice that only describe a narrow band of the 'average' normal.

Building on the connectivity described by complexity and systems theorists, an alternative to the linear view of scientific progress is that the process of knowledge development is essentially cyclical, as in Figure 3. Science works through cycles of observation and inductive thinking, theory development and testing, reflection and evaluation. Effective research proceeds by raising new and more informed questions as much as by seeking to provide answers. Analogies can be drawn between this approach and the operation of complex feedback mechanisms. The specific graphical example given in Figure 4, again related to social support in labour, may serve to illustrate the point.

Based on the arguments we have set out above, we assert that even the most apparently simple interventions in childbirth are framed by (and, crucially, dependent upon) the 'noise' of beliefs, skills and values. In claiming this, we are not suggesting that linear models, or indeed randomised controlled trials, do not have an important and powerful role in research. They work within certain parameters. What we do suggest is that they form important links within a wider cycle of knowledge development. We also suggest that even this cyclical view must be considered as taking place within complex systems. It does not necessarily proceed in an orderly manner, from lack of knowledge

Figure 3.
Science/knowledge development as a cycle

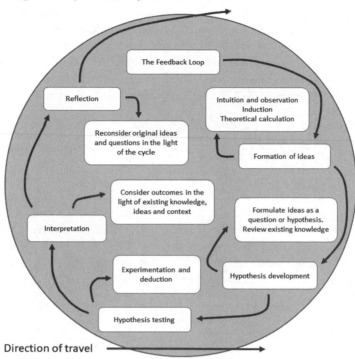

Figure 4.
Simplified example of influences on input and outcome in relation to social support and labouring women

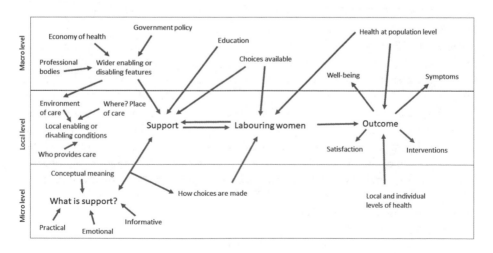

to enlightenment. As Bateson argues: 'all you have is the hope of simplicity, since the next fact may drive you to the next level of complexity'.[19] This implies a shift in thinking away from the notion of the randomised controlled trial as the 'gold standard' of evidence for medicine, to the notion of the trial as an important but partial aspect of the evidence base for care. To be effective, experimental research needs to build on considerable prior knowledge, much of which will need to be developed using a range of methodologies and taking into account a range of considerations. Its findings will need to be interpreted in the light of knowledge of the wider system of which it forms a controlled part.

In 2000, the UK Medical Research Council published guidelines for research on what it saw as the special case of overtly 'complex' interventions, such as the introduction of multicomponent systems.[85] While this is valuable, it does not take into account the possibility that the majority of the unanswered questions in healthcare provision and policy entails complexity, in the sense we are discussing. In order to examine the feasibility of taking this approach in practice, we turn next to a discussion of systems theory as a model for ways of encapsulating complexity in research, practice and care provision.[86] According to this theory, cause and effect involves uncertainty and contingency. Contingency means that effects are dependent on the situation, may be influenced by a range of factors and are, therefore, never absolutely predictable. Additionally, an action may have unintended as well as intended consequences. Again, key advocates of evidence-based medicine allow for this when they note that the 'best' evidence is always provisional, not certain. Instead of a linear relationship between cause and effect, this approach rests on the kind of web of connections, or connectivity, identified by complexity theorists. Systems analysis has played a major role in the thinking in economics and business modelling, and in more obviously scientific disciplines such as climatology.

To look at how this could be relevant to the understanding of normal birth, we want to look in detail at Hodnett's work on labour support. In reporting on this body of work to a conference on research in the area of normal childbirth, Hodnett noted how she had come full circle in her thinking. Her research career started with the question, based on her experience as a labour nurse, 'why do some women go out of labour after hospital admission?'. Through a series of classic trials and overviews of trials, which were based in positivist linear thinking and which were very well designed according to these tenets, she investigated the importance of the continuing presence of a support nurse in labour, seeing this as the active ingredient in preventing the problem of stalled labour, and its potentially adverse consequences. Despite nurses' perceptions of improved awareness and ability to provide support in her latest trial, following in-depth training,[87] the intervention was found to make no difference to almost all the outcomes assessed. To understand this paradox, Hodnett found herself returning to her original question about the environment of care: why, given the systematic review evidence on the effectiveness of labour support, did labour support apparently make no difference in practice in this trial? 'Bottom line: it's the environment. I've come full circle.'[88]

In acknowledging the contextual influences in this study, and in a subsequent Cochrane review of home-like settings for place of birth,[89] Ellen Hodnett and her colleagues have begun to incorporate the integral effect of context and 'noise' in trials of complex health interventions. Beyond this lesson from complex adaptive systems thinking comes another insight from emergence. Wilson and colleagues make the following claim: 'health can only be maintained (or re-established) through a holistic approach that accepts unpredictability and builds on subtle emergent forces with the overall system'.[83] Accepting this claim would allow us to move away from trying to understand and categorise every aspect of variation as potentially pathological. We could then spend our time trying to see how the system works as a whole for each individual. The next section picks up this possibility in the specific context of salutogenesis.

Salutogenesis

We have discussed above our claim that current systems of health care are rooted in pathology. This is despite the pronouncement by the World Health Organization that health is a state of wellbeing.[90] Outside of clinical research, there have been a number of psychological and sociological studies of the nature of wellbeing. Within the maternity services, however, as we have noted, most outcome measures are focused on morbidity.

We wish to propose that practice, research and policy development in the maternity services should instead be framed by the concept of salutogenesis, or the generation of wellbeing. This term was coined by an American researcher named Aaron Antonovsky in 1979.[91] We do not propose that all elements of Antonovsky's approach should be taken up. However, in order to set the framework for our application of the concept, we set out the basic principles of his thesis below.

Antonovsky developed his initial theories while researching survivors of Holocaust concentration camps. He expected to find high levels of pathology and social disintegration. However, to his surprise, he found that some survivors had high levels of optimism and social success. This phenomenon caused Antonovsky to ask the question: 'how is it that some people survive such terrible experiences apparently completely intact emotionally and spiritually, and others disintegrate entirely?'. His further studies indicated that the answer lies in connections: in the connectivity between individuals, their experience and their social histories. In this sense, the concept of salutogenesis differs markedly from other wellbeing theories, or, for example, concepts of mastery or self-efficacy, which see the essence of wellbeing in self-empowerment.

Antonovsky challenged the current biomedical discourse, arguing that: 'A salutogenic orientation, concerned with overall health, pressures one to think in systems terms... it leads one to seek to understand and deal with all the entropic [disorder-promoting] forces and... negentropic [order-promoting] forces...' (p115).[92] In the same paper, he goes on to pose the following fundamental question: 'We are all familiar with the concept of a risk factor. Can we not think of the concept of a salutary factor?' (p116).

As can be seen, Antonovsky's theories fit well with the complex, uncertain systems-orientated approach we have set out in the preceding sections. His philosophy opens the door to turning the concept of risk systems on its head. Rather than starting with a long list of conditions and social situations that rule women out of having a physiological birth, maybe in a stand-alone unit or at home, the idea of positive or order-promoting forces allows a woman to bring salutogenic aspects of her clinical, emotional, social, spiritual and family history to the table. For example, a woman who has a family history of prolonged gestation or long labours may not be entering the realms of pathology when her pregnancy reaches the 42nd week, or her active labour has gone on for 10 hours with only small apparent signs of progress, but with mother and baby coping well. A woman with a previous history of a stillbirth following a premature labour may be ideally suited to have her baby in a free-standing unit if she feels that, emotionally, this is one way to heal the trauma of her past experiences, and she is now at 38 weeks of gestation. A well-controlled diabetic may do better relaxed in the care of midwives she knows than tense in a highly monitored environment with highly skilled carers she does not know. All these situations may maximise the opportunity for normal birth. Some researchers suggest that maximising normal birth may even have unlooked-for consequences on maternal and, therefore, infant biochemistry and neurohormones.[93–95] Indeed, in his 1979 publication, Antonovsky was beginning to explore connections between his work and psychoneuroimmunology in adults. A 1999 German review of Antonovsky's own work and that of researchers associated with it demonstrated that the field appeared to be under-researched at the time.[96] A more recent review of nearly 500 studies, published in 2006, indicated associations between the so-called sense of coherence construct and perceived health across a range of population groups.[97] This was particularly striking for psychological wellbeing. The evidence was less clear for physical health.

Antonovsky proposed that individuals who score highly on the sense of coherence (SOC) construct tend to experience high levels of wellbeing, with a strong sense of positive health, even in apparently extreme circumstances. The SOC equates somewhat to the psychological concept of 'buffering',[98] but it is more than simply a protective barrier. It has three components: meaningfulness, manageability and comprehensibility:

1. Meaningfulness: the deep feeling that life makes sense emotionally; that life's demands are worthy of commitment. It is essentially seeing coping as desirable.
2. Manageability: the extent to which people feel they have the resources to meet the demands, or feeling that they know where to go to get help.
3. Comprehensibility: the extent to which a person finds or structures their world to be understandable, meaningful, orderly and consistent instead of random and unpredictable. Paradoxically, a strong sense of coherence appears to help individuals cope with chaos and uncertainty when they do encounter it.

Antonovsky held that the development of the sense of coherence is a product of infancy and childhood. He believed that if a sense of coherence was not well developed by the time an individual was a young adult (and, more precisely, before they reached their 30s), it was unlikely to develop further in later life. He emphasised that the components necessary for its occurrence included personal and familial elements, and community and societal factors.[91] He also held that societies (at least within small groupings) could exhibit a sense of coherence. This perspective reverberates with concepts of community capacity and social capital, which are gaining credibility in policy circles in a number of countries.[99]

We feel that the fundamental components of salutogenesis as proposed by Antonovsky are potentially powerful factors in optimal childbearing. We also concur with the overall concept of salutogenic wellbeing as the product of a complex personal and societal interaction, and with the reformulation of healthcare and health research towards a way of seeing that is salutary as opposed to pathogenic. However, we diverge from Antonovsky's view that a sense of coherence is largely fixed by the time of early adulthood. We contend that major life-changing events, such as childbirth, could have a profound effect, and that this, in turn, can have an impact on the social capital necessary to promote a positive sense of coherence in others, including children, the wider family and local communities.

One clear practice-based example of our contention is that of the La Paz project in Brazil. Brazil is a country with extremely high caesarean section rates. A recent population-based study in Sao Paulo state found rates of 32.9% in the public sector and 80.4% in the private sector in 2001–2003.[100] Levels have been high for at least a generation. In 2001, a collaborative group of Japanese and Brazilian researchers reported on a project that set out to make changes in practice with a view to influencing ways of birth in one particular Brazilian hospital.[101] Prior to the implementation of changes, women were in labour without privacy or companionship, and with routine pharmacological and technological intervention. Before starting the project, the researchers asked the local community what the most important health issues were. Childhood diarrhoea was at the top of the list. The implementation phase took two years. It involved simple changes, like installing curtains round labour beds for privacy, allowing companions for the women in labour and making the rooms warmer. At the end of the two years, members of the community were again asked what the most important health issues were for them. While childhood diarrhoea was still seen to be important, normal birth was at the top of the list. Beyond this, the researchers note: '"Project Luz" has given many women the feeling of strong confidence in a safe delivery and child rearing ... leading to self-transformation, which empowers them profoundly. This ... raises their concerns about society, their lives, and motivates their participation in community activities and development.' (pS1).[101]

While a sense of coherence was not assessed in the Project Luz study, there are elements of manageability, meaningfulness and comprehensibility in the above account. Beyond this, there are issues of social capital. The value of positive and respectful birth, then, may have implications for societal wellbeing. Again, these issues remain to be explored in the future.

As an example of a systems approach that is rooted in a salutogenic philosophy, the Ontario Women's Health Council (OWHC) of Canada took a conscious decision to look at positive (salutogenic in Antonovsky's terminology) factors in childbirth, by investigating units with low rates of caesarean section as opposed to those with high rates, in order to understand what made things go right.[102] The 12 characteristics identified in the four units studied included pride in a low caesarean section rate, one-to-one care in labour and belief that birth was a normal process. As noted above, one of us (SD) has previously discussed the potential of a salutogenic way of seeing as both a way of maximising the potential for optimal birthing and an outcome measure for birth.[2] This use of the concept, in synergy with acknowledgement of connectivity, would allow for the design of birth settings and of supportive care that consciously maximises a sense of coherence in the birthing woman.

Some aspects of this are pursued further in another chapter.* Such changes to the way of doing birth would not privilege either technological or physiological approaches. Instead, they would acknowledge that each woman and her baby enter pregnancy, childbirth and the postnatal period with a unique set of circumstances and 'initial conditions' in the complexity theory sense. In this context, the woman, baby and caregiver would be partners in a dynamic process, in which the mother feels emotionally as well as physically safe.

Salutogenesis gives us a new framework for understanding women's experiences of labour. It permits us an understanding of how we can base maternity care and research in this area on promoting positive wellbeing as a primary approach, with the identification and treatment of pathology as a component rather than a driver. Such an understanding can extend beyond individuals to systems and organisations, as is illustrated in the Brazilian and Canadian studies described above. This way of seeing may also maximise the contribution of childbearing women to the social capital of their community, as was evidenced in La Paz. This potential remains to be evaluated.

Implications of the new way of seeing for normal birth

As we said at the beginning of this chapter, the impetus to examine the sometimes rather obscure ideas and theories set out in the preceding sections arose from the difficulty one of us (SD) found in trying to define and understand 'normal birth'.[1,2,57,103,104] Throughout this book,** various authors have examined aspects of normality and, in one chapter, Beverley Beech and Belinda Phipps offer a useful account of different definitions in use currently. Our understanding of the nature of 'normality' has been profoundly influenced by the theories we have explored, and by the new framework of complexity, uncertainty, non-linearity and salutogenesis that we propose for healthcare in general, and for childbearing in particular. While Ann Oakley's discussion of birth as a normal process is relevant to our thinking in this area,[105] it is the brief discussion of 'normalising uniqueness' by Robbie Davis-Floyd and Elizabeth Davis that has captured our imagination.[60] The discussion takes place in the context of an examination of intuition in midwifery knowledge and home birth. The authors state: 'The midwifery normalization of uniqueness must be understood in the context of the technomedical pathologization of uniqueness' (p165).[60] Their chapter sets out numerous examples of midwives' responses to uncertainty, to connectivity in labour, to sensitivity to initial conditions and to recognition of edge-of-chaos, far-from-equilibrium and phase states. Examples are cited where the woman's sense of coherence is illustrated. Cyclical, non-linear patterns of care, support and decision-making are illustrated. These conceptual terms are not used in the chapter, and neither author makes reference to the theories we have expounded above. However, in their exposition of a midwife's 'intuitive' response to the 'unique normality' of labour, our theories appear to come together. Davis-Floyd and Arvidson[46] address the topic of intuition in depth and from a range of disciplinary perspectives, but it has rarely been explored rigorously in the midwifery literature. In a meta-synthesis of literature on maternity care expertise, intuition emerged as a component of what was termed 'enacted vocation'.[106] The authors did not

---

* Chapter 3 in Hall, 2008 'Birth and Spirituality', in: Downe, S. (Ed) *Normal Birth, evidence and debate*, 2nd ed. Elsevier, Oxford

** ibid, Chapter 4

see intuition as mysterious, but, following Benner,[107] as a process that is: 'built on the knowledge, understanding and experience that precedes the intuitive leap' (p136).[106]

This seems to describe a non-linear way of thinking, with a high level of dynamic connectivity between knowledge, understanding and experience. Expert practitioners with this orientation are likely to approach normal birth with an appreciation that it is a dynamic and non-linear process. In this construction, each woman's labour is unique to her and her baby, and to the interaction and connectivity between her personal and familial history, her biophysical processes and those of her foetus, the environment in which she labours, the attitude and response of the caregiver(s) and a multitude of other factors.

We are left, then, back in what appears to be some confusion. If we cannot define normality in precise terms, how can we measure and quantify it? Are we really saying that everything is relative, and that high rates of intervention and morbidity, and low rates of wellbeing, are acceptable?

No, we are not taking this position. Our stance is that wellbeing is maximised by a salutogenic approach to birth, in which a sense of coherence in the woman, baby and family is maximised. It is likely that, for most women, this outcome is promoted by maximising the possibility of physiological birth, while optimising the experience of necessary intervention for the few who need it, whether this need is clinical, psychological, emotional or spiritual. The promotion of the conditions for physiological birth is best achieved by the recognition of flexible definitions of normality, understood in the context of uncertainty, non-linearity and complexity. We believe that this recognition of the 'unique normality' of each woman should be a fundamental midwifery skill, and it should be recognised and supported by other health professionals and the healthcare systems within which caregivers operate.

Conclusions

As described by Rose,[108] the preferred philosophical stance for the underpinning science of normal birth is that which is generated from 'hand, brain and heart'. In an Egyptian context, this has been reinterpreted as 'skilled help from the heart'.[109] Without this understanding of the complexity of birth, the uncertainty of our knowledge in the area and the salutogenic potential of childbearing, we approach normality with very limited vision.

We believe that our exploration in this chapter of the recent history of scientific thought and of theories from fields as far apart as physics and psychology has been a positive move towards optimising birth.[110] What we are advocating is not a rejection of science, but a movement on from the 'art or science?' dichotomy. Science needs to be reclaimed from the narrow, positivist construction that has effectively dominated health research and the evidence-based health movement to date, and the artistry of clinical practice (in midwifery and obstetrics) needs to be reconstructed as a legitimate skill for dealing with contingency. In the process, we may come to acknowledge what most expert practitioners know: clinical artistry and science are not as distinct as we have tended to assume.

Perhaps we can learn something by looking back at Mendel's work on inheritance. Mendel was a monk, scientist and gardener. His studies, which formed the foundation for modern genetic theory, were virtually overlooked in the 19th century, perhaps because they did not fit the paradigm of his time and society. Mendel combined careful extended observation, intuition, inductive and deductive theory development and experimental testing. His work was rooted in the tacit knowledge of gardening, a complex ecological system, yet he was able to use theory to identify fundamental simple principles within that complex system. Research, by contributing to the development of knowledge, by providing evidence of various kinds and as part of decision-making for better healthcare, could be seen in a similar way.

We recognise that our proposal that childbirth should be framed by the concept of 'unique normality' is currently more of a manifesto than a reality. We are grateful to the many thinkers whose ideas and theories we have used as building blocks for our proposals. We hope that you, our readers, will find something of interest in what we have said, and that it will inspire you to explore further this fascinating and crucial topic, normal birth.

References

1   S Downe, 2000 A proposal for a new research and practice agenda for birth. *MIDIRS Midwif Digest* **10** 337–341.
2   S Downe, 2006 Engaging with the concept of unique normality in childbirth. *British Journal of Midwifery* **14** (6), 352–356.
3   C McCourt, 2005 Research and theory for nursing and midwifery: rethinking the nature of evidence. *Worldviews on Evidence-based Nursing* **2** (2), 1–9.
4   S Beake, C McCourt, L Page, 1998 The use of clinical audit in evaluating maternity services reform: a critical reflection. *J Eval Clin Pract* **4** 75–83.
5   J Berger, 1990 *Ways of seeing* Penguin: London
6   AL Cochrane, 1972 *Effectiveness and efficiency: random reflections on health services* Nuffield and Provincial Hospitals Trust: London
7   A Oakley, 1992 *Social support and motherhood. The natural history of a research project* Blackwell: Oxford
8   B Jordan, 1993 *Birth in four cultures: a cross-cultural investigation of childbirth in Yucatan, Holland, Sweden and the United States* Waveland Press: Champaign, IL
9   RE Davis-Floyd, CF Sargent, 1997 *Childbirth and authoritative knowledge; cross cultural perspectives* University of California Press: Berkeley, CA
10 J Weaver, 2002 Court ordered caesarean sections. In: A Bainham, S Day-Sclater, M Richards, Ed. *Body lore and laws* Hart: Oxford
11 T-A Samuels, H Minkoff, J Feldman, et al. 2007 Obstetricians, health attorneys, and court-ordered cesarean sections. *Womens Health Issues* **17** (2), 107–114.
12 N Hampson, 1968 *The enlightenment* Penguin: Harmondsworth
13 J Gribben, 2002 *Science. A history* Allen Lane: London
14 F Capra, 1983 *The turning point: science, society, and the rising culture* Fontana: London
15 K Popper, 1959 *The logic of scientific discovery* Harper and Row: New York
16 TS Kuhn, 1970 *The structure of scientific revolutions* University of Chicago Press: London
17 E Martin, 1989 *The woman in the body* Open University Press: Milton Keynes
18 S Yusuf, R Collins, R Peto, 1984 Why do we need some large, simple randomized trials?. *Stat Med* **3** 409–420.
19 G Bateson, 1985 *Mind and nature. A necessary unity* Fontana: London
20 M Jelinek, 1992 The clinician and the randomised controlled trial. In: J Daly, I McDonald, E Willis, Ed. *Researching health care: designs, dilemmas, disciplines* Tavistock Routledge: London 76–89.
21 D Sackett, W Rosenberg, J Muir Gray, et al. 1996 Evidence based medicine: what it is and what it isn't. *Br Med J* **312** 71–72.
22 DL Sackett, SE Straus, WS Richardson, et al. 2002 *Evidence based medicine. How to practice and teach EBM* Churchill Livingstone: Edinburgh
23 National Institute for Health and Clinical Excellence (UK) 2007 *The guidelines manual 2007: Chapter 7* Online.

Available http://www.nice.org.uk/page.aspx?o=422950 (accessed 13 August 2007)

24 Duff M, Winter C (In press) The progress of labour. Orderly chaos? In: McCourt C (ed.) Time and childbirth. Berghahn, Oxford.

25 Royal Australian and New Zealand College of Obstetricians and Gynaecologists 2006 Intrapartum fetal surveillance clinical guidelines. 2nd edn Online. Available http://www.ranzcog.edu.au/publications/womenshealth.shtml#IFSG (accessed 13 August 2007)

26 National Institute for Health and Clinical Excellence (UK) 2001 Inherited clinical guideline C. Electronic fetal monitoring: the use and interpretation of cardiotocography in intrapartum fetal surveillance. Online. Available http://guidance.nice.org.uk/CGC (accessed 13 August 2007)

27 Society of Obstetricians and Gynaecologists of Canada 2002 Fetal health surveillance in labour (Part II). Online. Available http://www.sogc.org/guidelines/index_e.asp#Obstetrics (accessed 13 August 2007)

28 Z Alfirevic, D Devane, GML Gyte, 2006 Continuous cardiotocography (CTG) as a form of electronic fetal monitoring (EFM) for fetal assessment during labour. *Cochrane Database Syst Rev* (Issue 3), Art. No.: CD006066. DOI: 10.1002/14651858.CD006066

29 D Macdonald, A Grant, M Sheridan-Pereira, et al. 1985 The Dublin randomized controlled trial of intrapartum fetal heart rate monitoring. *Am J Obstet Gynecol* **152** 524–539.

30 DS Walker, S Shunkwiler, J Supanich, et al. 2001 Labor and delivery nurses' attitudes toward intermittent fetal monitoring. *J Midwifery Womens Health* **46** 374–380.

31 AM Gülmezoglu, CA Crowther, P Middleton, 2006 Induction of labour for improving birth outcomes for women at or beyond term. *Cochrane Database Syst Rev* (Issue 4), Art. No.: CD004945. DOI: 10.1002/14651858.CD004945.pub2

32 Department of Health 2005 UK statistical bulletin. NHS maternity statistics: England 2003–04. Online. Available www.dh.gov.uk/en/Publicationsandstatistics/Publications/PublicationsStatistics/DH_4107060 (accessed 13 August 2007)

33 ED Hodnett, S Fredericks, 2003 Support during pregnancy for women at increased risk of low birthweight babies. *Cochrane Database Syst Rev* (Issue 3), Art. No.: CD000198. DOI: 10.1002/14651858.CD000198

34 R Mander, 2001 *Supportive care and midwifery* Blackwell: Oxford

35 C McCourt, 2003 Social support. In: C Squire, Ed. *The social context of childbirth* Radcliffe Medical Press: Oxford

36 JK Gupta, GJ Hofmeyr, R Smyth, 2004 Position in the second stage of labour for women without epidural anaesthesia. *Cochrane Database Syst Rev* (Issue 1), Art. No.: CD002006. DOI: 10.1002/14651858.CD002006.pub2

37 K O'Driscoll, D Meagher, 1980 *Active management of labour. Clinics in obstetrics and gynaecology* Saunders: London

38 K O'Driscoll, M Foley, D MacDonald, et al. 1984 Active management of labour as an alternative to cesarean section for dystocia. *Obstet Gynecol* **63** 485–490.

39 JG Thornton, RJ Lilford, 1994 Active management of labour: current knowledge and research issues. *Br Med J* **309** 366–369.

40 ME Foley, M Alarab, L Daly, et al. 2004 The continuing effectiveness of active management of first labor, despite a doubling in overall nulliparous cesarean delivery. *Am J Obstet Gynecol* **191** (3), 891–895.

41 R Davis-Floyd, 1994 The technocratic body: American childbirth as cultural expression. *Soc Sci Med* **38** 1125–1140.

42 ED Hodnett, S Gates, GJ Hofmeyr, et al. 2003 Continuous support for women during childbirth. *Cochrane Database Syst Rev* (Issue 3), Art. No.: CD003766. DOI: 10.1002/14651858.CD003766.pub2

43 D Kernick, 2002 The demise of linearity in managing health services: a call for post normal health care. *J Health Serv Res Policy* **7** 121–124.

44 DA Schon, 1983 *The reflective practitioner* Basic Books: New York

45 P Benner, CA Tanner, CA Chesla, 1996 *Expertise in nursing practice. Caring, clinical judgement and ethics* Springer: New York

46 R Davis-Floyd, PS Arvidson, 1997 *Intuition: the inside story* Routledge: New York

47 A Edwards, G Elwyn, K Hood, et al. 2000 Judging the 'weight of evidence' in systematic reviews: introducing rigour into the qualitative overview stage by assessing signal and noise. *J Eval Clin Pract* **6** 177–184.

48 M Bloch, 1967 From cognition to ideology. *Ritual, history and power. Selected papers in anthropology: London School of Economics Monographs on Social Anthropology No. 58* Athlone Press: London

49 EP Thompson, 1967 Time, work-discipline, and industrial capitalism. *Past Present* **38** 56–97.

50 EA Friedman, 1978 Labour: clinical evaluation and management. 2nd edn Appleton-Century-Crofts: New York

51 JW Studd, RH Philpott, 1972 Partograms and action line of cervical dilatation. *Proc R Soc Med* **65** 700–701.

52 In: R Frankenberg, Ed. *Time, health and medicine* 1992 Sage: London

53 W Simonds, 2002 Watching the clock: keeping time during pregnancy, birth, and postpartum experiences. *Soc Sci Med* **55** 559–570.

54 McCourt C (ed.) In press. Time and childbirth. Berghahn, Oxford.

55 GG Lennon, 1962 *Diagnosis in clinical obstetrics* John Wright & Sons: Bristol 196

56   MM Garrey, ADT Govan, C Hodge, et al. 1980 *Obstetrics illustrated, 3rd edn* Churchill Livingstone: Edinburgh

57   S Downe, 1996 Concepts of normality in the maternity services: application and consequences. In: L Frith, Ed. *Ethics and midwifery: issues in contemporary practice* Butterworth Heinemann: Oxford 86–103.

58   LL Albers, M Schiff, JG Gorwoda, 1996 The length of active labor in normal pregnancies. *Obstet Gynecol* **87** 355–359.

59   LL Albers, 1999 The duration of labor in healthy women. *J Perinatol* **19** 114–119.

60   R Davis-Floyd, E Davis, 1997 Intuition as authoritative knowledge in midwifery and home birth. In: R Davis-Floyd, PS Arvidson, Ed. *Intuition: the inside story: interdisciplinary perspectives* Routledge: New York 145–176.

61   In: P Troop, M Goldacre, A Mason, *et al* Ed. *Health outcome indicators: normal pregnancy and childbirth. Report of a working group to the Department of Health* 1999 National Centre for Outcomes Development: Oxford

62   D Kernick, 2006 Wanted – new methodologies for health service research. Is complexity theory the answer?. *Fam Pract* **23** (3), 385–390.

63   J Cornfield, 1969 The Bayesian outlook and its application. *Biometrics* **25** 617–657.

64   GRIT Study Group 2003 A randomised trial of timed delivery for the compromised preterm fetus: short term outcomes and Bayesian interpretation. *BJOG* **110** (1), 27–32.

65   GB Hazen, M Huang, 2006 Large-sample Bayesian posterior distributions for probabilistic sensitivity analysis. *Med Decis Making* **26** (5), 512–534.

66   ME Hannah, WJ Hannah, SA Hewson, et al. 2000 Planned caesarean section versus planned vaginal birth for breech presentation at term: a randomised multicentre trial. Term Breech Trial Collaborative Group. *Lancet* **356** 1375–1383.

67   KL Hogle, L Kilburn, S Hewson, et al. 2003 Impact of the international term breech trial on clinical practice and concerns: a survey of centre collaborators. *J Obstet Gynaecol Can* **25** 14–16.

68   GJ Hofmeyr, ME Hannah, 2003 Planned caesarean section for term breech delivery. *Cochrane Database Syst Rev* (Issue 2), Art. No.: CD000166. DOI: 10.1002/14651858.CD000166

69   JF Molkenboer, FJ Roumen, LJ Smits, et al. 2006 Birth weight and neurodevelopmental outcome of children at 2 years of age after planned vaginal delivery for breech presentation at term. *Am J Obstet Gynecol* **194** (3), 624–629.

70   O Kempthorne, 1969 Commentary on Cornfield J 1969 The Bayesian outlook and its application. *Biometrics* **25** 649

71   U Merry, 1995 *Coping with uncertainty: insights from the new science of chaos, self-organization and complexity* Praeger: Westport, CT

72   Department of Health 1993 *Report of the Chief Medical Officer's Expert Group on the sleeping position of infants and cot death* HMSO: London

73   M Willinger, HJ Hoffman, RB Hartford, 1994 Infant sleep position and risk for sudden infant death syndrome: report of meeting held January 13 and 14, 1994, National Institutes of Health, Bethesda, MD. *Pediatrics* **93** 814–819.

74   D Salsburg, 1990 Hypothesis versus significance testing for controlled clinical trials: a dialogue. *Stat Med* **9** 201–211.

75   J Gleick, 1998 *Chaos: the amazing science of the unpredictable* Vintage: London

76   MR Lissack, 2003 *Chaos and complexity – knowledge management?* Online. Available http://www.leader-values.com/content/detail.asp?ContentDetailID=47 (accessed 29 August 2007)

77   SM Pikkujamsa, TH Makikallio, LB Sourander, et al. 1999 Cardiac interbeat interval dynamics from childhood to senescence: comparison of conventional and new measures based on fractals and chaos theory. *Circulation* **100** 393–399.

78   C Haigh, 2002 Using chaos theory; the implications for nursing. *J Adv Nurs* **37** 462–469.

79   K Sweeney, F Griffiths, 2002 *Complexity and healthcare, an introduction* Radcliffe Medical Press: Oxford

80   C Winter, 2002 *Assessing the progress of labour: orderly chaos* South Bank University: London MSc Thesis

81   MM Gross, S Drobnic, MJ Keirse, 2005 Influence of fixed and time-dependent factors on duration of normal first stage labor. *Birth* **32** (1), 27–33.

82   I Prigogine, 1987 *From being to becoming: the new science of connectedness* Bantam Dell: New York

83   T Wilson, T Holt, T Greenhalgh, 2001 Complexity science: complexity and clinical care. *Br Med J* **323** 685–688.

84   RL Ackoff, 1980 The systems revolution. In: M Lockett, R Spear, Ed. *Organisations as systems* Open University Press: Milton Keynes

85   Medical Research Council Health Services and Public Health Research Board 2000 *A framework for development and evaluation of RCTs for complex interventions to improve health* MRC: London

86   J O'Connor, I McDermott, 1997 *The art of systems thinking* Thorsons: London

87   for the Nursing Supportive Care in Labor Trial Group 2002 ED Hodnett, N Lowe, ME Hannah, et al.Effectiveness of nurses as providers of birth labor support in North American hospitals: a randomized controlled trial. *J Am Med Assoc* **288** 1373–1381.

88   ED Hodnett, 2002 Comments made during keynote address: Is the hospital culture a major risk factor for abnormal labour and birth?. *The research evidence. First Normal Birth Research Conference* University of Central

Lancashire: Preston, UK 29 September 2003

89   ED Hodnett, S Downe, N Edwards, et al. 2005 Home-like versus conventional institutional settings for birth. *Cochrane Database Syst Rev* (Issue 1), Art. No.: CD000012. DOI: 10.1002/14651858.CD000012.pub2

90   World Health Organization 1992 Basic documents. 19th edn WHO: Geneva

91   A Antonovsky, 1979 *Health stress and coping: new perspectives on mental and physical well-being* Jossey-Bass: San Francisco

92   A Antonovsky, 1993 The implications of salutogenesis: an outsider's view. In: AP Turnbull, JM Patterson, SG Behr, *et al* Ed. *Cognitive coping: families and disability* Brookes: Baltimore, MD Ch. 8

93   A Soloman, 1985 The emerging field of psychoneuroimmunology: advances. *J Inst Adv Health* **2** 6–19.

94   G Chirico, A Gasparoni, L Ciardelli, et al. 1999 Leukocyte counts in relation to the method of delivery during the first five days of life. *Biol Neonate* **75** 294–299.

95   R Gitau, E Menson, V Pickles, et al. 2001 Umbilical cortisol levels as an indicator of the fetal stress response to assisted vaginal delivery. *Eur J Obstet Gynecol Reprod Biol* **98** 14–17.

96   J Bengel, R Strittmatter, H Willmann, 1999 *What keeps people healthy? The current state of discussion and the relevance of Antonovsky's salutogenic model of health* Online. Available http://www.bzga.de/bzga_stat/pdf/60804070.pdf (accessed 13 August 2007)

97   M Eriksson, B Lindstrom, 2006 Antonovsky's sense of coherence scale and the relation with health: a systematic review. *J Epidemiol Community Health* **60** (5), 376–381.

98   NK Grote, SE Bledsoe, 2007 Predicting postpartum depressive symptoms in new mothers: the role of optimism and stress frequency during pregnancy. *Health Soc Work* **32** (2), 107–118.

99   N Lin, 2001 *Social capital* Cambridge University Press: Cambridge

100 S Kilsztajn, MS Carmo, LC MachadoJr, et al. 2007 Caesarean sections and maternal mortality in Sao Paulo. *Eur J Obstet Gynecol Reprod Biol* **132** (1), 64–69.

101 C Misago, C Kendall, P Freitas, et al. 2001 From 'culture of dehumanization of childbirth' to 'childbirth as a transformative experience': changes in five municipalities in north-east Brazil. *Int J Gynecol Obstet* **75** S67S72.

102 Ontario Women's Health Council 2000 *Attaining and maintaining best practices in the use of Caesarean section: an analysis of four Ontario hospitals. Report of the Caesarean Section Working Group of the Women's Health Council* Online. Available http://www.womenshealthcouncil.on.ca/English/page-1-361-1.html2000 (Accessed 30 August 2007)

103 S Downe, 1994 How average is normality?. *Br J Midwifery* **2** (7), 303–304.

104 S Downe, C McCormick, BL Beech, 2001 Labour interventions associated with normal birth. *Br J Midwifery* **9** 602–606.

105 A Oakley, 1993 Birth as a normal process. In: A Oakley, Ed. *Essays on women and health* Edinburgh University Press: Edinburgh 2

106 S Downe, L Simpson, K Trafford, 2007 Expert intrapartum maternity care: a meta-synthesis. *J Adv Nurs* **57** (2), 127–140.

107 P Benner, 1984 *From novice to expert: excellence and power in clinical nursing practice* Addison-Wesley: Menlo Park, CA

108 H Rose, 1983 Hand, brain, and heart: a feminist epistemology for the natural sciences. *Signs: J Women Culture Soc* **7** 73–90.

109 A el-Nemer, S Downe, N Small, 2006 'She would help me from the heart': an ethnography of Egyptian women in labour. *Soc Sci Med* **62** (1), 81–92.

110 L Cragin, HP Kennedy, 2006 Linking obstetric and midwifery practice with optimal outcomes. *J Obstet Gynecol Neonatal Nurs* **35** (6), 779–785.

CHAPTER 7

Risk, safety, fear and trust in childbirth

Mandie Scamell, Nancy Stone and *Hannah Dahlen*

Introduction

Despite the international recognition that the concept of risk, and its minimisation through active management, has come to dominate almost every aspect of childbirth across the world (Bryers and Teijlingen, 2010; Smith, Devane and Murphy-Lawless, 2012; Maclean, 2014; Skinner and Maude, 2016), practitioners working in maternity services, who are those managing perinatal risk on a daily basis, tend to assume that a mutually shared techno-rational understanding to risk prevails across the multidisciplinary maternity care team (Skinner, 2008). In this chapter this tendency will be subjected to critical scrutiny, the links between risk and birth practices will be explored, and an opportunity for trust and practice development will be introduced.

The chapter will explore three interlinked propositions: the first is that the operations of the techno-rational approach to risk are not as self-evident as they appear, and that they do not necessarily coincide with an evidence-based approach to care. The second is that the contemporary understanding of risks in maternity care is intrinsically linked to increasing application of technology. The third proposition explored in this chapter is that critical evaluation and analysis of how risk operates in maternity care provides a unique opportunity for hope where birth can be reframed as a trustworthy physiological process worthy of protection.

The Emergence of Risk

The term risk is derived from the Italian *risco* and the Spanish *riesco*, both deriving from the Latin word resecum, meaning 'the one that cuts'. This 'cutting' referred to the rocky escarpments that were a danger to seafarers and ships since the beginnings of maritime adventure (Liuzzo, et al, 2014). In this sense, the term risk was initially associated with danger. Throughout the Enlightenment, with the emergence and development of probability to calculate beneficial and unfavourable outcomes for specific events, the belief in fate and divine law was replaced with the belief that the future could be influenced by basing choices on rational calculations (Bernstein 1996/1998). Hence, probability ushered in new ways of thinking about human agency and outcomes of events. According to Hacking, it is because of probability calculations that we live in a risk society (Hacking 1975/2007). Today, risk is predominantly associated with the possibility of loss or with danger. Douglas writes:

'Whereas originally a high risk meant a game in which a throw of the die had a strong probability of bringing great pain or great loss, now risk refers only to negative outcomes. The work has been preempted to mean bad risks' (1992/2003).

Risk theorists and their contribution to the risk discourse

Ulrich Beck contributed to the theory of the risk society in 1986 with his seminal work *Risk Society: Towards a new Modernity*, first published in translation in 1992. Beck believed that the scientific advancements and technologies that characterised modernity, and that had brought about the breakdown of traditional societies, had created uncontrollable and unmanageable side-effects. While Beck was originally concerned with environmental catastrophes, such as chemical pollution and acid rain, it will be shown in this chapter that the technological advancements in maternity care also come with unintended negative outcomes when they are unnecessarily implemented.

Mary Douglas developed a cultural theory of risk that grew out of her work on pollution in *Purity and Danger* (1966/2007). In *Purity and Danger*, she showed how primitive societies understood and constructed pollution, danger and risk within their social context. She concluded that primitive as well as modern societies uphold social order in part by defining danger and creating social structures and policies to contain it. She believed that lay people and experts define risk differently. Defining risk is thus not just about creating safety; risk becomes a tool in discourse concerning power, legitimation and authority (ibid). Stephen Lyng, in his work on voluntary risk-taking, shows that risk can also be associated with pleasure (1990). Lyng classified risk-taking in leisure activities as edgework, noting that these activities 'all involve a clearly observable threat to one's physical or mental well-being or one's sense of an ordered existence' (1990, p857). An important aspect of *edgework* according to Lyng is that the participants, whether they are skydiving or racing cars, believe that they have 'the ability to maintain control over a situation that verges on complete chaos... and (are able) to avoid being paralysed with fear...' (ibid, p859). Perceptions and consciousness are altered while they participate in an activity that they seemingly control through skills that they have developed to master the situation.

Definitions of risk, and what risk becomes associated with, are therefore culturally constructed. They help to maintain social structures, being at once a product of these structures and a tool by which social order is maintained.

Risk in maternity care

In modern care, risk aversion is an organising concept. In UK health policy, for example, effective risk management has been linked to the idea of 'an organisation with a memory' (DoH, 2000). This means that exceptional adverse events, where harm has occurred in the past, are used to plan care in the future. The organisation, as a part of the process of learning from its mistakes, tightens its risk adversity programme every time an adverse event takes place.

Replacement of evidence-based care with single-issue risk avoidance

The 'organisation with a memory' approach to risk management, though persuasive and pervasive, has significant limitations in relation to evidence-based decision-making in maternity care, as in other areas of health (Brown, 2008; Flynn, 2002). The focus on exceptional and singular incidents where harm has already occurred, in an effort to improve safety outcomes in the future for all women and their babies, is problematic. It means that routine care is planned around evidence collected from just a small number of exceptional cases. Or, as Heyman (2010) suggests, health service planning follows a *'closing the gate after the horse has bolted'* logic. Planning maternity care using hindsight to examine poor outcomes that have already occurred means that the avoidance of extremely rare risks of significant harm takes precedence over the much more common risks of morbidity (iatrogenic or otherwise) of over-use of 'just in case' intervention. Through institutional mechanisms, risk management becomes a focal point for strict behavioural restrictions on the woman, and on her caregivers during pregnancy and labour (Healey, 2017; Scamell, 2016). These beliefs enhance the notion that every pregnancy and birth harbours risk. As one of the authors (MS) wrote in her study on midwifery risk in the UK: 'There is low risk and there is high risk, but there is no such thing as no risk' (Scamell, 2011). Hence, in cultures and organisations that are extremely risk-averse, there can never be an assumption of a safe pregnancy or birth.

To provide one detailed example of how the 'organisation with a memory' approach to risk has been translated in maternity care, we will focus upon the example of the application of *Modified Early Obstetric Warning Systems (MEOWS)* into midwifery practice in the UK. This is a tool that was developed to enable staff working in busy intensive care units to recognise the deteriorating patient. It is based on regular recording of clinical symptoms, on the assumption that if a certain number of them are present, an alarm is triggered. While this seems to be useful in very sick patients at risk of rapid deterioration, it was not designed for, and has not been tested in, less acute patients, let alone largely healthy childbearing and postnatal women. Despite this, the 2003–05 UK Confidential Enquiry into Maternal and Child Health recommended the introduction of a modified version, the Maternity Early Warning System (MEOWS), for all maternity inpatients, regardless of presence of pathology, with no attempt to assess the potential benefits or adverse consequences. It was simply assumed that safety would be improved through the timely recognition of acute deterioration in the health of pregnant or postnatal women who were inpatients (Lewis, 2007). This clinical recommendation arose out of a maternal mortality inquiry that reports a 14:100,000 mortality rate. Put another way, the national implementation of the MEOWS arose out of a 0.0014% chance of occurrence. Some authors report that the tool is sensitive and specific (Quinn, 2016), particularly in acutely ill women in middle-income settings (Singh 2016), but there have been no studies comparing usual practice to use of the MEOWS, to see if the tool picks up deterioration any better than expert caregivers would do, and questions have been raised about its efficacy (Macintosh, 2014). As Mackintosh et al point out:

'Widespread policy support for the MEOWS is based on its intuitive appeal and no validated system for use in the maternity population currently exists.' (p26)

According to the Centre for Evidence Based Medicine, individual clinical cases that shape practitioners' practice can be interpreted as

'Expert opinion without explicit critical appraisal or based on physiology bench research or "first principles"' (CEBM, 2018)

As can be seen from the hierarchy of knowledge figure below, such exceptional cases that result in devastating outcomes should be considered to be the least reliable form of evidence for service planning. Despite this, however, lessons learned from maternal mortality reports in high-income countries are used to intensify the routine surveillance of all mothers.

Figure 1.
Level of evidence adapted from CEBM

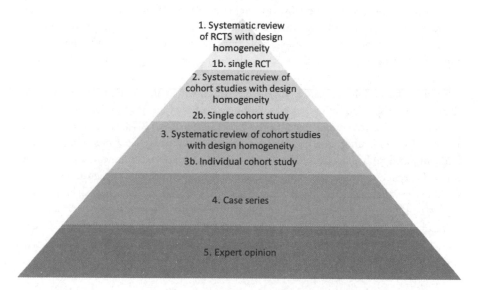

When risks of something as shocking as death are involved, emotions obscure the possibility for impartial, scientifically based decision-making. When the stakes are high and the level of harm extreme, a formal evidence-based approach to care tends to be seen as less critical.

Personal, institutional and professional abhorrence for the possibility of tragic outcomes, no matter how unlikely those outcomes might be, becomes the emotional driver underpinning routine care within a risk-averse society. These rare outcomes, which are considered calculable and quantifiable by policymakers (Luhmann, 2008), take centre stage with their shock value, and intensify fear. This results in the notion that *if the possibility of an event happening is calculable, then the avoidance of that event is also possible.* With correct action, an unwanted outcome can therefore be anticipated and averted (Lupton, 1999/2013). Through this process of meaning-making, it seems inevitable that technology for both surveillance and intervention will be privileged during the normal physiological process of pregnancy and childbirth.

Further, in contexts where the extremely rare risk of harm to a baby is valued over the much more common risks of morbidity (iatrogenic or otherwise) to the mother, 'risk management' becomes a lever for strict behavioural restrictions on the woman, both during pregnancy and labour. When risk is attached to the woman's behaviour, she is made responsible for disciplining herself. Ruhl writes:

> *Responsibility is equated with the capacity to behave rationally; the term presupposes a calculation of expected benefits and risks. … In the case of the contemporary regulation of pregnancy, the 'type of human life' that is to be enhanced is predicated on a specific definition of responsible behaviour, which is highly medicalised…and articulated in a vocabulary of risk management* (Ruhl 1999, p96).

For example, using this logic, women should choose to give birth in a hospital maternity unit since it is believed to inevitably improve adverse perinatal outcomes as a result of the possibility for obstetric specialists to intervene at a moment's notice. This is without regard to good quality evidence from a number of high-income countries that healthy women with uncomplicated pregnancies are safer giving birth outside of hospital in many contexts, with no extra risk to their babies unless they are having their first baby at home (Birthplace in England Collaborative Group 2011; De Jong 2017).

Unlike the notion of positive risk-taking (discussed in the examples of risky sports above), where risk might be embraced to improve quality of life, improve optimal outcome or even just add a bit of excitement (Lyng 1990, Lupton 1999/2013), risk in health policy and organisation is understood as something that is always bad. Far from being a neutral evidence-based probability calculation (a careful and impartial measurement of the pros and cons), the techno-rational approach to risk demands that low probability high-impact harms should be avoided at all costs regardless of the statistical probability of that harm occurring (Douglas, 1990). As Kotoska (2017) noted in his study on informed consent and refusal of obstetric treatment, the death rate of astronauts (1.8%) is considered acceptable; however, for women who want to have a vaginal birth after a caesarean section (0.05% foetal risk), court orders are sought in some countries to prohibit them from birthing vaginally.

This is because foetal rights are understood as clashing with women's autonomy and their right to decide where and how they choose to give birth. Chervenak, McCullough and Brent have published extensively in the USA on obstetric ethics, with the argument that intrapartum decision-making should not be based solely on a pregnant woman's rights model, but rather on an ethical principle of beneficence (Chervenak, McCullough et al

2011; Chervenak and McCullough 2017). In this model, the obstetrician is the arbiter of what is beneficent – they must balance paternalistic care with proper informed consent. According to Chervenak et al, the woman's rights model:

>...*requires the obstetrician to implement birth plans that unconditionally exclude cesarean delivery or the unconditional right to planned home birth. This model eliminates the obstetrician's beneficence-based obligations to both the pregnant and fetal patients and therefore reduces the obstetrician to a mere automaton. This model also has absurd implications* (Cherenak 2011, 315.e4)

The conviction that women endanger their unborn child by choosing to birth outside a hospital has been echoed in German obstetric journals (Arabin, Chervenak et al 2013; Rath and Schmidt, 2013). In addition, several countries in Europe have constitutionalised foetal rights, including Ireland and Hungary (de Londras, 2015).

Risk-management decisions, which are based on frequency distributions and statistical inferences, create boundaries between normal and deviant categories that have to be negotiated by individuals. Depending on the decisions they make (where the 'right' decision is for 'normalised' behaviour), these categories are used to judge the moral quality of that individual. In the context of healthcare, risk calculations are presented as if they are completely impartial, and as an unbiased basis on which healthcare practitioners can give counsel to pregnant women. While the numbers seem to convey a sense of neutrality, the actual construction and application of categories has its foundation in social mores. When confronted with uncertainty, risk-management decisions thus also become a matter of morality (Adams, 2003).

Intensification of technology in maternity routine care

Health policy across the world intrinsically promises increased safety through the intensification of risk management. As the World Health Organization (2018) points out:

>'*There has been a substantial increase over the last two decades in the application of a range of labour practices to initiate, accelerate, terminate, regulate or monitor the physiological process of labour, with the aim of improving outcomes for women and babies.*' (WHO, 2018:1)

In maternity care this means that the minimisation of risk through interventions is assumed to inevitably improve the outcomes for mother and baby. One of the risk surveillance techniques utilised during labour in many maternity units across the world, regardless of risk status, is continuous electronic foetal heart monitoring (EFM). This surveillance promises to minimise risk, in spite of evidence showing that the introduction of EFM has done little to improve neonatal outcomes. It is also associated with increased rates of operative birth and consequent iatrogenic morbidity (Alfirevic et al, 2017). Despite this evidence, the implied (but not actual) promise of reduced risk is considered more important than, for example, a woman's desire to move around unencumbered.

Once a surveillance device or technology such as EFM is introduced into routine care, it is rarely subject to evaluation, and almost inevitably comes to be seen as crucial.

Failure to carry out such a test or measurement is not only considered unreasonable, it also exposes those responsible for the failure to institutional scrutiny. As a result of this, maternity staff (midwives and obstetricians) are seen to be 'good' practitioners if they spend much of their time carefully applying the technologies of risk management, and therefore, identifying ever more subtle markers of what *might* indicate some unspecified future pathology (in the absence of any data that this is in fact so). This has an opportunity cost – it limits the time available for preserving and protecting physiological labour and birth in the present (Scamell and Alaszewski, 2012). With unquestioning faith in machines and technology, there is a loss of belief (self-belief and that of others) that healthcare practitioners have expertise in any other area of ensuring foetal wellbeing. When risk is understood in this way (in line with Beck's 'Risk Society', as discussed above), taking even unfounded precautionary actions to reduce very nominal or rare harms becomes an indication of good healthcare practice (Healey, 2017; Scamell, 2011) and responsible and even moral parenting (Lee et al, 2014).

All the developments undertaken in the context of the Risk Society can, however, also be understood as representing a troubling development in the unsettling of normal childbirth. The technologies that are used to manage childbirth – even the paperwork used to record it – shape the way birth is imagined. Importantly, a commitment to birth as a normal physiological process becomes framed as a potential dangerous ideology, threatening the successful management of risk. Any resistance to surveillance (by healthcare staff or service users) is thus seen as incompetent, incompliant, petulant or irrational.

Where the focus is on possible physical harms, other important aspects of wellbeing, such as psychological, social, cultural and spiritual needs, and even longer-term adverse clinical effects for mother or baby, become less relevant. The irony is that by ignoring these important aspects of what makes us human, other unexpected risks emerge as women try to circumnavigate the trauma inflicted by their depersonalised and dehumanised care (Powell, Kennedy & Shannon, 2004; Regan & Liaschenko, 2007; Jackson, Dahlen et al, 2012; Dahlen, 2014). Understood in this critical way, the management of risk through the intensification of dependence on technology does not fulfil the promise of increased personal safety for labouring women, a proposition often overlooked in a world focused on risk management (Dahlen, 2014).

Erosion of confidence in birth through the expansion of fear

The translation of uncertainties of childbirth into risks means apportioning blame becomes a normative organisational practice. This means that healthcare staff involved in a case with a poor outcome will not only fear the event itself, but also the subsequent risk-management interrogation (Copeland, Dahlen et al, 2013; Dahlen & Caplice, 2014). Furthermore, when maternity care personnel are threatened with accountability for poor or tragic outcomes, they will knowingly or unknowingly influence women to make the institutionally sanctioned choice (Plested & Kirkham, 2016). This fear undermines professional and community confidence in normal birth, encouraging defensive maternity practices that are defined by their reliance on technological surveillance and intervention (Scamell, 2016). Plested and Kirkham

(2016) write that the maternity system is experienced by women as permeated by fear, and that:

'Fearful behaviours of practitioners for themselves created a situation where participants felt that midwives and institutional safety was prioritised over their personal circumstances…' (Kirkham, p31).

When midwives and obstetricians act out of past fear for current care provision, they miss the particular moment for each particular woman and baby, with all of its current and future possibilities. Accepting this results in the capacity to work with what is in the present – seeing what is now at hand, as opposed to projecting scenarios out of past experiences or singular tragic events.

Trust as an antidote to fear

In the last section of the chapter, we want to examine the potential of reframing maternity care provision around notions of trust, in the context of uncertainty.

One of the most effective ways to moderate the influence of fear and put risk into perspective is to increase relationship-based models of care, such as continuity of midwifery care. Relationships between midwives and linked obstetricians lead to trust: women feel safe to trust in their midwife/midwives and themselves, and midwives and obstetricians learn to trust each other to maximise wellbeing for all women and babies. Concurrently, maternity care staff become invested in women they get to know, and advocate for them. Over time, they see benefit from this approach, and they learn to trust the abilities of women to give birth physiologically. This is manifested in the encouraging outcomes seen in the many randomised controlled trials of continuity of midwife-led care models (Sandall, Soltani et al, 2015). Trust is the antidote to fear, and relationships build trust.

When women are able to enter into trusting relationships with their caregivers, a culture of compassion can ensue, and care at birth can have a loving and authentically caring component that mitigates fear. Compassion is a quality of companionate love, defined by Hatfield et al (1993) as *'the affection and tenderness men and women feel for those with whom their lives are deeply entwined'* (p583). For Oakley, *'love is a scientific concept…and is as important as science – technical knowledge, monitoring and intervention'* (2004, p327). Love is rendered through midwifery (and maternity) care that promotes self-confidence and enhances normality. Rather than surveillance technologies becoming the sole arbiter of safety, connection enhanced through listening and watching can strengthen communication between midwives (and others) and women, and empower women to co-create a safe environment (Smythe, 2010).

Conclusion

In this chapter, the culture of risk avoidance has been subjected to critical scrutiny. We have critiqued the assumption that risk management in childbirth is wholly benevolent as it is currently undertaken in maternal health practice across the world. This exposes some of the deeply troubling consequences of the prioritisation of standardised protocol-driven 'learning from mistakes' above other elements of care, such as respect for autonomy, and the preservation of physiological birth where this is of benefit to the mother and baby. We have argued that risk management can operate to subsume evidence-based care and professional expertise, and that it can intensify the application of technology (with all of the iatrogenic harms such intensification inevitably introduces). We also consider two crucial areas for maternity practice development. The first is that the meaning and implications of risk management should never be taken as given. Instead the technologies of risk should be applied with caution, and with an understanding of the significant limitations inherent in this approach to practice. The second is the unique opportunity provided by a shift to a culture of trust, properly balanced with safety. The multidisciplinary maternal health team already has the knowledge, skills and values necessary to rebalance the scales of risk in such a way that respect, autonomy, evidence-based care, trust and physiological birth can all be seen as equally important components of safe, positive maternity care provision.

Suggestions for practitioners for dealing with fear

- Identify the fear
- Take responsibility for it (it's your fear)
- Do an obstetric emergency course
- Don't forget to breathe
- Visualisation
- Watch the self-talk and practise thought-stopping
- Talk to someone about how you feel
- Move (take a break from the situation, ask someone else's opinion)
- Have a cup of tea
- Knitting at birth can reduce adrenaline and keep anxious hands out of mischief
- Write about how you are feeling and reflect on it
- Get some evidence to support or refute your fear
- Centre yourself with affirmations such as 'trust in birth'
- If the fear will not go away or gets stronger then take note, it may be real. While birth should be trusted, it also needs to be respected
- Shed the fear and do not carry it into the next birth

Dahlen & Caplice (2010)

Key points for consideration for practitioners

- Personalising your care will increase the wellbeing of women, families, and yourself as the healthcare practitioner.
- Implementing safe care means deepening the connection between yourself and the women you care for and includes professional, yet also warm, heartfelt communication. This aids in discovering and strengthening the emotional and physical resources that each woman has to accomplish birth.

- Take time to reflect on the various ways that you sense how women are feeling during pregnancy, and how you perceive what is going on in labour. Incorporate these other ways of knowing into your care.
- Treat each moment of care as significant. These moments can be spent building trust and supporting hope. Keep in mind that women will remember their birth experience for the rest of their lives. Make it special.
- Be honest with yourself about what your strengths and weaknesses are in your care of labouring women and get the appropriate training where needed.

References

Adams, J. (2003). Risk and Morality: Three Framing Devices. *Risk and Morality*. R. Ericson and A. Doyle. Toronto University of Toronto Press: 87-103.

Alfirevic, Z., Gyte, G.M., Cuthbert, A. and Devane, D., 2017. Continuous cardiotocography (CTG) as a form of electronic fetal monitoring (EFM) for fetal assessment during labour. *Cochrane database of systematic reviews*, (2).

Arabin, B., et al. (2013). "Die geplante Hausgeburt in industrialisierten Landern: Burokratische Traumvorstellung vs. professionelle Verantwortlichkeit." *Z Geburtshilfe Neonatol* **217**(1): 7-13.

Beck, U. (1992). *Risk society : towards a new modernity*. London ; Newbury Park, Calif., Sage Publications.

Bernstein, P. L. (1996/1998). *Against the gods: The Remarkable Story of Risk*. New York, John Wiley & Sons.

Birthplace in England Collaborative Group, Brocklehurst P, Hardy P, Hollowell J, Linsell L, Macfarlane A, McCourt C, Marlow N, Miller A, Newburn M, Petrou S, Puddicombe D, Redshaw M, Rowe R, Sandall J, Silverton L, Stewart M. 2011 Perinatal and maternal outcomes by planned place of birth for healthy women with low risk pregnancies: the Birthplace in England national prospective cohort study. BMJ.23;343:d7400. doi: 10.1136/bmj.d7400)

Brown, P., 2008. Legitimacy chasing its own tail: Theorizing clinical governance through a critique of instrumental reason. *Social Theory & Health*, 6(2), pp.184-199.

Bryers and Teijlingen, 2010 - Bryers, H.M. and Van Teijlingen, E., 2010. Risk, theory, social and medical models: a critical analysis of the concept of risk in maternity care. *Midwifery*, 26(5), pp.488-496.

Chervenak, F., et al. (2011). "The professional responsibility model of obstetrical ethics: avoiding the perils of clashing rights." *American Journal of Obstetrics and Gynecology* **205**(4): 315.e311-315.e315.

Chervenak, F. A. and L. B. McCullough (2017). "Ethical dimensions of the fetus as patient." *Best Practice & Research Clinical Obstetrics and Gynaecology* **43**: 2-9.

Copeland F, et al. (2013). "Conflicting Contexts: Midwives interpretation fo childbirth through photo elicitation." *Women and Birth* Available online 25th December 2013.

Dahlen HG (2014). "Managing Risk or Facilitating Safety?" *International Journal of Childbirth* **4**(2): 66-68.

Dahlen HG and Caplice S (2014). "What do midwives fear?" *Women and Birth* **Online** http://dx.doi.org/10.1016/j.wombi.2014.06.008.

de Jonge A, Peters L, Geerts CC, van Roosmalen JJM, Twisk JWR, Brocklehurst P, Hollowell J. 2017 Mode of birth and medical interventions among women at low risk of complications: A cross-national comparison of birth settings in England and the Netherlands. PLoS One. 2017 Jul 27;12(7):e0180846. doi: 10.1371/journal.pone.0180846. eCollection 2017.

de Londras, F. (2015). "Constitutionalizing Fetal Rights: A Salutary Tale from Ireland." *Michigan Journal of Gender and Law* **22**(2).

Department of Health (2000) An Organisation with a Memory: Report of an Expert Group on Learning from Adverse Events in the National Health Service. webarchive.nationalarchives.gov.uk/ukgwa/20130107105354/http://www.dh.gov.uk/prod_consum_dh/groups/dh_digitalassets/@dh/@en/documents/digitalasset/dh_4088948.pdf

Douglas, M. (1966/2007). *Purity and Danger: an Analysis of Concept of Pollution and Taboo*. London; New York, Routledge.

Douglas, M. (1992/2003). *Risk and blame: essays in cultural theory*. London; New York, Routledge.

Douglas, M., (1990). *Risk as a forensic resource*. Daedalus, pp.1-16

Flynn, R., 2002. Clinical governance and governmentality. *Health, risk & society*, 4(2), pp.155-173.

Hacking, I. (1975/2007). *The Emergence of Probability: A Philosophical Study of Early Ideas about Probability, Induction and Statistical Inference*. New York, Cambridge University Press.

Hatfield, E., Cacioppo, J. T., & Rapson, R. L. (1993). Emotional contagion. *Current Directions in Psychological Science*, 2(3).

Healy, S., Humphreys, E. and Kennedy, C., 2016. Can maternity care move beyond risk? Implications for midwifery as a profession. *British Journal of Midwifery*, 24(3), pp.203-209.

Heyman, B., Alaszewski, A., Shaw, M. and Titterton, M., 2010. *Risk, safety and clinical practice: health care through the lens of risk*. Oxford University Press

Howick, J., Chalmers, I., Glasziou, P., Greenhalgh, T., Heneghan C., Liberati, A., Moschetti, I., Phillips, B., and Thornton, H. (2011) Explanation of the 2011 Oxford Centre for Evidence-Based Medicine (OCEBM) Levels of Evidence (Background Document). *Oxford Centre for Evidence-Based Medicine*. Available at at www.cebm.ox.ac.uk/resources/levels-of-evidence/ocebm-levels-of-evidence. Accessed January 2018.

Jackson, M., et al. (2012). "Birthing outside the system: Perspectives of risk amongst Australian women who have high risk homebirths." *Midwifery* **28**(5): 561-567.

Kotaska A. (2017). Informed consent and refusal in obstetrics: A practical ethical guide. *Birth*, DOI: 10.1111/birt.12281, 1-5

Lee, E., Bristow, J., Faircloth, C. and Macvarish, J., 2014. *Parenting culture studies*. Springer.

Lewis, G. (2007) The Confidential Enquiry into Maternal and Child Health (CEMACH). Saving mothers' lives: Reviewing maternal deaths to make motherhood safer–2003-2005. *The Seventh Report on Confidential Enquiries into Maternal Deaths in the United Kingdom*. CEMACH, London.

Liuzzo, G., Bentley, S., Giacometti, F., Serraino, A. (2014). The Term Risk: Etymology, Legal Definition and Various Traits. *Ital J Food Saf*, 3(1): 2269.

Luhmann, N. (2008). *Risk : a sociological theory* (Fourth printing ed.). New Brunswick, N.J.: Transaction Publishers.

Lupton, D. (1999/2013). *Risk*. London; New York, Routledge.

Lyng, S. (1990). "Edgework: A Social Psychological Analysis of Voluntary Risk Taking." *The American Journal of Sociology* **95**(4): 851-886.

Mackintosh N, Watson K, Rance S, Sandall J. 2014 Value of a modified early obstetric warning system (MEOWS) in managing maternal complications in the peripartum period: an ethnographic study. BMJ Qual Saf. 2014 Jan;23(1):26-34. doi: 10.1136/bmjqs-2012-001781. Epub 2013 Jul 18.

Maclean, E., 2014. What to expect when you're expecting? Representations of birth in British newspapers. *British Journal of Midwifery*, 22(8), pp.580-588.

Oakley, 2004. 'Who Care for Women? Science Versus Love in Midwifery Today' in *Midwifery and the Medicalization of Childbirth: Comparative Perspectives*. Eds. Van Teijlingen E., Lowis G., Mccaffery P. and Porter M. New York: New Science Publishers.

Plested, M., & Kirkham, M. (2016). Risk and fear in the lived experience of birth without a midwife. *Midwifery*, 38, 29-34

Powell Kennedy H and Shannon M (2004). "Keeping birth normal: research findings on midwifery care during childbirth." *Journal of Obstetrics and Gynecology* **33**(5): 554-560.

Quinn AC, Meek T, Waldmann C. 2016 Obstetric early warning systems to prevent bad outcome. Curr Opin Anaesthesiol. 2016 Jun;29(3):268-72. doi: 10.1097/ACO.0000000000000338.

Rath, W. and S. Schmidt (2013). "Out-of-Hospital Obstetrics." *Z Geburtsh Neonatol* **217**: 1-2.

Rath, W., and Schmidt, S. (2013). Out-of-Hospital Obstetrics. *Z Geburtsh Neonatol*, 217, 1-2. doi:10.1055/s-0033-1333703

Regan M and Liaschenko J (2007). "In the mind of the beholder: Hypothesized effect of intrapartum nurse's cognitive frames of childbirth caesarean section rates." *Qualitative Health Research* **17**(5): 612-634.

Ruhl, L. 1999. Liberal governance and prenatal care: risk and regulation in pregnancy. *Economy and Society*, 28(1), 95-117. Doi:10.1080/03085119900000026

Sandall J, et al. (2015). "Midwife-led continuity models versus other models of care for childbearing women . ." *Cochrane Database of Systematic Reviews* **Issue 9. Art. No.: CD004667. DOI: 10.1002/14651858.CD004667.pub4.**

Scamell, M., 2016. The fear factor of risk–clinical governance and midwifery talk and practice in the UK. *Midwifery*, 38, pp.14-20.

Scamell, M., 2011. The swan effect in midwifery talk and practice: a tension between normality and the language of risk. *Sociology of health & illness*, 33(7), pp.987-1001

Scamell, M. and Alaszewski, A., 2012. Fateful moments and the categorisation of risk: Midwifery practice and the ever-narrowing window of normality during childbirth. *Health, risk & society*, 14(2), pp.207-221

Singh A, Guleria K, Vaid NB, Jain S. 2016 Evaluation of maternal early obstetric warning system (MEOWS chart) as a predictor of obstetric morbidity: a prospective observational study. Eur J Obstet Gynecol Reprod Biol. 2016 Dec;207:11-17. doi: 10.1016/j.ejogrb.2016.09.014. Epub 2016 Oct 8.

Skinner, J., 2008. Risk: Let's look at the bigger picture. *Women and Birth*, 21(2), pp.53-54.

Skinner, J. and Maude, R., 2016. The tensions of uncertainty: Midwives managing risk in and of their practice. *Midwifery*, 38, pp.35-41.

Smith, V., Devane, D. and Murphy-Lawless, J., 2012. Risk in maternity care: a concept analysis. *International journal of childbirth*, 2(2), p.126.

mythe, E. (2010). Safety is an interpretive act: A hermeneutic analysis of care in childbirth. *International Journal of Nursing Studies*, 47, 1474-1482. doi:10.1016/j.ijnurstu.2010.05.003

World Health Organization, 2018. *Intrapartum care for a positive childbirth experience*. Geneva: World Health Organization

CHAPTER 8

The role of emotion, empathy, and compassion in organisations

Susan Crowther, Cary L. Cooper, Fiona Meechan and Neal M. Ashkanasy

Introduction

In this chapter, we address the 'feel', 'mood' or 'affectivity' of an organisation. There is always one mood or another in any situation that human beings find themselves working and living in; maternity organisations are no different. Mood in this context may or may not be an affective state. In terms of organisational mood, de Rivera[1] offers the following definition: *'an objective group phenomenon that can be palpably sensed – as when one enters a party or a city and feels an attitude of gaiety or depression, openness or fear'* (p197). Taking this as our starting point, we contend that maternity organisations around the world tend to be attuned to moods of fear and anxiety. These moods are likely to lead to risk-averse behaviours that act against human connectedness and compassionate interactions between people working in and being cared for within these organisations. We contend that this has consequences, not only for maternity care staff, but also for outcomes in maternity care.

Theories of organisational culture and climate

In 1975 Schneider[2] defined organisational climate as a mutually agreed description of an organisation's practices and procedures. Ashkanasy[3] notes further that culture refers to deeply embedded values and assumptions, while climate refers to organisational factors that are consciously perceived. As such, climate is a constituent of culture amenable to managerial control. Ashkanasy and Härtel[4] emphasise that affective culture and climate can be either positive or negative, with the positive forms associated with compassion and wellbeing, while the negative forms are associated with stress and malpractice. In this regard, Ashkanasy[5] notes that affective climate represents a culmination of affective processes that begin with the manner with which employees react emotionally to 'affective events' that occur in the workplace on a day-to-day basis.[6-7] For example, a midwife who is abused by a supervisor (i.e. s/he experiences an 'affective event') is likely to harbour negative feelings that s/he then communicates to others though 'emotional contagion';[8] eventually resulting in a negative affective climate.

Empathy and compassion in healthcare

Given that the delivery of compassionate care can lead to improved health outcomes,[9-10] health systems have a vested interest in ensuring that care is delivered compassionately. In addition, given the association with positive culture and climate, the delivery of compassionate care might be an ethical issue across cultures;[11] simply the right moral approach. This is reflected in the UK NHS Constitution, which emphasises compassion (DoH, 2015:2). In addition, compassion is identified as one of the '6 Cs' developed by the UK Chief Nursing Officer in relation to nursing and midwifery. Importantly, the UK 'Compassion in Practice' strategy document[12] highlights that in order to deliver compassionate care to people using NHS services, leaders and managers in the NHS need to create cultures in healthcare organisations that are based on supporting and caring for staff. As part of the '6 Cs', DoH[12] defines compassion as:

> '...how care is given through relationships based on empathy, respect and dignity – it can also be described as intelligent kindness and is central to how people perceive their care.' (p13)

Similarly, in the United States, compassion is a '...first principle of medical ethics across the health professions'.[13] Further, compassion has been identified as one of the five core human values set out in the International Charter for Human Values in Healthcare, which was developed by an international partnership of healthcare professionals using a range of qualitative research methods; the Charter has now been endorsed by a range of organisations from various countries within Asia, Australasia, Africa, Europe and North and South America.[14]

The definition and operationalisation of compassion is not without its difficulties.[15] In this regard, scholars also use the terms 'compassion' and 'empathy' interchangeably (as it is in the '6 Cs' definition). Yet, as with the differentiation of culture and climate, it is important to be clear about what is meant, because the different concepts can have different outcomes for both staff and service users.

Empathy

The concept of empathy relates to the ability to understand and resonate with someone else's emotions and experiences, and communicate that understanding,[16,17] and when this is demonstrated by clinicians, it has been found to have many benefits for patients, including improved compliance with treatment plans, improved physiological outcomes, improved satisfaction and reduced stress.[18]

However, research from the field of neuroscience has shown that empathising with another person can also lead to negative affect, a physical sensation of discomfort, or even pain.[19] Klimecki et al claim that empathy has the potential to lead to distress and emotional burnout, and they further found that empathy training (where the focus is on resonating with the suffering of another) leads not only to stronger sharing of distressing emotions with those experiencing suffering, but also to generally more negative affect in response to day-to-day life occurrences.[20]

Other research has shown that people find it easier to empathise with some people (i.e. people who are like themselves), rather than others dissimilar to themselves.[21,22] This leads in turn to a potential for some people to receive more empathetic care than others, which could have implications within a maternity organisation, particularly because such organisations are populated with multiple professional groups with vastly different aspirations, perspectives, philosophies and differing psychosocial and cultural worldviews.

In order to preserve the health of clinicians and ensure that patients experience equity in their treatment it has been argued that compassion may be a more appropriate concept.

Compassion

Compassion builds on the concept of empathy in that there is similarly a recognition of the emotions of the other person; the difference is that compassion also includes the motivation to act to alleviate the circumstances of the other.[17-23] Rather than being only an emotional reaction, compassion arguably entails a rational decision to help another, based on the premise that all life is of value.[24]

Compassion can be demonstrated in the smallest of gestures of care, such as a reassuring touch,[25] or the care demonstrated by a nurse ensuring that a patient had a smooth journey between departments:

> 'At the junction between two hospital buildings, there is a joint in the floor. Mindful of Chloe's broken neck, this wonderful nurse stopped the trolley and carefully lifted each wheel over the join in the floor to prevent any painful jolting of her injuries. Compassion is revealed in the smallest of acts.' Youngson[26]

In theory then, it is possible to deliver truly compassionate care to all – and relatively easily, through empathising (understanding the circumstances of the other) and acting to alleviate those circumstances. However, although compassion is the focus in current healthcare policy, the wider organisational context in maternity care specifically (and in healthcare in general) does not tend to allow for compassionate organisational climates.[27]

The current situation in maternity care

Maternity services around the world are under pressure to provide ever higher quality services to societies whose expectations are growing. Despite the rhetorical focus on person-centred care and informed choice,[28,29] rising acuity and centralisation of services into bigger units is leading to closure of small and personal units.[30-33] This paints a picture of global organisational activity which is at odds with the very strong evidence from around the world that childbearing women desire more relational models of care.[34,35] Maternity care should be about positive relationships, and attunement to the most intimate of human experiences.[35-37] However, the move away from organisational conditions that can foster this atmosphere is exacerbated by a drive towards a more technocratic, fragmented, task-orientated impersonal service, despite strong policy statements in the opposite direction.[28,29,38] In such a situation, maternity work becomes mundane and exhausting – instead of fulfilling, spiritually energising and transformative.

As an example of this kind of effect on organisational climate, the UK Royal College of Midwives 2016 report *Why midwives leave – Revisited,*[39] a follow-on report from 2002,[40] continues to highlight concerns related to morale, overwork, staffing issues, bullying, risk averse cultures and ongoing turf disputes between professional groups. The main reason midwives give for leaving or wanting to leave is an inability to work in a way congruent with providing quality midwifery care to women and families.[41-44] Possible causes for this are unacceptable models of delivering care, organisational demands, increasing acuity, poor managerial support or increasingly unworkable staffing ratios. This situation was reported at least a decade ago.[45,46] According to the RCM report, when midwives were asked what they would need to stay or return to practice, their response was organisational cultural change and improvements in working conditions. This situation is not isolated to UK midwifery. In a 2016 WHO global survey[47] of 2,500 midwives from 93 countries, *Midwives' voices, midwives' realities*, professional and social economic barriers were highlighted as influencing delivery of quality safe care. Issues of staff shortages, overwork, bullying, power issues, gender inequalities, poor pay, lack of respect and paucity of professional development are evident globally. Equally these concerns are not solely about midwifery. Some of these concerns also beset obstetricians.[48] Moreover, midwives in Australia and New Zealand are similarly challenged by organisational and practice demands.[49-52]

Bringing compassion into maternity organisations

Birth is a time in human life that has spiritual meaning and is a rite of passage for mothers and new families. Healthy relationships in maternity care require compassion and emotional wellbeing among staff.[53] When maternity care becomes transformed into a biomedical risk-avoidance process by the organisations that host birth, the spiritual quality and joyful emotions of childbirth can be lost.[37] Despite widespread acknowledgement of this risk, contemporary maternity organisations seem to be moving away from systems that encourage human connection and the expression of purpose and meaning in the process of pregnancy and childbirth.[54,55] In this context spirituality may or may not relate to any religious faith, and is a quality of care that acknowledges the existential need to find and make meaning, which foregrounds a sense of purpose and provides feelings of connectedness that help individuals and communities integrate experiences.[56] When midwives and other maternity care workers become drained of their emotional reserves, sense of purpose and ability to find meaning in what they do, their ongoing ability to provide compassionate care diminishes. Thomas and Wilson named this phenomenon 'compassion fatigue'.[57] The expectation that maternity care workers should 'cope and be resilient' in what is often a harsh organisational environment does not allow staff to thrive[58] or compassion to flourish.

One of the main issues for healthcare organisations is to recognise the relational aspect of actively engaging with the 'other'.[15] Critically, this involves organisations fostering a culture of compassion[59] and positivity.[4] This necessitates the need for compassion towards staff, for example by showing staff that their lives and contributions are of value. When management are person-centred and afford compassion, caregivers are more likely to deliver compassionate care to service users.[59,60] This also requires a generosity of spirit among colleagues, especially when the unpredictability of childbirth challenges healthcare providers professionally and personally.[61] This means listening to and caring for staff (i.e. having 'caring conversations' as a matter of course), celebrating acts of compassion and supporting staff to act in a compassionate way.[15]

Building compassion also requires implementing models of maternity care so that relationships are at the core of the changes. For example, the 2017 Scottish Government review of maternity and neonatal services[62] placed continuity of carer at the start of all its recommendations (along with community hubs that will provide care in communities nearer to where people live to improve services). This message is filtering through to policy that big is not necessarily better, that relationships matter, and that care should be focused around the needs of people, not institutions. But we need to be cautious. Despite the appearance of positive maternity policies, changes are not actually happening in practice. On the contrary, for many services there is a sense of moving away from community-focused and personalised relational care as maternity institutions become further entrenched in standardised processes. The challenge will be to bring innovative policy recommendations into practice reality so that all women and maternity care providers can benefit.

Supporting staff to deliver compassionate practice might also include providing compassion training. Drawing on their own and others' research, Klimecki et al found that compassion training (focusing on '...extending caring feelings...to other human beings' p873) allows people to recognise the negative circumstances that others experience.[20] This contrasts with empathy training, insofar as it activates different neural networks, also encouraging pro-social, helping behaviour and strengthening positive affect more generally, with the added benefit of naturally strengthening resilience. At the same time, it is crucial that midwives and other members of the maternity care team are not expected to become excessively resilient and 'always cope' in increasingly adverse working conditions. A positive organisational climate does not expect practitioners to engage in unhealthy patterns of behaviour because they are expected to 'toughen up'.[58] There will come a point when providers will 'snap', resulting in burn-out, cynicism and reckless, unsafe, and disrespectful behaviours and attitudes.[63] An organisational climate that depletes and exhausts the emotional responsiveness of staff is more likely to engender such consequences.

In addition, organisations need to support staff to practise self-compassion (including being kind to oneself and reducing self-judgement). This also fosters individual resilience in the face of stress, particularly the types of stress experienced by healthcare providers, including, for example, traumatic births and stillbirths.[50,64,65] Initiatives such as Compassionate Mind Training and mindfulness practice[66-68] can help individuals to meet their own needs so they are then better placed to meet the needs of others. This again recognises the concept that caregivers' lives are of value in the same way that service users' lives are. As Kanov et al assert, compassion is not only necessary for individual and organisational effectiveness in healthcare, but also for organisational resilience and sustainability.[9] Indeed, this is arguably now of more interest than ever following the global financial challenges over the last decade and the resultant organisational strain experienced by many maternity services around the world.

Discussion

If maternity organisations fail to attend to the impact and nature of what we discuss in this chapter, then services become unsustainable and the staff working in them learn to cope in unrealistic and harmful ways. Maintaining the status quo is therefore not an option; the situation will worsen, and both staff and service users will suffer. The expectation to be resilient in an organisation that does not promote psychosocial and spiritual wellbeing is untenable and brutish. In such a toxic environment, compassion retreats into darkness leaving fragmented and disconnected individuals surviving the demands imposed on them each day. This effect is exacerbated by processes of emotional contagion that translate individual experiences of negative affect into a more general negative affective climate. The end result is problems with staff recruitment and retention, bullying, turf wars and horizontal violence. Consequently, staff (midwifery and medical) simply do not enjoy coming to work. The result of this situation is unforgiveable for all involved. Women, families and society begin to attune to childbirth as a life experience that is unsafe, technologically determined and sterile in terms of relationships, resulting in a loss of expectation that childbirth is a profoundly important event of great social, psychological, emotional and spiritual significance.

When the organisational mood of maternity care is attuned to fear, routinised risk-avoidance strategies become morally and practically essential, and childbirth becomes an industrial process in which cost efficiency and risk management are prioritised regardless of unique individual needs and wishes. The opportunity for all staff members working in maternity to feel professionally and personally inspired by the care they provide depends on the development of positive organisational climates. This is important for everyone, healthcare professionals and families. Maternity services need to attune in a particular way that honours sensitive compassionate care so all using them and working in them feel safe. Families need to be at the centre of decisions about their care at a significant and transformative time in their lives. Likewise, healthcare professionals need to provide their professional and vocational services in a supportive, positive organisational environment. This is possible when staff feel cherished, heard, respected and managed compassionately.

Conclusion

Compassion in maternity services leads to safer care and more enjoyable working conditions. Models of maternity care that enable compassionate relationships are therefore to be encouraged. This requires managers to appreciate the power of relationships and how they build compassionate organisations. Attuning in this way is essential if we are all to flourish spiritually, psychologically and physically in maternity organisations. In sum, we have attempted to show in this chapter that compassion requires organisations to attune to the right mood.

Key points for consideration

- There is a distinction between empathy and compassion
- Organisations should foster a culture of compassion and positivity, for example, by valuing staff
- When managers are person-centred and afford compassion, caregivers are more likely to deliver compassionate care to service users
- Promoting compassionate services does not include supporting unhealthy work patterns
- Self-care is crucial and fosters individual resilience, which in turn creates a healthier, happier workforce

References

1   De Rivera J. Emotional climate: Social structure and emotional dynamics. International Review of Studies on Emotion. 1992;2:197-218.
2   Schneider B. Organizational climates: An essay. J Personnel psychology. 1975;28(4):447-79.
3   Ashkanasy NM. Organizational climate. In: Clegg SR, Bailey JR, editors. International Encyclopedia of organization studies2007. p. 1028-30.
4   Ashkanasy NM, Härtel CEJ. Positive and negative affective climate and culture: The good, the bad, and the ugly. In: Schneider B, Barbera K, editors. The Oxford handbook of organizational climate culture2014. p. 136-52.
5   Ashkanasy NM. Emotions in organizations: A multi-level perspective. Multi-level issues in organizational behavior and strategy: Emerald Group Publishing Limited; 2003. p. 9-54.
6   Ashkanasy NM, Dorris AD. Emotions in the workplace. Annual Review of Organizational Psychology and Organizational Behavior 2017;21(4):67-90.
7   Weiss HM, Cropanzano R. Affective Events Theory: A theoretical discussion of the structure, causes and consequences of affective experiences at work. In: B.M. Staw, Cummings LL, editors. Research in organizational behavior: An annual series of analytical essays and critical reviews: Elseveier Science/JAI Press; xxxx. p. 1-74.
8   Hatfield E, Cacioppo JT, Rapson RL. Emotional contagion. Curr Dir Psychol Sci. 1993;2(3):96-100.
9   Kanov JM, Maitlis S, Worline MC, Dutton JE, Frost PJ, Lilius JMJABS. Compassion in organizational life. 2004;47(6):808-27.
10 Fotaki M. Why and how is compassion necessary to provide good quality healthcare? J International journal of health policy management. 2015;4(4):199.
11 Opdebeeck H, Habisch A. Compassion: Chinese and western perspectives on practical wisdom in management. J Journal of Management Development. 2011;30(7/8):778-88.
12 Department of Health. Compassion in Practice: Nursing, Midwifery and Care Staff – Our Vision and Strategy. London: DH; 2012.
13 Lown BA. Compassion is a necessity and an individual and collective responsibility: comment on" Why and

how is compassion necessary to provide good quality healthcare?". International journal of health policy and management. 2015;4(9):613.

14 Rider EA, Kurtz S, Slade D, Longmaid III HE, Ho M-J, Pun J, Kwok-hung,, et al. The International Charter for Human Values in Healthcare: an interprofessional global collaboration to enhance values and communication in healthcare. J Patient education counseling Psychologist. 2014;96(3):273-80.

15 Dewar B, Adamson E, Smith S, Surfleet J, King L. Clarifying misconceptions about compassionate care. J Journal of Advanced Nursing. 2014;70(8):1738-47.

16 Flickinger TE, Saha S, Roter D, Korthuis PT, Sharp V, Cohn J, et al. Clinician empathy is associated with differences in patient–clinician communication behaviors and higher medication self-efficacy in HIV care. J Patient education counseling Psychologist. 2016;99(2):220-6.

17 Post SG, Ng LE, Fischel JE, Bennett M, Bily L, Chandran L, et al. Routine, empathic and compassionate patient care: definitions, development, obstacles, education and beneficiaries. J Journal of evaluation in clinical practice. 2014;20(6):872-80.

18 Wilkinson H, Whittington R, Perry L, Eames C. Examining the relationship between burnout and empathy in healthcare professionals: A systematic review. J Burnout Research. 2017;6:18-29.

19 Bernhardt BC, Singer T. The neural basis of empathy. J Annual review of neuroscience. 2012;35:1-23.

20 Klimecki OM, Leiberg S, Ricard M, Singer TJSc, neuroscience a. Differential pattern of functional brain plasticity after compassion and empathy training. 2013;9(6):873-9.

21 Wiseman T. Toward a holistic conceptualization of empathy for nursing practice. J Advances in Nursing Science. 2007;30(3):E61-E72.

22 García-Rabines DJP. Bloom, P.(2016) Against Empathy. The Case for Rational Compassion. Londres: Penguin Random House UK, 285 pp. 2017(020):160-5.

23 Fotaki M. Why and how is compassion necessary to provide good quality healthcare? J International journal of health policy management and Compliance Series. 2015;4(4):199.

24 Von Dietze E, Orb A. Compassionate care: a moral dimension of nursing. J Nursing Inquiry. 2000;7(3):166-74.

25 Sinclair S, Beamer K, Hack TF, McClement S, Raffin Bouchal S, Chochinov HM, et al. Sympathy, empathy, and compassion: A grounded theory study of palliative care patients' understandings, experiences, and preferences. 2017;31(5):437-47.

26 Youngson R. Compassion in healthcare—the missing dimension of healthcare reform. J Caregiver stress staff support in illness, dying, bereavement. 2011:49-61, page 39

27 Valizadeh L, Zamanzadeh V, Dewar B, Rahmani A, Ghafourifard M. Nurse's perceptions of organisational barriers to delivering compassionate care: a qualitative study. J Nursing ethics. 2018;25(5):580-90.

28 WHO. WHO recommendations: intrapartum care for a positive childbirth experience. Geneva: World Health Organization; 2018.

29 World Health Organization. WHO recommendations on antenatal care for a positive pregnancy experience. Geneva, Switzerland 2017.

30 Hung P, Kozhimannil KB, Casey MM, Moscovice ISJHsr. Why are obstetric units in rural hospitals closing their doors? 2016;51(4):1546-60.

31 Walsh D. Improving maternity service. Small is beautiful: Lessons for maternity services from a birth centre. Oxford: Radcliffe Publishing; 2007a.

32 Combier E, Charreire H, Le Vaillant M, Michaut F, Ferdynus C, Amat-Roze J-M, et al. Perinatal health inequalities and accessibility of maternity services in a rural French region: closing maternity units in Burgundy. 2013;24:225-33.

33 Monk AR, Tracy S, Foureur M, Barclay LJW, Birth. Australian primary maternity units: past, present and future. 2013;26(3):213-8.

34 Jenkins M, Ford J, Morris JM, Roberts C. Women's expectations and experiences of maternity care in NSW - What women highlight as most important. Women and Birth. 2014:2014-219.

35 Downe S, Finlayson K, Oladapo O, Bonet M, Gülmezoglu AM. What matters to women during childbirth: a systematic qualitative review. PLoS One. 2018;13(4):e0194906.

36 Hunter B, Berg M, Lundgren I, Ólafsdóttir ÓÁ, Kirkham M. Relationships: The hidden threads in the tapestry of maternity care. Midwifery. 2008;24(2):132-7.

37 Crowther S, Smythe L, Spence D. Mood and birth experience. Women and birth : journal of the Australian College of Midwives. 2014;27(1):21-5.

38 Grant J. The Best Start: A Five-year Forward Plan for Maternity and Neonatal Care in Scotland: Scottish Government; 2017.

39 Royal College of Midwives. Why midwives leave – Revisited. In: RCM, editor. London2016.

40 Ball L, Curtis P, Kirkham M. Why Do Midwives Leave?: Talking to Managers: Royal College of Midwives; 2002.

41 Hildingsson I, Gamble J, Sidebotham M, Creedy DK, Guilliland K, Dixon L, et al. Midwifery empowerment: National surveys of midwives from Australia, New Zealand and Sweden. 2016;40:62-9.

42 Dixon L, Guilliland K, Pallant J, Sidebotham M, Fenwick J, McAra-Couper J, et al. The emotional wellbeing of New Zealand midwives: Comparing responses for midwives in caseloading and shift work settings. 2017(53).

43 Creedy D, Sidebotham M, Gamble J, Pallant J, Fenwick JJBp, childbirth. Prevalence of burnout, depression, anxiety and stress in Australian midwives: a cross-sectional survey. 2017;17(1):13.

44 Stoll K, Gallagher JJW, Birth. A survey of burnout and intentions to leave the profession among Western Canadian midwives. 2018.

45 Curtis P, Ball L, Kirkham M. Ceasing to practise midwifery: Working life and employment choices. British journal of midwifery. 2006;14(6).

46 Curtis P, Ball L, Kirkham M. Management and morale: Challenges in contemporary maternity care. British journal of midwifery. 2006;14(2).

47 WHO. Midwives' voices, midwives' realities. In: WHO, editor. Geneva: WHO; 2016.

48 Govardhan L, Pinelli V, Schnatz PF. Burnout, depression and job satisfaction in obstetrics and gynecology residents. Connecticut Medicine. 2012;76(7):389-95.

49 Young C, Smythe L, McAra-Couper J. Burnout: Lessons from the lived experience of case loading midwives. International Journal of Childbirth. 2015;5(3):154-65.

50 Calvert I, Benn C. Trauma and the Effects on the Midwife. International Journal of Childbirth. 2015;5(2):100-12.

51 Cooke GPE, Doust JA, Steele MC. A survey of resilience, burnout and tolerance of uncertainty in Australian general practice registrars. BMC Med Educ. 2013;13.

52 Pallant JF, Dixon L, Sidebotham M, Fenwick J. Adaptation and psychometric testing of the Practice Environment Scale for use with midwives. Women and Birth. 2015.

53 Moloney S, Gair S. Empathy and spiritual care in midwifery practice: Contributing to women's enhanced birth experiences. Women Birth. 2015;28(4):323-8.

54 Crowther S, Smythe E, Spence D. Kairos time at the moment of birth. Midwifery. 2015;31(4):451-7.

55 Crowther S, Hall J. Spirituality and spiritual care in and around childbirth. Women and Birth. 2015;28(2):173-8.

56 Puchalski CM, Blatt B, Kogan M, Butler A. Spirituality and health: the development of a field. Academic medicine Journal of the Association of American Medical Colleges. 2014;89(1):10-6.

57 Thomas RB, Wilson JP. Issues and controversies in the understanding and diagnosis of compassion fatigue, vicarious traumatization, and secondary traumatic stress disorder. J International Journal of Emergency Mental Health. 2004.

58 Crowther S, Hunter B, McAra-Couper J, Warren L, Gilkison A, Hunter M, et al. Sustainability and resilience in midwifery: A discussion paper. Midwifery. 2016;40:40-8.

59 Bramley L, Matiti M. How does it really feel to be in my shoes? Patients' experiences of compassion within nursing care and their perceptions of developing compassionate nurses. J Journal of clinical nursing. 2014;23(19-20):2790-9.

60 Deery R, Fisher P. Professionalism and person-centredness: developing a practice based approach to leadership within NHS maternity services in the UK. Health Sociology Review. 2016.

61 Hunter M, Crowther S, McAra-Couper J, Gilkison A, MacGregor D, Gunn J. Generosity of spirit sustains caseloading Lead Maternity Carer midwives in New Zealand. 2016.

62 Scottish Executive Health Department (SEHD). A Framework for maternity services in Scotland. In: Department SEH, editor. Edinburgh: Tactica Solutions; 2001.

63 Knapp R. Wellbeing and resilience: 1. The resilient midwife The Practising Midwife. 2017;20(3):26-8.

64 Beaumont E, Durkin M, Hollins Martin CJ, Carson J. Compassion for others, self-compassion, quality of life and mental well-being measures and their association with compassion fatigue and burnout in student midwives: A quantitative survey. Midwifery. 2015.

65 Rice H, Warland J. Bearing witness: Midwives experiences of witnessing traumatic birth. Midwifery. 2013.

66 Beaumont E, Irons C, Rayner G, Dagnall N. Does compassion-focused therapy training for health care educators and providers increase self-compassion and reduce self-persecution and self-criticism? J Contin Educ Health Prof. 2016;36(1):4-10.

67 Germer CK, Neff KD. Self-compassion in clinical practice. J Journal of clinical psychology. 2013;69(8):856-67.

68 Beaumont E, Martin CJH. Heightening levels of compassion towards self and others through use of compassionate mind training. British Journal of Midwifery. 2016;24(11):777-86.

CHAPTER 9

Progressive understanding of human rights in maternity care: from individual rights to systemic issues

Nicola Philbin and *Rebecca Schiller*

Introduction

Recognition and understanding of human rights in maternity care has been developing over the last decade. The initial focus of this global movement has been the necessary and important work of articulating what human rights are, why and how they apply in maternity care, and in tackling individual issues of abuse and disrespect.

As progress in these specific areas is made by activists, healthcare practitioners, organisations and academics, the broad scope and potential wider application of human rights in maternity systems are beginning to be appreciated. There remains a great deal of scope for new ideas to be elaborated, different legal directions to be explored and varying approaches to be analysed, to assess their utility in moving human rights concepts into reality.

It is our aim that this chapter will provoke further conversations as to how human rights language and ideas can be used to influence policy and practice in maternity services around the world for the better.

In the first part of this chapter Nicola Philbin will introduce some human rights tools which have yet to be fully explored in a maternity context, such as the right to health and the right to benefit from scientific progress, and consider their potential scope to tackle systemic birth rights issues.

Rebecca Schiller will then give a personal account of the approach of Birthrights to these issues in the UK. Through this case study she will suggest ways to build in future on the work that is being done to ensure human rights are recognised and understood in maternity care. She will track how the charity has evolved beyond helping individuals with specific human rights issues to develop a layered organisational model that aims to address systemic cultural and practice issues within maternity care systems, using human rights language and concepts.

Part 1: Progressive realisation of social human rights in childbirth

Human rights law is a field that is constantly evolving. Many of the underlying principles have been established by cases brought to human rights courts by individuals, and much of the development by the courts of human rights concepts is influenced by the work of the UN treaty bodies, reporting by NGOs and academic debate and research.

It is therefore interesting to take a look at the basis of recognition and realisation of human rights in maternity care so far – and comforting to know that this young movement still has far to go. There remains much scope and potential for new ideas to be elaborated and varying approaches to be analysed as to their helpfulness in moving human rights concepts into reality.

The work so far – civil and political rights

Human rights fall into two categories – civil and political rights, and economic, social and cultural rights. Much of the recognition of human rights in the birth field so far has been in the first category.

Internationally, organisations such as the White Ribbon Alliance and World Health Organization have focused on highlighting issues of disrespect and abuse during childbirth, based on the human rights principles of autonomy, dignity and equity.[1,2]

In parallel, the concept of obstetric violence has been developed,[3] particularly in South America. In Venezuela, this concept is enshrined in law.[4] It is important to note that, in Spanish, 'obstetrics' refers to what is done by maternity nurses and midwives as well as by medical staff, so that the term 'obstetric violence' refers to abusive and disrespectful behaviour by all maternity providers. It is another means of addressing structural/systemic violence against women within maternity care.

Many of the UN bodies working on maternity care have focused largely on the urgent need to improve stillbirth and infant and maternal mortality rates in developing countries. This work has been based on the Right to Life[5] and specific wording on this issue in the relevant treaties.[6]

Article 8 of the European Convention on Human Rights,[7] the 'Right to Respect for Private and Family Life', has been a central focus of efforts to date within Europe to improve choice in maternity care using human rights arguments in court. Each of the applicants in the cases Ternovszky[8] and Dubska[9] relied on the argument that the right to choose the circumstances of childbirth is inherent in the right to a private life under Article 8.

Scope for future development – economic, social and cultural rights

The rights set out in the International Covenant on Economic, Social and Cultural Rights,[11] such as the right to health and the right to benefit from scientific progress, seem equally relevant to maternity care. These have so far received less attention from lawyers or activists in the maternity field, and offer untapped potential as tools to address the complex systemic issues highlighted in this book.

For human rights of an economic, social or cultural nature, all individual countries have a responsibility to be working on an ongoing basis towards the fullest possible realisation of those rights, to the maximum of their available resources at the time. This is the particular human rights concept of 'Progressive Realisation' – there should be an ongoing process of improvement in respect of each right, including that there should be no 'regression' or undoing of previous progress.[12]

Human-rights based approaches to maternity issues have also mainly to date focused on behaviour by individual care-providers, rather than outcomes produced by the maternity system in which those individuals work. The Dubska judgement[9] illustrates this well – the court affirmed the Article 8 rights of individual women during childbirth, but failed to consider in detail the quality requirements placed on maternity systems by the human right to health.

The human right to health

Under the human right to health, all states are required, through their maternity systems, to respect, protect and fulfil the rights of both women and babies during childbirth to the enjoyment of the highest attainable standard of physical and mental health (Article 12, ICESCR).[13]

The notion of the highest attainable standard of health takes into account both an individual's biological and socio-economic circumstances, and a state's available resources. It cannot guarantee a 'right to be healthy', but instead is the right to the enjoyment of a variety of facilities, goods, services and conditions necessary for the realisation of the highest attainable standard of health, including underlying determinants of health.

More detail on what a state is required to provide to enable enjoyment of this right has been set out in the Availability, Accessibility, Acceptability, Quality (AAAQ) framework described in General Comment 14.[14] Facilities, goods and services have to be available in sufficient quantity, without discrimination, physically accessible, and affordable. Information and ideas around relevant health issues must be readily available. Facilities, goods and services must be respectful of medical ethics, culturally appropriate, and designed to respect confidentiality and improve the health status of those concerned, while being scientifically and medically appropriate and of good quality.

To what extent can individual countries be said to be sufficiently implementing the AAAQ requirements in maternity care? Many of the issues discussed in this book would seem to raise questions as to whether individuals giving birth or babies born in modern maternity systems move into family life having achieved their highest attainable standard of health during childbirth.

The human right to benefit from scientific progress

The scope of the right to share in scientific advancement and its benefits[15] is considerably less developed than the right to health, but includes access to the benefits of science and scientific knowledge, without discrimination; opportunities to freely contribute to scientific research; opportunities to participate in decision-making; and development of an enabling environment to foster the development and diffusion of science and technology.

In the sphere of maternity care, it seems feasible that arguments could be made that this right requires states to implement evidence-based maternity policies, to include provision for individual decision-making ability within such policies, to pay attention to the equity, provenance, funding and conduct of ongoing research in the field (such as provision for midwifery-led research alongside obstetric-led research), particularly within the private sector, and take steps to prevent the use of technology or interventions without scientific basis.

Indeed, although the traditional focus in maternity research has been on pathology and pre-empting/treating it, as scientific research increasingly shows the benefits to women and babies of continuous midwifery care, the importance of supporting hormone flow in labour, and the psychosocial and emotional benefits of respectful, supportive physiological birth, as discussed elsewhere in this book, the right to benefit from scientific progress may provide useful arguments when putting the case for changes to maternity policies to introduce such care.

Other relevant human rights

A number of other human rights also appear relevant to various common current maternity care practices, although there is no relevant case law or legal discussion around them yet. A policy of standard episiotomy during birth, still applied in many hospitals around the world despite the evidence of harm caused, seems only a step away from the female genital mutilation which breaches a number of human rights.[16] Constraining women to labour and give birth supine or in lithotomy position, with no consent, explanation and for no good reason, does not fulfil the right to be free from torture or other cruel, inhuman or degrading treatment, or scientific experimentation.[17] It seems reasonable that the Right to Education[18] should include applicability to education about evidence-based healthcare including childbirth. The right to freedom of thought/opinion[19] potentially offers protective arguments to women who wish to give birth on their own terms, but are offered only standardised interventions.

Greater role for rights-holders – reporting mechanisms and accountability

There has also over recent years been growing recognition of some maternity care issues by human rights monitoring bodies such as CEDAW (the body monitoring the Convention on the Elimination of all Forms of Discrimination Against Women).[20] In 2013, CEDAW criticised Greece for its high caesarean rates.[21] In 2017, it took Ireland to task for over-medicalised birth practices.[22] This focus has been catalysed by in-depth reporting of maternity care issues to the treaty bodies by human rights activists, working with in-country NGOs to produce country reports for submission to CEDAW.

Similarly, the other various human rights highlighted above all have associated Special Rapporteurs, individuals officially responsible for monitoring progress in implementing the rights, and regular reporting mechanisms, giving scope for birth activists and NGOs to bring issues to other relevant human rights bodies, who can hold individual states accountable for the practices in their country.

This was illustrated recently by the success of birth activist group RODA in highlighting maternity rights issues in Croatia to the Special Rapporteur to Health, who incorporated them into his recent report on progress in Croatia.[23] Once incorporated into a report, progress in addressing the issues raised will be monitored by the relevant Special Rapporteur or Human Rights Committee, as part of regular timetabled reviews.

Introduction of the global Sustainable Development Goals (SDGs) for 2015–30 has brought increased recognition of the importance of monitoring and accountability for the implementation of the SDGs and the human rights they represent.[24] There is vital ongoing work to develop suitable practical indicators, benchmarks and accountability mechanisms to track compliance with the relevant human rights that are implicit in the SDGs.

The right to health also positively requires the active and informed participation of rights-holders in health system planning at community, national and international levels.[25] This should include the views of parents in development of maternity services and feedback on quality, availability, accessibility or acceptability of services. However, service-user involvement often seems to be lacking, and this is therefore an area ripe for increased attention from activists and for collaboration about successful models both within and between countries.

The range of applicable human rights concepts relevant to maternity care appears to offer considerable scope both to strengthen arguments seeking to influence maternity policy-making, and to hold individual governments to account for the quality and type of maternity care they choose to offer. As research continues to illustrate the improved quality and acceptability to women of continuity of care/midwifery models, there are increasingly strong arguments that individualised, compassionate, respectful, evidence-based care should be realised by all states, in order to respect, protect and fulfil their obligations under human rights to health, to benefit from scientific progress, and many others.

This also raises interesting questions as to why these rights are not better known and upheld more widely among healthcare practitioners? The work of Birthrights in the UK shows what can be done to improve maternity care through increased awareness and understanding of human rights issues. The second section of this chapter describes some of these activities from the personal perspective of Rebecca Schiller.

Part 2: Birthrights: a case study of the progressive development of human rights in childbirth

Since its inception in January 2013, Birthrights (the UK human rights in childbirth organisation) has played a part in the progress made by the human rights in childbirth movement. In this section I will outline the organisational model that Birthrights has evolved as one example of how human rights and the law can be used to effect positive changes in maternity care, moving beyond tackling individual injustices and towards attempting to make an impact on frontline practice, service provision and local and national policies.

Birthrights, much like human rights in general, is a living, evolving organisation. Our impact is still to be tested by the passing of time and formal evaluation. Our model may not be applicable in some situations or locations and there are certainly other models, ideas and organisations to learn from. Nevertheless I hope that this brief outline of Birthrights' approach can spark ideas for others looking to use the law and human rights in innovative ways to improve maternity care.

Birthrights is a registered charity founded in January 2013 by human rights barrister Elizabeth Prochaska and backed by a group of lawyers, healthcare professionals and services users united by the belief that all women matter during childbirth. We aim to improve women's experiences of pregnancy and childbirth by promoting respect for their fundamental rights to dignity, autonomy, privacy and equality.

Initially an entirely volunteer-run organisation, our primary focus in 2013 was to achieve some visibility and recognition of the existence and relevance of human rights in the childbirth context. We set out to do so through the provision of free legal advice to women and their families on issues connected with lawful maternity care in the UK, alongside accurate, website-based factsheets on key issues, underpinned by the important ECHR Ternovzsky and Dubska judgements on human rights in maternity care. We also aimed to offer explanation and interpretation of the UK's Human Rights Act (1998)[26] and other key judgements in the English and UK courts, as relevant to the pregnancy and childbirth context.

We developed an ambition to look to a deeper understanding of these issues and a desire to engage with the media, medical and midwifery establishment and policy-makers. Our Dignity Survey[27] sought to discover more about the real-life human rights experiences of women in England alongside midwives' understanding of, and attitudes to, ideas of dignity in childbirth. Through the launch of this report at a sold-out conference, and the interest from high-profile speakers and the media, it became clear that something about the work we were doing was striking a chord with a range of voices. It engaged people from very different birth groups and interests, and from the reproductive rights movement, frontline workers and policy-makers and importantly, women themselves. This unifying potential of the human rights model in the often-fractured birth world is yet, I believe, to be fully exploited.

The intervening three years have seen us evolve a circular model with four interrelated parts, by both design and happy accident.

The first quarter of the circle entails the provision of free advice on lawful maternity care to women and their families and to healthcare professionals. We elevate the most egregious, frequent or puzzling issues that we hear as a consequence of undertaking this work into the other sections of our work. This frontline advice service provides an important feedback loop to drive and check our other activities and help us adapt them as necessary.

The next quarter of the circle is made up of research and campaigning work, which may include strategic legal intervention if necessary. An example of this is our recent partnership with the University of Bournemouth to investigate disabled women's experiences of dignity in maternity care.[28]

Moving further around the circle, the research and advice work then feeds directly into our policy and media activities, which have developed partly in response to our desire to effect change at a systems level, but also because of the willingness of policy-makers and the media to engage with our organisation. I firmly believe that it is important to continue to tackle individual cases, but that we also need to complement this by carving out a channel to policy-makers to allow women's voices to be amplified and presented in terms that policy-makers will engage with.

I have also concluded, with a mixture of frustration and pragmatism, that the perceived authority that the law provides can give a legally-focused birth organisation access to a seat at the policy table that may be denied to other groups representing women's interests. This may be partly to do with the dominance of the legal profession in a society that is still strongly influenced by patriarchy. By harnessing the deference to (or, at least, recognition of) the law we can use it to reframe issues that have previously been brushed aside at a policy level as 'women's issues'. This then provides an ethical and legal imperative for engagement.

In 2017 Birthrights was invited to review and comment on the operational guidance for the new A-EQUIP model of midwifery supervision in England.[29] The guidance was of key importance, not only to midwives, but also to the women they care for. Prior to the new model, Supervisors of Midwives filled an important role advocating for women's rights and bridging the gap between the needs of individuals and what the system could provide. This system has recently been changed by the UK government,[30] creating the potential to leave women without their advocates.

While the impact of these changes is only just beginning to be tested and felt, we were delighted that the final guidance[31] is strongly grounded in human rights principles and case law. Those carrying out the role of Professional Midwifery Advocate are instructed to work with women to safeguard their rights, flowing from the European Court of Human Rights (ECHR) and the Human Rights Act 1998, to be treated with dignity, respect and as autonomous individuals from whom informed consent is required for any intervention undertaken.'[32]

The final part of the circle that makes up our organisational model, is perhaps our most influential area of work: education and training. This strand emerged because of demand for Birthrights to provide training on human rights and respectful care to NHS teams, or to deliver existing training on topics such as the creation of documentation inspired by a human rights sensibility. While this was initially a small and tangential area of our work, we soon felt that it could provide a powerful mechanism for Birthrights to make an impact on frontline maternity workers, altering their practice and making a bigger difference to women than our advice work could.

Aware of our resource limitations, we have also secured funding to produce free training videos and online learning programmes with partners such as the Royal College of Midwives. We now deliver a mixture of free, open sessions (funded by our supporters and trusts and foundations) and paid-for training that helps cover the costs associated with our small staff team.[34]

In some circles we have made enough progress that we are able to move beyond a basic insistence that these rights exist, to beginning to work with others to realise their potential in education, policy, campaigning, research and the media. Going forward we are aware that Birthrights is still at the beginning of its organisational journey. As we realise the potential that the human rights framework has in maternity care, we intend to invest in more pro-active policy work tackling examples of unlawful maternity policy that our advice services highlights, and addressing these at local to national level. We plan to undertake more research to understand how human rights violations impact on those suffering severe and multiple disadvantage, on disabled women and on those with mental health and mental capacity issues, recognising that these groups may suffer disproportionately. We intend to prioritise collaborative working to empower other organisations, grassroots, voluntary sector and women's organisations to use human rights in their maternity focused work, believing that our small organisation will have the greatest impact if we share our tools with others.

Discussion

Our experience shows that using a human rights approach has the potential to unite different maternity interest groups behind a common belief system. Indeed, almost all working in the field would support the human rights principles outlined above. There is considerable scope for using human rights law and concepts as tools to achieve progress in improving maternity care around the world, and this approach uses the law in a completely different way to the more common legal involvement in liability and litigation issues. However, the vast majority of lawyers have not studied human rights in depth and are unfamiliar with these tools – there is a need to improve awareness among lawyers as well as medical staff and policy-makers.

There are undeniably difficulties in enforcement of individual human rights, particularly economic, social and cultural rights. The legal processes are time-consuming and costly. However, they offer scope to underpin a change of mindset and ethical approach to policy-making, increasing the focus of policy-makers on evidence-based maternity care. They support the contention that both mother and child have the human right not to be damaged, in pregnancy or during birth, by either negligent or unsafe care, or through the universal application of standardised conveyor-belt maternity care.

Conclusion

The unexplored human rights applications set out in the first half of this chapter provide further avenues for examination and debate, particularly in relation to the impact they may have on behaviour change, maternity professionals' education, research priorities, and policy and service provision. As the human rights in childbirth movement makes progress towards a full realisation of women's human rights in maternity care, it may become apparent that the work done away from the direct legal channels, but inspired and underpinned by their power and values, could be the most effective in promoting a culture of safe, respectful, quality care that treats all women as individuals who matter.

Key points for consideration

Care should be:

- Rights-based and evidence-based.
- Respectful of a woman's rights to dignity, autonomy, privacy and equality.
- Individualised to each woman and baby, not conveyor-belt care.
- Fully respectful of a woman's right to choose the right care provider and care for her and her baby.
- Aimed at the realisation of the highest attainable standard of health for women and babies.

References

1   White Ribbon Alliance (2011) *RESPECTFUL MATERNITY CARE: THE UNIVERSAL RIGHTS OF CHILDBEARING WOMEN*. Available at: https://www.whiteribbonalliance.org/wp-content/uploads/2017/11/Final_RMC_Charter.pdf (Accessed: 10 January 2019).

2   World Health Organization (2015). *The prevention and elimination of disrespect and abuse during facility-based childbirth*. Available at: http://apps.who.int/iris/bitstream/10665/134588/1/WHO_RHR_14.23_eng.pdf?ua=1&ua=1. (Accessed: 10 January 2019).

3   Sadler, M., Santos, M.J., Ruiz-Berdún, D., Rojas, G.L., Skoko, E., Gillen, P. and Clausen, J.A. (2016) 'Moving beyond disrespect and abuse: Addressing the structural dimensions of obstetric violence', *Reproductive Health Matters*, 24(47), pp. 47–55. doi: 10.1016/j.rhm.2016.04.002.

4   Pérez D'Gregorio, R. (2010). Obstetric violence: A new legal term introduced in Venezuela. *International Journal of Gynecology & Obstetrics*, 111(3), pp.201-202.

5   Ohchr.org. (1966). OHCHR | International Covenant on Civil and Political Rights, Article 6 [online] Available at: http://www.ohchr.org/en/professionalinterest/pages/ccpr.aspx (Accessed 10 January 2019).

6   Ohchr.org. (1966). *OHCHR | International Covenant on Economic, Social and Cultural Rights, Article 12.2(a)*. [online] Available at: http://www.ohchr.org/EN/ProfessionalInterest/Pages/CESCR.aspx (Accessed 10 January 2019).

7   European Convention on Human Rights, Article 8. (1950). [ebook] European Court of Human Rights/ Council of Europe. Available at: https://www.echr.coe.int/Documents/Convention_ENG.pdf (Accessed 10 January 2019).

8   CASE OF TERNOVSZKY v. HUNGARY (Application no. 67545/09) ECHR 2010. Available at: http://hudoc.echr.coe.int/eng?i=001-102254. (Accessed: 10 January 2019)

9   *Dubská and Krejzová v. The Czech Republic* nos. 28859/11 and 28473/12, ECHR 2016. Available at: http://hudoc.echr.coe.int/eng#{"itemid":["001-168066"]} (Accessed: 10 January 2019)

11   United Nations (1966). *International Covenant on Economic and Social Rights*. Available at: http://www.ohchr.org/Documents/ProfessionalInterest/cescr.pdf. (Accessed: 10 January 2019)

12   Ohchr.org. (2018). *OHCHR | International Covenant on Economic, Social and Cultural Rights, Article 2.1*. [online] Available at: http://www.ohchr.org/EN/ProfessionalInterest/Pages/CESCR.aspx (Accessed 10 January 2019).

13   Ohchr.org. (2018). *OHCHR | International Covenant on Economic, Social and Cultural Rights, Article 12.1*. [online] Available at: http://www.ohchr.org/EN/ProfessionalInterest/Pages/CESCR.aspx (Accessed 10 January 2019).

14   Office of the High Commissioner Human Rights United Nations (2000) *CESCR General Comment No 14: The Right to the Highest Attainable Standard of Health (Art 12)*. Available at: http://tbinternet.ohchr.org/_layouts/treatybodyexternal/Download.aspx?symbolno=E%2fC.12%2f2000%2f4&Lang=en (Accessed: 10 January 2019).

15   Ohchr.org. (2018). *OHCHR | International Covenant on Economic, Social and Cultural Rights, Article 15*. [online] Available at: http://www.ohchr.org/EN/ProfessionalInterest/Pages/CESCR.aspx (Accessed 10 January 2019).

16   Un.org. (2018). *Eliminating Female Genital Mutilation*. [online] Available at: http://www.un.org/womenwatch/daw/csw/csw52/statements_missions/Interagency_Statement_on_Eliminating_FGM.pdf (Accessed 10 January 2019).

17   Ohchr.org. (2018). *OHCHR | International Covenant on Civil and Political Rights, Article 7*. [online] Available at: http://www.

ohchr.org/en/professionalinterest/pages/ccpr.aspx (Accessed 10 January 2019).

18   Ohchr.org. (2018). OHCHR | *International Covenant on Economic, Social and Cultural Rights, Article 13.* [online] Available at: http://www.ohchr.org/EN/ProfessionalInterest/Pages/CESCR.aspx (Accessed 10 January 2019).

19   Ohchr.org. (2018). *OHCHR | International Covenant on Civil and Political Rights, Article 18.* [online] Available at: http://www.ohchr.org/en/professionalinterest/pages/ccpr.aspx (Accessed 10 January 2019).

20   Ohchr.org. (2018). *OHCHR | Committee on the Elimination of Discrimination against Women.* [online] Available at: http://www.ohchr.org/EN/HRBodies/CEDAW/Pages/CEDAWIndex.aspx (Accessed 10 January 2019).

21   Concluding Observations on the Seventh Periodic Report of Greece. (2013). [ebook] United Nations: CEDAW. Available at: https://www.google.com/url?sa=t&rct=j&q=&esrc=s&source=web&cd=1&ved=2ahUKEwjFqM bcrOXaAhWL3VMKHSM-B88QFjAAegQIABAo&url=http%3A%2F%2Fwww2.ohchr.org%2Fenglish%2Fbodies %2Fcedaw%2Fdocs%2Fco%2FCEDAW.C.GRC.CO.7.doc&usg=AOvVaw0rLGC6bGeD1MBsDNIOrtk5 (Accessed 10 January 2019).

22   Concluding observations on the combined sixth and seventh periodic reports of Ireland. (2017). [ebook] CEDAW. Available at: http://tbinternet.ohchr.org/_layouts/treatybodyexternal/Download.aspx?symbolno=C EDAW%2fC%2fIRL%2fCO%2f6-7&Lang=en (Accessed 10 January 2019).

23   *Report of the Special Rapporteur on the right of everyone to the enjoyment of the highest attainable standard of physical and mental health on his visit to Croatia.* [online] Available at: https://documents-dds-ny.un.org/doc/ UNDOC/GEN/G17/107/70/PDF/G1710770.pdf?OpenElement (Accessed 10 January 2019).

24   Seeking accountability for women's rights through the Sustainable Development Goals. (2017). [ebook] Centre for Economic and Social Rights/UN Women. Available at: http://www.cesr.org/sites/default/files/sdgs_ accountability_womens_rights.pdf (Accessed 10 January 2019).

25   Office of the High Commissioner Human Rights United Nations (2000) *CESCR General Comment No 14: The Right to the Highest Attainable Standard of Health (Art 12).* Available at: http://tbinternet.ohchr.org/_ layouts/treatybodyexternal/Download.aspx?symbolno=E%2fC.12%2f2000%2f4&Lang=en (Accessed: 10 January 2019).

26   Legislation.gov.uk. (2018). Human Rights Act 1998. [online] Available at: https://www.legislation.gov.uk/ ukpga/1998/42/contents (Accessed 10 January 2019).

27   Birthrights. (2018). *Dignity Survey.* [online] Available at: http://www.birthrights.org.uk/campaigns/dignity-in-childbirth/dignity-survey/ (Accessed 10 January 2019).

28   Hall, J., Collins, B., Ireland, J. and Hundley, V. (2018). [online] Birthrights.org.uk. Available at: http://www. birthrights.org.uk/wordpress/wp-content/uploads/2018/03/Birthrights-Bournemouth-Liverpool-Human-Rights-and-Dignity-Experiences-of-Disabled-Women-during-Pregnancy-Birth-and-Early-Parenting-1.pdf (Accessed 10 January 2019).

29   NHS England (2017). *NHS England » A-EQUIP - a model of clinical midwifery supervision.* [online] England.nhs.uk. Available at: https://www.england.nhs.uk/publication/a-equip-a-model-of-clinical-midwifery-supervision/ (Accessed 10 January 2019).

30   GOV.UK. (2017). *Changes to Nursing and Midwifery Council governing legislation.* [online] Available at: https:// www.gov.uk/government/consultations/changes-to-nursing-and-midwifery-council-governing-legislation (Accessed 10 January 2019).

31   NHS England (2017). *NHS England » A-EQUIP - a model of clinical midwifery supervision.* [online] England.nhs.uk. Available at: https://www.england.nhs.uk/publication/a-equip-a-model-of-clinical-midwifery-supervision/ (Accessed 10 January 2019).

32   NHS England (2017). *NHS England » A-EQUIP - a model of clinical midwifery supervision.* [online] England.nhs.uk. Available at: https://www.england.nhs.uk/publication/a-equip-a-model-of-clinical-midwifery-supervision/, page 17 (Accessed 10 January 2019).

33   Birthrights. (2018). *Training.* [online] Available at: http://www.birthrights.org.uk/resources/training-and-education/ (Accessed 10 January 2019).

CHAPTER 10

Media representation of childbirth

Lesley Kay, Vanora Hundley and Nadezhda Tsekulova

Introduction

Childbirth is a profoundly personal experience which normally takes place in a very public sphere. In pregnancy women's bodies and lives become almost unwittingly part of accepted societal discourse. In most societies, without invitation, people comment on and touch women's abdomens, speculate on the baby's gender, ask intimate questions about how the woman is experiencing her pregnancy, offer unsolicited advice about birthing, and share stories of their own experiences (Raskoff, 2013). As a consequence, women do not experience pregnancy and birth in seclusion, but as a member of the society in which they live; a society which dictates conventions and in which a profoundly personal event becomes part of the collective experience. This process, which Bainbridge identifies as the pregnant woman becoming *'public property'* (2006), is also reflected in the way that the media represent pregnancy and childbirth. In recent years the media has become fascinated with birth and there has been a growth in the number of reality television programmes (Roberts et al, 2017). In this chapter we will explore how childbirth has been described in the media, with specific focus on two European countries, Bulgaria and the United Kingdom (UK). We will look at how media portrayals affect women, their partners and wider society, and how this might impact on expectations and service provision.

Case studies of childbirth and the media

The Bulgarian situation

Until the middle of the 20th century Bulgaria had a predominantly rural population, with most births taking place at home (Slaychev, 1942). There are still young mothers whose grandmothers tell them how they were born '*on the field*', at home or in unusual conditions and circumstances. In the second half of the 20th century Bulgaria became a communist state. Fundamental laws of that time restricted the rights of citizens to move about freely, to own property, to freely express their ideas, to access and exchange information and also denied them the right to privacy and bodily integrity. For example, the 1973 Law on Public Health stated that: '*Every Bulgarian citizen has the right to receive free medical assistance from the respective health care facility*' (Article 26.1). The corresponding '*health care facility*' was the state and municipal hospital in the larger settlements and the health service in the smaller ones. This system meant that it would not have occurred to most women that they could be involved in any choice about birthplace. Maria Georgieva, a nurse, who was interviewed by Tsekulova for a radio programme in 2013, gave birth to her daughter in 1980 in the Regional Hospital in Bourgas. When asked about how she chose where to deliver she answered, with laughter:

'*Who then would even think to have a choice? That was inconceivable! Pregnant women were followed up in the district polyclinic, and women's counselling was obligatory and a subject to a fine. The births were conducted in the district hospital with the medical team on the shift.*'

The media environment at the time was strongly influenced by political propaganda and women's choice was minimal, meaning that in practice the media could have no influence on their decisions. The psychologist Aaronson Elliot defines propaganda as '*the communication of a point of view with the ultimate goal of having the recipient of the appeal come to "voluntarily" accept this position as if it was his or her own*' (2009, p103). This definition reflects precisely the totalitarian idea of the functions of the media during the period of the communist regime (Deenichina, 2005; Mindova, 2014). The content of periodicals and books was controlled by an institution called 'Glavlith'. Glavlith is the abbreviation of the Headquarters for Literature and Publishing. Literature on health topics, including textbooks for medical professionals such as doctors and midwives, as well as popular literature for citizens, was published only by the public publishing house Zdravizdat (Health Publishing), and practice shows that this communication strategy achieved the goals of the regime. Women generally were not able to choose who cared for them during pregnancy or who assisted them during the birth. This affirmed the role of the medical specialist – whether a doctor or a midwife – as a holder of absolute power in the process of childbirth. Women were completely deprived of decision-making and access to quality information was hampered and, in some cases, impossible.

The health system gradually started to open up following a change in the political system in 1989. There was an opportunity for private initiatives among physicians, and patients had the right to choose their healthcare facility and their health expert. However, pregnancy and childbirth remained under the authority of the state medical facilities, meaning that the opportunity to participate in decisions about where and how to give birth was not yet on the agenda. The new millennium has brought many changes, but birth is still rarely seen in the mainstream media. Instead it is a topic that is usually only discussed in relation to the traditional Bulgarian holiday on 21 January that celebrates childbirth. This is a time when midwives and obstetrician-gynaecologists are formally recognised. Occasionally, it also appears in relation to other matters. Usually, when that happens, it is related to cases with poor outcomes such as maternal or infant deaths and violence against the mother and infant.

In the minds of the majority, birth is not a natural physiological process, but a dangerous procedure in which '*everything can happen*' and '*the woman is one foot in the grave*' and '*does not understand*' (Tzekulova, 2017). Despite social media being used more and more frequently to open up discussion about birth, this form of communication (and its potential to make women question their options), is not yet prevalent enough to bring about a real change in processes and practices. Further there is no responsibility as yet for journalists to seek out up-to-date and scientifically substantiated information rather than merely representing and reinforcing outdated stereotypes.

However, new technologies and the Internet have impacted all aspects of life, including childbirth and child-raising, quickly and significantly changing opportunities for women to receive information and exchange opinions. In 2002 the first Bulgarian pregnancy and maternity portal (bg-mamma.com) was created in response to the need for information. The site rapidly became the largest community of mothers in Bulgaria, and a social network for sharing personal and professional opinions, experiences and recommendations between parents and qualified professionals. By 2010 it contained over 2,000,000 topics related to conception, motherhood and parenting (CSD, 2010). Thus in Bulgaria the media, once an instrument to restrict women's choice to medical options, can now be seen a mechanism for facilitating greater choice in childbirth.

As well as enabling choice, the media is also becoming more instrumental in enabling women and their families to question medicalised and outdated birth practices in the country, and to debate the wider issue of human rights in childbirth. An example of this is evident in reports surrounding the death of a woman who died after giving birth in Sliven Hospital in August 2018 (EUSCOOP, 2018). The hospital claimed the woman suffered from chronic diseases that had led to a difficult labour and reported the cause of her death as 'unspecified'. According to the family, however, the woman had an uncomplicated pregnancy and expected an easy labour and smooth delivery. The family suggested that the woman died because of poor treatment and outdated birth practices. Harnessing the power of both social media and the wider media, the family were able to mount a 200-strong protest outside the hospital and to initiate an investigation into the circumstances around the woman's death by the Prosecutor's office.

The UK situation

In the UK, there is a debate about the role the media plays in inciting fear of childbirth among women of childbearing age and in society more generally (Hundley et al, 2014). Birth is currently depicted in English language media as a dramatic and high-risk event that needs to be 'managed' in hospital under the careful eye of highly trained professionals (Luce et al, 2016). The absence of 'normal' birth in the media could be argued to be restricting choice regarding place of birth by influencing women's decisions, despite expectations that women in the UK, unlike Bulgaria, will be offered this choice (NICE,

2017). However, the existing literature is not definitive in this regard. The systematic review by Luce et al found no studies that looked at the impact of media representations of birth on women's attitudes or decision-making (2016). It is necessary therefore to look elsewhere to understand the impact of media representations on women.

Kay et al (2017) explored how women from two different generations (1970s–1980s and 2012) came to understand birth in the milieu of other women's stories. Kay defined a birth story as a story which encompassed personal oral stories as well as media and other representations of contemporary childbirth, all of which had the potential to elicit emotional responses and generate meaning in the interlocutor. The study grew from a sense that the way people talk about and portray birth must surely be significant, having a positive or negative influence on audiences, and potentially steering women either towards or away from different models of care.

The study revealed the experience of 'being-in-the-world' of birth for two generations of women, and their way of communicating within that world. It showed that women experience aspects of the birth world in relation to other people who are in the same space, looking for and building connections with women in the same situation as them.

Kay et al found that women interpreted the birth accounts in popular UK media as primarily '*horror*' stories. These accounts stress the inherent 'dangers' of birthing and the need for expert and interventionist care. The stories describe, in typical narrative form, what happened and when, telling of who was there and what they did; they portray stages and interventions (often used to accelerate birth and/or to dispense with pain) rather than describing how the experience felt, as lived by the women, and any sense of what birth meant to them. The stories tell of or show birth as managed by the people and institutions around women rather than by the women themselves.

The situation appears to have parallels in Bulgaria where occasional media reports, when they do appear, concentrate on cases with poor outcomes such as maternal or infant deaths and violence against the mother and infant. Kay et al's findings suggest that the 'lifeworld' of birth being sustained is overwhelmingly one of product and process; concentrating on the birth of a healthy baby as the only significant outcome. The circulation of these media stories is a form of hidden 'authority' within the world of birth with the ability to dominate and oppress; making the medical model of birth the default 'setting' of birth and making women who birth outside the '*drama of birth*' (or who tell a positive story of birthing) feel ostracised. Further, women who choose to birth outside the accepted models of care as determined by the shared media stories may be labelled as difficult patients and/or 'bad mothers' for putting themselves and their unborn babies at unnecessary 'risk'.

The portrayal of birth as a commodity, for instance, and the favouring of negative stories over positive ones, has the potential to accentuate childbirth as a medical event which needs to be managed. Indeed, Luce et al found that this was the predominant portrayal of birth within the media (2016). Viewing childbirth as a medical event places a natural event into '*a pathological illness model*', which undoubtedly has ramifications for the ways in which women experience and make sense of their own birth (Miller, 2000, p309). The inference is that if women expect their birth to be medically managed and their experience to be negative, then it is likely to be so.

Similarly, the messages women receive from the stories shared may have a 'disciplining' effect; constraining them to behave compliantly, to follow accepted traditions and practices and 'perform' in a 'ladylike' fashion. Martin (2003, p56) suggests that *internalised technologies of gender* have a disciplinary effect on birthing women's behaviours. Martin (2003) argues that internalised technologies of gender *produce who we are* even during primal experiences such as birth. Certainly a number of the women interviewed by Kay and who were birthing in 2013 were conscious of behaving *appropriately* and spoke about not *screaming* (Isabel), following perceived hospital procedures (Stephanie), being *polite* (Mary), being a *good patient* and not embarrassing themselves by being out of control (Ruth).

In a world where the public way of understanding birth, the *drama* of birth as described by Isabel, is disseminated so widely, what is extraordinary, in other words the *horror*, is seen to be made ordinary through familiarity. In this way the appearance of *horror* in a story is accommodated and then made invisible by that accommodation, and other interpretations are effectively 'closed off' (Kay et al, 2017). One could argue that this phenomenon is evident on the television (TV) in the UK where birth representations are prolific and where childbirth is becoming *routinely witnessed and represented in more graphic and public ways* (Tyler and Baraitser, 2013, p1). Reality TV shows such as Channel 4's *One Born Every Minute*, for instance, with a remit to depict the 'drama and emotion' of a maternity unit, have led some feminist scholars to express concern about the exaggerated, medicalised portrayal of televised birth, which includes representations of women's bodies as inadequate and which positions technology and pain relief as effective remedies (Tyler and Baraitser, 2013; De Benedictis et al, 2018). In their content analysis of nine episodes of *One Born Every Minute* De Benedictis et al (2018, p13) demonstrate the *dominance of the medical model of birth that overwhelmingly represents women as passive subjects, visualised through representations of women on their backs, with limited if any input in decision-making during labour*. Interestingly the analysis challenges the assumption that caesarean section and emergencies are over-represented in reality TV; determining instead that their representation reflects national statistics. What is deemed significant, however, is the repetitive representation of other interventions such as the use of foetal scalp electrodes as a means to continuously monitor foetal wellbeing, with the researchers arguing that in their repetition the interventions are seen as routine and/or unexceptional and by inference inevitable parts of the childbirth process.

Arguably alternative representations of labour and birth such as those depicted in *Call the Midwife*, a BBC historical drama series based on a midwife's memoirs of working in East London in the 1950s–60s, can function as a means of destabilising accepted and pervasive discourses (Takeshita, 2017). In the series midwives are portrayed as the principal caregivers at births, with pregnancy and childbirth depicted as part of *the fabric of everyday life of the community* as opposed to being problematised medicalised events (Takeshita, 2017, p340). In this sense *Call the Midwife* appears to work as a counter-narrative, using storytelling to strengthen the notion of midwifery-led childbirth as normal and healthy.

The impact of horror stories of birth

The sharing of 'horror' stories, as in both the UK and Bulgarian examples, does not give women any understanding of themselves as capable of birthing or of mothering; rather they portray women as somehow lacking. Ultimately they frighten women. Cultural events (such as distressing stories) are recognised as a cause of fear for childbearing women (Fenwick, Gamble, Nathan, Bayes and Hauck, 2009). Lowe (1993) suggests that the current dominant worldview of reproduction challenges women's belief in their ability to labour effectively. Further Otley (2011, p216) argues that '*escalating intervention and operative rates are seen by women as proof that birth is dangerous and frightening*'. It is not surprising, therefore, that pregnant woman today may be frightened about the prospect of labour and childbirth.

Kay et al found that women in their UK study expressed more fear about giving birth than those in the generation before. The women pregnant in the 1970s–80s, unlike women in 2013, had some anxieties about giving birth, but were not overly fearful. Significantly these women were not continually confronted with dramatic media representations of childbirth. Indeed, when discussing such representations most of the women in the earlier generation were thankful that these 'resources' had not been available when they were pregnant as they could see that they could induce fear. Jean, for example, said:

> '*You didn't see childbirth on the telly, you know? Didn't have kind of all these pictures of screaming women and things like this on television....I think it puts in people's minds how painful it's going to be*'.

Evidence and discussion about a possible relationship between media representations and anxiety about labour and childbirth is slowly starting to emerge. For instance, in their study on media representations of pregnancy and childbirth in the United States (USA), Morris and McInerney maintained that the reality-based birth television shows they analysed made childbirth events '*much more dramatic and perilous than they are in reality*' (2010, p139), perhaps explaining why in the second USA *Listening to Mothers* report:

> '*32% of first-time mothers reported that they felt more worried about their birth after watching the shows.*' (Declercq et al, 2006, p24)

Similarly, in her commentary, Bak discusses how the popular media present birthing as a '*dramatised caricature*' which:

> '*Overwhelmingly both censors the natural ability of women's bodies to birth and distorts the process to reflect birth as a clinical event from which women need to be saved by medical representatives*' (Bak, 2004, p65)

Kay et al found that the women birthing today took great care to seek out information to prepare them for birth; frightened by what they heard and saw in popular stories, the women sought knowledge as a means of reducing their anxiety. Information-seeking for them could be framed as an attempt to secure a '*protective homeostatic function*' (Maslow, 2013, p61). However, in the event, given vast amounts of information via various mediums such as the Internet and television, the women in the study actually became overloaded and saturated with information, to the extent that it had a paralysing effect.

Kay et al argue that by engaging with media stories women come to expect birth to be a certain way and this expectation and '*cultural shaping*' is '*internalised*' and played out by individual women in their consequent maternity care choices (Reiger and Dempsey, 2006, p368). Further, it is possible that the social construction of birth in these media stories may have a direct effect on the physiological processes of childbearing, affecting the actual 'doing' of birth (Bordo, 1993). This follows because if birth is portrayed as something to be feared, as something excruciatingly painful which women will want to ultimately forget, then the very thought of it and the actual 'doing' of it is likely to promote adverse psychological responses. These responses will then be expressed through the role of oxytocin in the neural pathways in the brain and in hormonal responses through the nervous system affecting the complex physiological processes which need to be in motion to initiate, sustain and progress birth (Uvnäs Moberg, 2003) (see Chapter 2).

Alternative media sources

An understanding that positive stories need to be shared is finally being recognised at a grassroots level within the childbearing community and fostered within organisations such as the Positive Birth Movement, a movement initially spreading positivity about childbirth locally and now doing so on a global level via free groups and social media. The movement was set up as a means of questioning and challenging the accepted socially constructed and often negative portrayal of birth. The group defines a positive birth as the following:

> '*A positive birth means a birth in which a woman feels she has freedom of choice, access to accurate information, and that she is in control, powerful and respected. A birth that she approaches, perhaps with some trepidation, but without fear or dread, and that she then goes on to enjoy, and later remember with warmth and pride. A positive birth does not have to be 'natural' or 'drug free' – it simply has to be informed from a place of positivity as opposed to fear.*' (Positive Birth Movement, 2018).

Also of note is the Positive Birth Stories webpage, which aims to encourage the telling of real-life positive birth stories and in doing so to encourage and nurture confidence in women about their ability to birth. The webpage uses a powerful metaphor to describe the dangers of engaging with negative stories and of living in a world where the mode of being is portrayed in a particular light:

> '*Imagine you are preparing for the Olympics and your aim is gold. In the daily lead up to the games during conversations and in newspapers you read and television & films you watch you are exposed to detailed accounts of other athletes losing and dreadful past accidents in your particular race. Your mind starts to fill with these images and fear becomes a regular visitor. Your many consultations with professionals (supposed experts) are filled with the dire consequences of possible problems especially if you don't adhere to*

their way of competing. You leave their offices feeling powerless and worried. Eventually you stop training deciding to rely solely on their guarantee of assistance. Friends and family only confirm your fears with their own regaling of hideous accounts of the same race. The day comes and you feel extremely stressed and apprehensive about it and your ability. The race begins and the muscles designed to power you, falter because your tension and fear constrict them. Your coach and manager decide its best if they take over for you.' (www.positivebirthstories.com/about)

This metaphor is powerful because it is hugely reminiscent of the context of birth for women today; surrounded by negative stories, images and portrayals of birth, none of which are easily avoided and many of which are seemingly reinforced by the professionals who should be encouraging and supporting women and letting them know how powerful and able they are to birth their babies.

Conclusion

It has been 20 years since Clement described how television was often the only opportunity that most women had to view birth before experiencing it for themselves (1997). With increasing numbers of women turning to the media as a source of information about childbirth there is the potential, and some would argue a responsibility (Hundley et al, 2015), for maternity care providers to influence the messages that are shared. Professionals in the UK are recognising the value of social media as a mechanism for information-sharing (Byrom and Byrom, 2017). Similarly, as in Bulgaria, as the digital environment is enriched by communication platforms and the availability of specialised information, there are the beginnings of a new format for information exchange among women. This will undoubtedly become an influential factor in most countries in making important decisions about pregnancy and maternity. However, a recent UK study found that midwives, in particular, are reluctant to engage with more traditional forms of media such as television and newspapers (Luce et al, 2017). Since these traditional forms of media continue to attract the largest and broadest range of viewers, there is a need for better dialogue between midwives, other maternity care providers, and media producers to ensure that more representative portrayals of childbirth are available.

Key points for consideration

- Encourage the sharing of positive stories that reinforce women's capacity to birth.
- Offer help and guidance to women and families to 'unpack' and understand negative stories and portrayals of birth, in order to mitigate the damaging effects of expectant fear.
- Signpost women to good quality information throughout pregnancy, which they can choose to access when they need it and in a format they are comfortable with.
- Support women to use their embodied knowing as they birth.
- Increase dialogue between maternity care workers and media producers to encourage varied representative portrayals of childbirth.

References

Bainbridge, J. (2006) Unsolicited advice: A rite of passage through your first pregnancy. *British Journal of Midwifery* 14(5): 265.

Bak, C. (2004). Cultural lack of birth experience empowers media representations not women. *Midwifery Today - International Midwife.* Winter 2004, 44.

Bordo, S. (1993). *Unbearable weight: Feminism and the politics of childbirth in the United States.* Berkeley: University of California Press.

Byrom, S & Byrom, A. (2017). Around the world in 80 tweets – social media and midwifery. In: Luce, A., Hundley, V. and van Teijlingen, E (Eds). *Media and Midwifery.* London: Palgrave

Call the Midwife. 2012-2015. Directed by Heidi Thomas. Television Series. BBC.

Center for the Study of Democracy, Civil Society in Bulgaria (CSD) (2010) *Trends and Risks.* Available from: http://www.csd.bg/artShow.php?id=15423

Clement, S. (1997). Childbirth on television. British Journal of Midwifery 5(1): 37-42.

De Benedictis, S., Johnson, C., Roberts, J., Spiby, H. (2018). Quantitative insights into televised birth: a content analysis of 'One Born Every Minute'. Critical Studies in Media Communication, DOI: 10.1080/15295036.2018.1516046.

Declercq, E., Sakala, C., Corry, M., Applebaum, S. (2006). *Listening to Mothers II: Report of the Second National U.S. Survey of Women's Childbearing Experiences.* New York: Childbirth Connection. Available from: http://www.nationalpartnership.org/research-library/maternal-health/listening-to-mothers-ii-2006.pdf

Deenichina, M (2005). *Institutions of Hidden Media Censorship in Bulgaria (1956-1989).* // Yearbook of the Sofia University "St. Kliment Ohridski ", Sofia, Univ. Ed. St. Kliment Ohridski.

Elliot, A. (2009). *The Social animal.* Sofia: Damyan Yakov.

EUSCOOP, News from Bulgaria, 2018. Available at: https://www.euscoop.com/en/2018/8/20/woman-died-giving-birth-investigation-ongoing

Fenwick, J., Gamble, J., Nathan, E., Bayes, S., & Hauck, Y. (2009). Pre- and postpartum levels of childbirth fear and the relationship to birth outcomes in a cohort of Australian women. *Journal of Clinical Nursing, 18*(5), 667-677. Doi:10.1111/j.1365-2702.2008.02568.x

Hundley, V., Duff, E., Dewberry, J., Luce, A., van Teijlingen, E. (2014). Fear in childbirth: are the media responsible? *MIDIRS Midwifery Digest* 24:4:444-447.

Hundley V., van Teijlingen E., & Luce A. (2015). Do midwives need to be more media savvy? *MIDIRS Midwifery Digest* 25:1:5-10.

Kay, L., Downe, S., Thomson, G. & Finlayson, K. 2017, "'Engaging with birth stories in pregnancy: a hermeneutic phenomenological study of women's experiences across two generations'", *BMC Pregnancy and Childbirth,* vol. 17, pp. 283.

Lowe, N. (1993). Maternal confidence for labor: Development of the childbirth self-efficacy inventory. *Research in Nursing & Health,* 16(2), 141-149.

Luce A,. Hundley V. & van Teijlingen E. (2017). Midwives' Engagement with the Media. In: Luce, A., Hundley, V. and van Teijlingen, E (Eds) *Media and Midwifery.* London: Palgrave.

Martin, K. (2003). Giving birth like a girl. *Gender and Society,* 17(1), 54-72.

Maslow, A. (2013). *Toward a psychology of being.* London: Start Publishing LLC.

Miller, T. (2000). Losing the plot: Narrative construction and longitudinal childbirth research. *Qualitative Health Research,* 10(3), 309-323.

Mindova, V. (2014). *The speech of the totalitarian regime - the (not) heard truth or the unfortunate excommunication of the novel "Tobacco"* // Media and public communications. Ed., UNWE; Alma communication. 2014, No. 19. Available from: [www.media-journal.info]

Morris, T., & McInerney, K. (2010). Media representations of pregnancy and childbirth: An analysis of reality television programs in the United States. *Birth: Issues in Perinatal Care,* 37(2), 134-140. Doi:10.1111/j.1523-536X.2010.00393.x.

NICE (2017) *Intrapartum care for healthy women and babies [CG190]* Available at: https://www.nice.org.uk/guidance/cg190/chapter/recommendations

One Born Every Minute. 2010-2018. Television Series. Channel 4 Television Corporation. Otley, H. (2011). Fear of childbirth: Understanding the causes, impact and treatment. *British Journal of Midwifery,* 19(4), 215-220.

Positive Birth Movement. (2018). *What is a positive birth?* Retrieved from http://www.positivebirthmovement.org/what-is-positive-birth.html

Positive birth stories. (2018) Retrieved from http://www.positivebirthstories.com/

Raskoff, S. (2013) Pregnancy and Social Interactions. Everday Sociology. Available at: https://www.everydaysociologyblog.com/2013/07/pregnancy-and-social-interactions.html

Reiger, K., & Dempsey, R. (2006). Performing birth in a culture of fear: An embodied crisis of late modernity. *Health Sociology Review,* 15(4), 364-374.

Roberts J., De Benedictis, S., & Spiby, H. (2017). Love Birth, Hate One Born Every Minute? Birth community discourse around televised childbirth. In: Luce, A., Hundley, V. and van Teijlingen, E (Eds) *Media and Midwifery.* London: Palgrave

Slavchev, M, The development of obstetrics in Bulgaria in the last 50 years, Central Medical Library, // Chronicles of the Bulgarian Medical Association, Jubilee speech by Dr. Metodi Slavchev to the medical community, January and February XXXV, Book 1 & 2, Sofia, 1942

Takeshita, C. (2017) Countering technocracy: "natural" birth in The Busines of Being Born and Call the Midwife. *Feminist Media Studies,* 17 (3), 332-346.

Tyler, I., & Baraitser, L. (2013). Private view, public birth: Making feminist sense of the new visual culture of childbirth. *Studies in the Maternal,* 5 (2), 1-27.

Tzekulova, N. (2017). Unpublished quotes from the Bulgarian forums, groups and social media.

Uvnäs Moberg, K. (2003). *The oxytocin factor: Tapping the hormone of calm, love and healing.* USA: Da Capo Press.

CHAPTER 11

Choice, continuity and control: a clarion call to putting women at the centre of their care, and supporting normal birth

Sally Tracy and Lesley Page

Introduction

This chapter addresses notions of choice, continuity and control in the UK, Australia, and New Zealand. The clarion call of choice, continuity and control (also termed 'The three Cs'), served as organising concepts and a slogan to capture the profound change that was envisioned by the UK policy document *Changing Childbirth*[1] in 1993. Such slogans are important. The notion of the Three Cs points clearly to the need to give women choices; choices about where their baby should be born, where their care should be, and what kind of treatment they will consent to. Choice points to the personal autonomy that is fundamental to the rights and wellbeing of women. This right to choose is linked closely to being in control of your own body, your own plan of care, informed by knowledge and discussions with your known and trusted caregivers. Continuity, the comfort of a familiar face, is the lynchpin holding choice and control together. But rallying cries like this may become meaningless, unless system structures, culture and values of care are transformed. Indeed, slogans belie the complexity of change. *Changing Childbirth* provides a nuanced description of woman-centred, appropriate, accessible care. This is in contrast to neoliberal consumerist concepts of choice as a limited and constrained option to be chosen from a pre-determined menu.

However, despite the ground-breaking insights of the *Changing Childbirth* agenda, the difficulty of making a genuine choice in services where the dominant culture values medical intervention over holistic care, over therapeutic relationship, over more midwifery oriented interventions such as water for pain relief[2] was badly underestimated. This chapter examines some of the issues arising from experiences in the 25 years since the publication of *Changing Childbirth*, in three specific contexts, and some of the lessons that have been learned in this field.

The view from the UK

Some would say that the societal obsession with choice has led healthcare down a path of self-interest and economic rationalism, to the extent that, as health consumers, the value of compassionate care and connectedness is overlooked in demands for immediate self-gratification. The choice of elective caesarean section for convenience, to fit in with a busy business schedule (in the absence of any physical, psychological or social need), could be seen as an example of this.

Two decades after its publication, the principles of *Changing Childbirth* still form a common language, but the real changes have occurred on the fringes of maternity, rather than in the mainstream. There are many words 'missing' from *Changing Childbirth*. Words like 'normal birth', although there is a recognition of the importance of supporting physiology. It was assumed that normal birth would be supported and encouraged by continuity, and that women would be able to choose normal (physiological) pregnancy and birth. Developing midwifery through continuity of carer was seen to be critical, as the loss of autonomy in midwifery had been swept away in a tide of increasing medicalisation and institutionalisation. The need for teamwork and collaboration was also emphasised. It has become clear over time that a continuous relationship with a maternity care provider (a midwife), and an underlying philosophy of the importance of supporting normal birth, are both necessary to underpin high levels of normal birth. Indeed, it is interesting to note that where there is medical continuity in private practice the caesarean section rate is almost invariably higher than in public sector provision, and much higher than in midwifery-led continuity of care models.

Retrospectively it is easy to see why the shift of power, to put women at the centre of care, and to involve users of the maternity services in monitoring and creating the change that *Changing Childbirth* envisioned in the UK, might take some time to embed. Ten years after the report was published, Tricia Anderson wrote: *'were we naive to believe that this humanistic charter for change to woman centred individualised maternity care … would succeed without challenging the ruling hegemony … the supremacy of technology over women's voices?'* (pp259).[3]

From the start, there was a general perception that midwife-led care should only be offered to women without identified risk factors ('low-risk' women). This inadvertently conferred authority to medicine in the management of all pregnancies through a mandate to define risk and, through this mechanism, to override the decision-making of the woman or the midwife (though it should be noted that midwives have a legal duty to attend women labouring at home in the UK, no matter what their risk profile). The focus on midwifery care for 'low-risk' women (only) limits the value of midwifery as a discrete profession separate to and working collaboratively with medicine. All women benefit from midwifery care – and some women may need the professional skill of a doctor in parallel with the care of the midwife.[4] The care given by a midwife does not negate that offered by medicine, nor should it be set up in competition with medical care. Furthermore, health systems designed like factory production lines pose real difficulties for midwives trying to provide individualised woman-centred care. Sociologists describe the way these rigid bureaucratic structural factors affect the dynamics of power in the midwife/woman relationship as being 'with the bureaucracy' rather than being 'with women'.[5]

Twenty years on from *Changing Childbirth,* two new government policy reports for maternity care have been produced in the UK. *Better Births – A five year forward plan for maternity services* was published by NHS England in 2016,[6] and *The Best Start: A Five-Year Forward Plan for Maternity and Neonatal Care in Scotland* was issued by the Government of Scotland in 2017.[7] Consequent targets for continuity of carer in the 2019 NHS plan promise to build on the achievements in these reports. These recent reports incorporate the global evidence that has emerged slowly in support of midwives taking the lead in providing midwifery care for women regardless of their 'risk' status.[8] This involves coordinating care with other health professionals where needed in the interests of the woman or infant, without detracting from the practice of midwifery.[9,10]

The recent maternity services review in England, *Better Births,*[6] and in Scotland *The Best Start*[7] reported that women preferred to be cared for by one midwife or a small group of midwives. The report recommended that midwives who work in a continuity of care caseload group practice need their time to be 'ring-fenced', and not diverted to other services. This allows for flexible working where midwives manage their own diary, in conjunction with the rest of their colleagues.

The report also recommended that a scheme called the NHS Personal Maternity Care Budget, aimed at providing a simple mechanism to enable women to make a choice in selecting their chosen accredited provider, would be trialled in several areas in 2016–17, supported by NHS England.[6] In New Zealand a similar scheme has been working since 1990, giving women the choice of their lead maternity carer and a choice about place of birth.[9] The Independent Hospital Pricing Authority in Australia is currently considering a bundled maternity payment which would allow for health boards to offer innovative maternity models, including more midwifery-led care. Midwifery group practice models will play a major role in the future, reducing the public health burden by increasing normal outcomes and promoting more efficient use of funds.

The view from New Zealand and Australia

During the time the reforms discussed above were materialising in the UK, on the opposite side of the planet other reforms were taking shape in the form of legislation supporting the autonomy of midwives in New Zealand. They have had a profound effect on childbearing women in that country for the past 25 years.[9] The legislative changes introduced in New Zealand in 1990 recognised the rights of women to have both choice and control in maternity care irrespective of the complexity of their pregnancies. In the preamble to the legislation, Helen Clark, the then Minister for Health (and later Prime Minister of NZ) stated:

'The implementation of the Nurses Amendment Act 1990 should increase the choices available to women and their families in childbirth services. The Act restores autonomy to midwives, who were previously limited by legislation which allowed medical practitioners only to take full responsibility for the care of women. Statistics reflect the benefit of a commitment to natural childbirth, of continuity of care of the client and the rejection of unnecessary intervention. The majority of women have been socialised to perceive birth as an illness. The challenge of this legislation is to change that perception'.[9]

This wide-reaching reform resulted in a major reorganization of the maternity services, giving midwives the opportunity to provide continuity of care to women who could now choose both their caregiver and their place of birth.[9] New Zealand is the only country that has achieved nationwide reform leading to woman-centred services, through a profound change in legislated infrastructure. The government vision for continuity of care was set out under Section 88 of the Public Health and Disability Act 2000:

'Each woman, and her whanau, will have every opportunity to have a fulfilling outcome to her pregnancy and childbirth, through the provision of services that are safe and based on partnership, information and choice. Pregnancy and childbirth are a normal life-stage for most women, with appropriate additional care available to those women who require it. A Lead Maternity Carer chosen by the woman with responsibility for assessment of her needs, planning her care with her and the care of her baby and being responsible for ensuring provision of Maternity Services, is the cornerstone of maternity care in New Zealand.[75]

In contrast to the system in New Zealand, in most countries the provision of continuity of carer is difficult to achieve in maternity services in which most midwives have become accustomed to working shifts.[72,76] However, this is not impossible. For example, in Australia, caseload midwives who are funded through the government public hospital system are offered employment contracts for an annualised salary agreement. This method of remuneration has significant enabling effects that support women and midwives to work in partnership. In any system where the institution no longer dictates the movements of midwives, it allows them to respond to the women booked in their caseload. To achieve a sustainable level of flexibility, Australian midwifery group practice midwives might work within practices of four to six midwives, employed under an industrial award. However, only a few midwives are able to take up this option.

Choice in childbirth amid the cascade of interventions

Though there has been some public acknowledgement of the value of physiological birth processes, official recognition of healthy pregnancy and childbirth states and of unusual normal progress in labour remains elusive. The constant surveillance and scrutiny for risk has resulted in rising rates of medico-technical intervention, in particular caesarean section. Notwithstanding the deference to consumer choice as the gold standard, in most maternity systems women's ability to plan their options for care (exercise a real choice) and make informed decisions is severely restricted by the persuasive argument that hospital is the best and safest place for babies to be born. This message is reinforced relentlessly via the media, policy-makers and the medical establishment. It is very likely that this is associated with women choosing interventions in childbirth (see Chapter 7 for a discussion of the nature and consequences of the risk society on childbearing women).

The worldwide and rising prevalence of caesarean sections correlates strongly with socioeconomic status. In resource-poor countries even medically indicated caesarean sections are rarely available to many women, though levels in private hospitals, and for wealthy women, are high even in these settings. In contrast, lower middle-income countries have some of the highest rates in the world, again, especially among the more affluent women who seek more 'medicalised' health care within private delivery systems.[11] There has been a dramatic increase in the caesarean section rates in countries following political reform, for example in much of Eastern Europe in the shift from communism to capitalism, and in particular in the emerging economies of Brazil, India and China. Notwithstanding, in 2016 a sentinel ecological study examining all globally available data on caesarean sections found no corresponding improvement in perinatal outcomes associated with caesarean section rates greater than 10%.[12]

The *Lancet* series on optimising caesarean section examines the global epidemiology of use and disparities in caesarean sections[13] and the short and long-term effects of caesarean section on the health of women and children.[14] It describes interventions to reduce unnecessary caesarean sections in healthy women and babies[13] accompanied by a FIGO position paper[15] and WHO recommendations on non-clinical interventions to reduce unnecessary caesarean section.[16]

Compared with spontaneous vaginal birth, caesarean births carry the risk of morbidity[13,17] and mortality;[13,18] complications in subsequent pregnancies for mothers (e.g. uterine rupture, placenta praevia, and placenta accreta)[13,17,19-23] and infants.[14,24,25] Operative birth increases risks to the neonate such as respiratory distress syndrome,[26] persistent pulmonary hypertension[27] and admission to special care or neonatal intensive care nurseries, particularly if the caesarean section is performed before the onset of labour.[26,28-30] The risk of chronic diseases such as type 1 diabetes,[31] asthma,[32,33] and obesity[34] have all been identified through meta-analyses of cohort and case-control studies of caesarean sections (see Chapter 13 and 14).

The *Lancet* series[13] emphasises the importance of access to caesarean section being available while preventing the use of unnecessary caesarean section. The discussion of non-clinical interventions to reduce unnecessary caesarean section shows just how embedded the overuse of caesarean section is in all parts of the world.

A collateral consequence of the trend towards hospital birth is a corresponding increase in the use and reliance on a wide range of obstetric gadgets and technology; often introduced in a policy vacuum and within minimal attention to best evidence.[35] Although it is difficult to tease out the level of women's choice involved, linked population-based data in Australia revealed that among women with uncomplicated pregnancies, a third of all women had some form of intervention such as an induction or augmentation of their labour, combined with an epidural[36] and that this trend has continued to increase.[37,38] Cost modelling of these interventions showed a relative cost increase of up to 50% for low-risk primiparous women and up to 36% for low-risk multiparous women as labour interventions accumulate.[39] Additionally, there is emerging evidence that children born by spontaneous vaginal birth have fewer short and long-term health problems, compared with those born after birth interventions.[40] Currently many women are experiencing excessively high rates of caesarean section and other interventions that are not medically justifiable.[41]

A worldwide trend towards private healthcare, not only in high-income countries, but also in middle and low-income settings[12, 42-44] is partly responsible for this over-servicing. In the poorest settings, where ineffective, scientifically unwarranted care seems to account for close to about one-quarter to one-third of the total volume of procedures, it is important to address overuse as well as underuse, so that the resources recovered from the former can be reinvested in reducing the latter.[45]

In his *Lancet* commentary[46] on the power of midwifery, Richard Horton asserts that midwifery is about much more than assisting in childbirth. Midwifery is

'skilled, knowledgeable, and compassionate care for childbearing women, newborn infants, and families across the continuum throughout pre-pregnancy, pregnancy, birth, postpartum, and the early weeks of life….Midwifery includes family planning and the provision of reproductive health services. The services provided by midwives are best delivered not only in hospital settings but also in communities—midwifery is not a vertical service offered as a narrow segment of the health system. Midwifery services are a core part of universal health coverage. A re-evaluation of midwifery and midwifery services matters because progress in reducing child and maternal mortality is now revealing critical new obstacles to further success.' (p1057)

At a policy level there appears to be general agreement that increasing access to choice for continuity of midwifery care or midwifery-led care will play a major part in reducing intervention rates in pregnancy and childbirth, and in increasing the 'normal' birth rate. The question is, how to strengthen the role of midwives in a world where the potential of midwifery is not realised and even oppressed and eradicated? Moreover, even in countries with strongly progressive woman-centred policies, increase in access has been difficult to sustain, and the evidence is still treated as though it were contentious. For example, a pernicious backlash was seen in England in 2017, from a few individuals, press, and a government minister, that amounted to a campaign against normal birth, even as government sought to put new policy into practice.[47] It is hard to see how 'normal birth' policies can succeed within techno/medical environments that act as powerful agents of social control, shaping individual values, beliefs and behaviours.[48] In short, women experience very little choice or control when pregnancy is treated as a disease, safety is tied to being born in hospital and risk is managed by the experts.

Choice within contemporary consumerist societies

During the heady days of the women's health movement 50 years ago, the slogan 'a woman's right to choose' was coined, in a strategic effort to move the locus of control away from a paternalistic patient/doctor relationship to one of a market-based consumer.[49] In the struggle to convince legislators and policy-makers that women should have the right to choose midwifery care, the assumption was that situating women as 'consumers' of maternity care would place them in a more powerful position to balance the scales of power with the medical profession in dictating financial arrangements and public policy decisions. Consumer activism of the 1980s and 90s did achieve greater representation for women, and ostensibly achieved greater choices through market ideology and competition.[50] However, it could be argued that today's consumerist society is not so much aimed at meeting women's needs and interests than at generating profit. The emphasis is much more about choice for the individual (i.e. for those who can already afford it) than for generating community good(s).[51] Today's feminists protest for more choice for women in their daily lives: more opportunities, more freedom, less restraint and less-constricted roles to play. 'Choice' has become the most significant word in a world of unconstrained consumerism. However, as Joseph Stiglitz, the Nobel prize-winning economist, cautioned:

'We have created a society in which materialism overwhelms moral commitment ... market fundamentalism has eroded any sense of community and has led to rampant exploitation of unwary and unprotected individuals'.[52]

In neoliberal societies the power of individuals to care for themselves and navigate complex systems is often overestimated, and the need for the development of systems and resources to support individual users of resources, and to enable professionals (including midwives) to practise fully and effectively, is often underestimated.

Just as successful advertising shapes consumer choice in a market economy, today's focus on individual choices in maternity care is shaped by social media, medical professionals and other repositories of 'authoritative' information,[53] including the 'menu' of service providers.[54] The highly pervasive modern discourse of neo-liberalism is built on a single, fundamental principle: the superiority of the individual in market-based competition over other modes of organisation.[55]

Not only does a market-centric discourse elevate the notion of individual consumer power, but the 'politics' of the market also drive the privatisation of healthcare and lower the protection afforded to public health systems from the forces of private market competition.[55] Perkins (2003) argues that the medicalisation of birth is an institutionalised 'market strategy' allowing doctors to reclassify physiological processes that will require medical solutions.[56] The uncontrolled variation in caesarean section rates, for example, reflects the manner in which differences in the organisation of healthcare and methods of payment can also influence choice of mode of birth,[42,43,57-64] with higher rates in the private sector.[65, 66] Hospitals today reflect the pressures of commodification and consumer 'choice' through their competitive funding plans and the expansion of medical technologies.[50]

As an example, in Australia, with the exception of the midwifery group practice providers noted above, and some independent midwives, the Australian system reflects the motivating interests of powerful professional stakeholders, especially those of medical associations and doctors.[67] By contrast, in some other health systems (e.g. the Netherlands, Britain, and since the 1990s, New Zealand and Canada) primary healthcare policy funds primary providers such as midwives in community-based services as the first contact point for healthy pregnant women and acknowledges home birth to be a viable option.[9,68]

How models of continuity of care support normal childbirth

Although continuity of care may manifest in different circumstances with various caregivers, this section will examine the sole domain of continuity of midwifery care and the effect it has on childbirth. The latest Cochrane review of midwife-led continuity models versus other models of care for childbearing women found that women who received midwife-led continuity of care were more likely to be cared for in labour by midwives they already knew.[8] They were less likely to need epidural analgesia to help them to cope with labour pain. In addition, fewer women had episiotomies or instrumental births. Women's chances of a spontaneous vaginal birth were also increased and there was no difference in the number of caesarean births. Women were less likely to experience preterm birth, and they were also at a lower risk of losing their babies.

A recent trial of caseload continuity of midwifery care found it both safe and cost-effective when offered to women irrespective of 'risk' factors.[10] It has been proposed that one of the mechanisms that could affect these outcomes is that midwives working in partnership with women help to disrupt the techno-scientific approach to birth.[71] Continuity of care recognises a woman's sense of her own experience of giving birth as unique and singularly important. It increases the opportunity for women to experience birth without the use of drugs and anaesthesia promising to reduce pain. The essence of one-to-one care is a close and trusting relationship between the woman and her midwife based on kind, personal, sensitive and respectful care.[72]

However, if continuity of care is to become 'mainstream', through which all women achieve a stronger level of control in their birth experience, major clinical and system redesign is required within health systems. This may involve reconfiguring existing birth suite staff, services and management structures. It will also involve rearranging birth spaces to allow less emphasis on technological apparatus; giving consideration to the woman's inherent, mammalian need to feel safe and secure in the space in which she is about to give birth.[73] In addition to this, it is apparent that the way midwives working in continuity models are funded is pivotal to the success of continuity of care. As noted above, funding models provide powerful barriers or enablers to the opportunities women experience in choosing continuity of care with a midwife and a place to give birth. Funding maternity services for example through a 'fee for service' may not always produce the best outcomes and may engender grave unintended consequences in maternity care.[74]

Caseload care for women of all risk involves the midwife becoming the *named* midwife for 35–40 women per year and coordinating each woman's care in collaboration with the other members of her group practice. Ideally, a designated collaborating obstetrician that is supportive of the philosophy of woman-centred care should be appointed to work closely with two to three practice groups (usually about 8–12 midwives). A strong collaborative relationship between the group midwives and their nominated consultant obstetrician is integral to promoting physiological normal birth with a minimum of medical intervention, and the maximum optimal outcomes for mother and baby.[77] This arrangement provides women with continuity of care and carer during pregnancy, birth and postnatally with a named midwife or one of her partner midwives within the midwifery group practice, and with the linked obstetrician if she needs this extra input. Clear plans of care, including referral to specialist services, should be negotiated and documented with input from the women, the caseload midwife and the obstetrician.

Continuity of midwifery care is a complex intervention that consists of multifaceted components that can act independently and interdependently. These complex networks of components can have powerful and pervasive effects on how systems actually perform and function.[78,79] Performance and function are affected by factors such as enhanced senior management support, clear governance structures and communication, clinical engagement, and give and take between professionals.[80] Maternity care is unique because the services support predominantly healthy women through a natural life event that does not always require a doctor-led intervention.[81]

Continuity of midwifery care not only offers the best experience and outcomes for women who are giving birth,[8] it is also cost-effective.[10,82,83] Reducing costs through reorganising the delivery of midwifery care in the public hospital system could play a major part in reducing public health expenditure. Many small differences in most clinical outcome measures in favour of continuity of midwifery care account for the lower median cost for caseload midwifery than for standard care.[10,83]

The future – moving from 'consumer choice' to 'people power' on the strength of data

Data-driven solutions could drive a powerful health revolution that promises new possibilities for insight and change. However, the voices of women (along with other service users) have been absent in the domain of data extraction and analysis, which is largely directed by specialised professionals and researchers. Increasingly, data are generated, collected and analysed by users using a variety of wearable sensors such as smartphone apps. A new level of accessibility and transparency is possible through social media that has the *potential* to give women a much greater control of their own healthcare decisions.[69] As citizens rather than consumers women have the opportunity to be engaged and involved in evaluating the impact of interventions and shaping the modifications and plans for ongoing improvement and sustainability. When research is embedded in communities it enhances the ability of women to co-lead research and shape choices that are meaningful for them. Moving from 'consumer' to 'citizen' in the 21st century promises to ultimately reshape women's choices. In the words of economist and ecologist, Kate Raworth:

'...unlike the citizen, the consumer's means of expression is limited: while citizens can address every aspect of cultural, social and economic life...consumers find expression only in the market place' [70] (p102)

Conclusion

The importance of vision and national leadership in policy and funding cannot be overestimated in the provision of continuity, choice and control for women in childbirth. One-to-one midwifery care appears to work in the maternity system by intercepting some of the pathways that can contribute to unnecessary intervention. It works on the assumption that women will labour more effectively, need to stay in hospital less time and feel a stronger sense of satisfaction and personal control if they have the opportunity to get to know their midwife in a partnership relationship[71,72] rather than rely on unfamiliar hospital staff during their pregnancy and maternity care. Relationship-based continuity of carer improves safety and quality by bridging the gaps in fragmented services, by helping navigate complex systems of care.[84]

While the precise aspects are not fully understood, mechanisms that make continuity or relationship-based care work could include advocacy, trust, choice, control and listening to women. These are important processes that could link relational continuity with improved outcomes and experience.[84] Continuity models have an impact on improving safety, reducing preterm birth and providing a better experience for women.[8] There is also compelling evidence that women with identified risk factors during pregnancy and birth have improved outcomes where their care is coordinated as required between midwifery, specialist and obstetric services under a midwifery-led model of midwifery care, regardless of risk.[10] Indeed, the evidence on the benefits of relationship-based continuity of carer are so compelling that it is increasingly unethical not to move to this approach, by enabling models of continuity of care that offer authentic choice and control to childbearing women, and that are sustainable, woman-centred and midwife friendly.

Key points for consideration

- The model of care must allow for the creation of a relationship built up over time so women and their midwives may get to know and trust each other.
- The management of midwives providing relationship-based continuity of carer must be enabling not controlling, care should be flexible and woman-centred and midwife friendly.
- There should be one named midwife for each woman who coordinates and provides most of her care supported by partner or buddy midwives, working in groups of 6 to 8.
- Midwives should self-roster and be paid an annualised salary to include on-call commitments.
- Women should be supported to make their own decisions working together with their midwife/midwives through a therapeutic relationship, in which the woman is supported in considering high-quality information, considered in the light of her and her baby's health, values, personal circumstances and preferences.

References

1   Department of Health. *Changing Childbirth: the Report of the Expert Maternity Group*. HMSO. London., 1993.
2   Newnham E, McKellar L, Pincombe J. *Towards the Humanisation of Birth: A study of epidural analgesia and hospital birth culture*. Australia: Palgrave McMillan, 2018.
3   Tricia Anderson. The misleading myth of choice: the continuing oppression of women and childbirth. In: Mavis Kirkham, ed. *Informed Choice in Maternity Care*. London: Palgrave MacMillan, 2004:257-263.
4   Sandall J. Every woman needs a midwife, and some women need a doctor too. *Birth* 2012;39(4):323-326.
5   Finlay S, Sandall J. "Someone's rooting for you": continuity, advocacy and street-level bureaucracy in UK maternal healthcare. *Soc.Sci.Med* 2009;69(8):1228-1235.
6   NHS. *Better Births: Improving outcomes of maternity services in England*. London UK: NHS, 2016.
7   Scottish NHS Forth Valley Scotland. *The Best Start: A Five-Year Forward Plan for Maternity and Neonatal Care in Scotland*. Scottish NHS 2017.
8   Sandall J, Soltani H, Gates Set al. Midwife-led continuity models versus other models of care for childbearing women. *Cochrane Database Syst.Rev* 2016;4:CD004667.
9   Grigg CP, Tracy SK. New Zealand's unique maternity system. *Women Birth* 2013;26(1):e59-e64.
10   Tracy SK, Hartz DL, Tracy MB, Allen J, Welsh A, Kildea S.et al Caseload midwifery care versus standard maternity care for women of any risk: M@NGO, a randomised controlled trial. *The Lancet* 2013; 382 November 23: 1723-1732
11   Betran AP, Ye J, Moller ABet al. The Increasing Trend in Caesarean Section Rates: Global, Regional and National Estimates: 1990-2014. *PLoS.One.* 2016;11(2):e0148343.
12   Ye J, Zhang J, Mikolajczyk Ret al. Association between rates of caesarean section and maternal and neonatal mortality in the 21st century: a worldwide population-based ecological study with longitudinal data. *BJOG.* 2016;123(5):745-753.
13   Boerma T, Ronsmans C, Melesse DYet al. Global epidemiology of use of and disparities in caesarean sections. *Lancet* 2018;392(10155):1341-1348.
14   Sandall J, Trabe RM, Avery Let al. Short-term and long-term effects of caesarean section on the health of women and children *Lancet.* 2018 Oct 13;392(10155):1349-1357.
15   Visser GH, Campos DA, Barnea ERet al. FIGO position paper: how to stop the caesarean section epidemic. *Lancet* 2018. Oct 13;392(10155):1286-1287
16   *WHO recommendations: intrapartum care for a positive childbirth experience*. Geneva: World Health Organization, 2018.
17   Lydon-Rochelle M, Holt VL, Martin DPet al. Association between method of delivery and maternal rehospitalization. *JAMA* 2000;283(18):2411-2416.
18. Deneux-Tharaux C, Carmona E, Bouvier-Colle MHet al. Postpartum maternal mortality and cesarean delivery. *Obstet.Gynecol.* 2006;108(3 Pt 1):541-548.
19   Caughey AB, Cahill AG, Guise JMet al. Safe prevention of the primary cesarean delivery. *Am.J Obstet.Gynecol.* 2014;210(3):179-193.
20   Green L, Knight M, Seeney FMet al. The epidemiology and outcomes of women with postpartum haemorrhage requiring massive transfusion with eight or more units of red cells: a national cross-sectional study. *BJOG.* 2016;123(13):2164-2170.
21   Lydon-Rochelle M, Holt VL, Easterling TRet al. Risk of uterine rupture during labor among women with a prior cesarean delivery. *N Engl J Med* 2001;345(1):3-8.
22   Lydon-Rochelle M, Holt VL, Easterling TRet al. First-birth cesarean and placental abruption or previa at second birth(1). *Obstet Gynecol* 2001;97(5 Pt 1):765-769.
23   Yang Q, Wen SW, Oppenheimer Let al. Association of caesarean delivery for first birth with placenta praevia and placental abruption in second pregnancy. *BJOG.* 2007;114(5):609-613.
24   Gray R, Quigley MA, Hockley Cet al. Caesarean delivery and risk of stillbirth in subsequent pregnancy: a retrospective cohort study in an English population. *BJOG.* 2007;114(3):264-270.
25   Jackson S, Fleege L, Fridman Met al. Morbidity following primary cesarean delivery in the Danish National Birth Cohort. *Am.J Obstet.Gynecol.* 2012;206(2):139-5.
26   Morrison JJ, Rennie JM, Milton PJ. Neonatal respiratory morbidity and mode of delivery at term: influence of timing of elective caesarean section. *Br J Obstet Gynaecol* 1995;102(2):101-106.
27   Jain L, Dudell GG. Respiratory transition in infants delivered by cesarean section. *Semin.Perinatol.* 2006;30(5):296-304.
28   Kolas T, Saugstad OD, Daltveit AKet al. Planned cesarean versus planned vaginal delivery at term: comparison of newborn infant outcomes. *Am J Obstet Gynecol* 2006;195(6):1538-1543.
29   Kupari M, Talola N, Luukkaala Tet al. Does an increased cesarean section rate improve neonatal outcome in term pregnancies? *Arch.Gynecol.Obstet.* 2016;294(1):41-46.
30   Tracy SK, Tracy MB, Sullivan E. Admission of term infants to neonatal intensive care: a population-based study. *Birth* 2007;34(4):301-307.
31   Cardwell CR, Stene LC, Joner Get al. Caesarean section is associated with an increased risk of childhood-onset

type 1 diabetes mellitus: a meta-analysis of observational studies. *Diabetologia* 2008;51(5):726-735.

32   Black M, Bhattacharya S, Philip Set al. Planned Cesarean Delivery at Term and Adverse Outcomes in Childhood Health. *JAMA* 2015;314(21):2271-2279.

33   Thavagnanam S, Fleming J, Bromley Aet al. A meta-analysis of the association between Caesarean section and childhood asthma. *Clin.Exp.Allergy* 2008;38(4):629-633.

34   Li HT, Zhou YB, Liu JM. The impact of cesarean section on offspring overweight and obesity: a systematic review and meta-analysis. *Int.J Obes.(Lond)* 2013;37(7):893-899.

35   King JF. A short history of evidence-based obstetric care. *Best.Pract Res.Clin.Obstet.Gynaecol.* 2005;19(1):3-14.

36   Roberts CL, Tracy S, Peat B. Rates for obstetric intervention among private and public patients in Australia: population based descriptive study. *BMJ* 2000;321(7254):137-141.

37   Dahlen HG, Tracy S, Tracy Met al. Rates of obstetric intervention among low-risk women giving birth in private and public hospitals in NSW: a population-based descriptive study. *BMJ Open.* 2012;2(5).

38   Tracy SK, Sullivan EA, Wang YAet al. Birth outcomes associated with interventions in labour amongst low risk women: A population based study. *Women and Birth* 2007;(2):41-48.

39   Tracy SK, Tracy MB. Costing the cascade: estimating the cost of increased obstetric intervention in childbirth using population data. *BJOG.* 2003;110(8):717-724.

40   Peters L, Thornton C, Anke de Jongeet al. The effect of medical and operative birth interventions on child health outcomes in the first 28 days and up to 5 years of age: A linked data population-based cohort study. *Birth* 2018;45:347-357.

41   Souza JP, Betran AP, Dumont Aet al. A global reference for caesarean section rates (C-Model): a multicountry cross-sectional study. *BJOG.* 2016;123(3):427-436.

42   Lee Yeun Yi, Roberts CL, Patterson JA et al. Unexplained variation in hospital caesarean section rates. *Medical Journal of Australia* 2013;doi: 10.5694/mja13.10279(199):348-353.

43   Macfarlane AJ, Blondel B, Mohangoo ADet al. Wide differences in mode of delivery within Europe: risk-stratified analyses of aggregated routine data from the Euro-Peristat study. *BJOG.* 2016;123(4):559-568.

44   Miller S, Abalos E, Chamillard Met al. Beyond too little, too late and too much, too soon: a pathway towards evidence-based, respectful maternity care worldwide. *Lancet* 2016;388(10056):2176-2192.

45   Berwick DM. Avoiding overuse-the next quality frontier. *Lancet* 2017;390(10090):102-104.

46   Horton R, Astudillo O. The power of midwifery. *Lancet* 2014;384(9948):1075-1076.

47   Page L. Women and babies need protection from the dangers of normal birth ideology: AGAINST: Support for normal birth is crucial to safe high-quality maternity care. *BJOG.* 2017;124(9):1385.

48   Davis-Floyd R. Consuming Childbirth: The Qualified Consumption of Midwifery Care. In: Janelle S.Taylor, Linda L.Layne, Danielle R Wozniak, eds. *Consuming Motherhood*. Pp . New Brunswick, NJ : Rutgers University Press , 2004:211-248.

49   Boston Women's Health Book Collective. *Our Bodies Ourselves*. Boston: New England Free Press, 1971.

50   Markella Rutherford, elina Gallo-Cruz. "Selling the ideal birth: Rationalization and re-enchantment in the marketing of maternity care". 2015. In Susan M. Chambré, Melinda Goldner (ed.) *Patients, Consumers and Civil Society (Advances in Medical Sociology, Volume 10)* Emerald Group Publishing Limited, pp.75 – 98

51   Matthew Hilton. *The Death of a Consumer Society*. In: Royal Historical Society, ed. Cambridge, UK: Cambridge University Press on behalf of the Royal Historical Society, 2008:211-236.

52   Stiglitz J. Moral Bankruptcy: Why are we letting Wall Street off so easy? 2010. www.motherjones.com/politics/2010/01/joseph-stiglitz-wall-street-morals

53   Jordan B. Authoritative Knowledge and Its Construction. In: Robbie Davis-Floyd, Carolyn F.Sargent, eds. *Childbirth and Authoritative Knowledge*. Berkeley, CA: University of California Press, 1997:55-59.

54   Bryant J, Porter M, Tracy SKet al. Caesarean birth: consumption, safety, order, and good mothering. *Soc.Sci. Med.* 2007;65(6):1192-1201.

55   Stephanie Lee Mudge. The State of the Art: What is neo-liberalism? *Socio-Economic Review* 2008;6:703-731.

56   Perkins C.B. *The medical delivery business: Health reform, childbirth and the economic order.* New Brunswick, NJ: Rutgers University Press., 2003.

57   Bragg F, Cromwell DA, Edozien LCet al. Variation in rates of caesarean section among English NHS trusts after accounting for maternal and clinical risk: cross sectional study. *BMJ* 2010;341:c5065.

58   Coulm B, Blondel B, Alexander Set al. Potential avoidability of planned cesarean sections in a French national database. *Acta Obstet.Gynecol.Scand.* 2014;93(9):905-912.

59   Di Lallo D, Perucci CA, Bertollini Ret al. Cesarean section rates by type of maternity unit and level of obstetric care: an area-based study in central Italy. *Prev.Med.* 1996;25(2):178-185.

60   Lutomski JE, Morrison JJ, Lydon-Rochelle MT. Regional variation in obstetrical intervention for hospital birth in the Republic of Ireland, 2005-2009. *BMC.Pregnancy.Childbirth.* 2012;12:123.

61   Paranjothy S, Frost C, Thomas J. How much variation in CS rates can be explained by case mix differences? *BJOG.* 2005;112(5):658-666.

62   Betran AP, Merialdi M, Lauer JAet al. Rates of caesarean section: analysis of global, regional and national estimates. *Paediatr.Perinat.Epidemiol.* 2007;21(2):98-113.

63 Glantz JC. Obstetric variation, intervention, and outcomes: doing more but accomplishing less. *Birth* 2012;39(4):286-290.

64 Grytten J, Monkerud L, Hagen TP et al. The impact of hospital revenue on the increase in Caesarean sections in Norway. A panel data analysis of hospitals 1976-2005. *BMC.Health Serv.Res.* 2011;11:267.

65 Hoxha I, Syrogiannouli L, Luta X et al. Caesarean sections and for-profit status of hospitals: systematic review and meta-analysis. *BMJ Open.* 2017;7(2):e013670.

66 Lutomski JE, Murphy M, Devane D et al. Private health care coverage and increased risk of obstetric intervention. *BMC.Pregnancy.Childbirth.* 2014;14:13.

67 Donnellan-Fernandez R, Newman L, Reiger K. Identifying better systems design in Australian maternity care: a Boundary Critique analysis. *Health Systems* 2013;2:213-225.

68 De Vries R, Benoit C, Van Teijlingen E et al. *Birth by Design: Pregnancy, Maternity Care and Midwifery in North America and Northern Europe.* New York: Routledge, 2001.

69 Wilbanks JT, Topol EJ. Stop the privatization of health data. *Nature* 2016;535(7612):345-348.

70 Kate Rayworth. *Doughnut Economics: Seven Ways to Think Like a 21st Century Economist.* London: Random House, 2017.

71 Guilliland K, Pairman S. *The Midwifery Partnership: A model for practice.* In: Victoria University of Wellington, NZ , 1995.

72 Page L. One-to-one midwifery: restoring the "with woman" relationship in midwifery. *J Midwifery Womens Health* 2003;48(2):119-125.

73 Stenglin M, Foureur M. Designing out the Fear Cascade to increase the likelihood of normal birth. *Midwifery* 2013;29(8):819-825.

74 The Centre for Health Economics Research and Evaluation (CHERE). Public and provider views – Supporting document for the Extended Medicare Safety Net Review Report 2009. In: Australia: Commonwealth of Australia, 2009.

75 New Zealand Ministry of Health (MOH). *Maternity Services. Notice Pursuant to Section 88 of the New Zealand Public Health and Disability Act 2000 .* In: 2000.

76 Page L, McCourt C, Beake S et al. Clinical interventions and outcomes of One-to-One midwifery practice. *J Public Health Med.* 1999;21(3):243-248.

77 Beasley S, Ford N, Tracy SK et al. Collaboration in Maternity Care is achievable and practical. *Aust.N.Z.J.Obstet Gynaecol.* 2012;52:576-581.

78 Braithwaite J, Runciman WB, Merry AF. Towards safer, better healthcare: harnessing the natural properties of complex sociotechnical systems. *Qual.Saf Health Care* 2009;18(1):37-41.

79 UK MRC. *Developing and evaluating complex interventions: new guidance.* In: London UK: Medical Research Council, 2008.

80 Macfarlane F, Greenhalgh T, Humphrey C et al. A new workforce in the making? A case study of strategic human resource management in a whole-system change effort in healthcare. *J Health Organ Manag.* 2011;25(1):55-72.

81 Redshaw M, Henderson J. *Safely Delivered: a national survey of women's experience of maternity care, 2014.* Oxford UK : NPEU, 2015.

82 McCourt C, Page L. *Report on the evaluation of One-to-One midwifery.* London: Thames Valley University, 1996.

83 Tracy SK, Welsh A, Hall B et al. Caseload midwifery compared to standard or private obstetric care for first time mothers in a public teaching hospital in Australia: a cross sectional study of cost and birth outcomes. *BMC. Pregnancy.Childbirth.* 2014;14:46.

84 Sandall J, Coxon K, Mackintosh N, et al. *Relationships: the pathway to safe, high-quality maternity care. Report from the Sheila Kitzinger symposium at Green Templeton College October 2015.* Oxford UK: Green Templeton College, Oxford., 2016.

CHAPTER 12

Sustainability of maternity care in a neoliberal health environment: the potential of the midwifery model

Lorna Davies

Introduction

'The global scale, interconnectedness and economic intensity of contemporary human activity are historically unprecedented as are many of the consequent environmental and social changes. The global changes, fundamentally influence patterns of human health, international healthcare and public health activities. A.J. McMichael, 2013, p1335

Like many other areas in healthcare, maternity services appear to be at crisis point in various parts of the world. In the UK, midwives have taken strike action in the last few years in an historically unprecedented move. Midwives in New Zealand have taken their government to the steps of the High Court in a gender-based pay claim case (Small, 2016), while midwife/obstetrician Agnes Gereb, in Hungary, has been imprisoned for offering to attend women who wish to birth at home (Grace, 2018). In Sweden, maternity clinics are closing down and rates of birth-related injury are considered to be unacceptably high (Avdic, Lundborg and Vikström, 2018). It would seem that maternity services are malfunctioning at a systemic level. Many have argued that the root cause is the free market focused ideology of neoliberalism, which has influenced almost every aspect of life in many countries in the last 40 years or so, including healthcare (Glynos, 2014; Humpage, 2014; Murphy-Lawless, 2018). This chapter does not attempt to undertake an in-depth analysis of the impact of neoliberalism in maternity care. Nonetheless, those working within the field need to recognise that the resolution of political, socio-economic and infrastructural issues is imperative if countries are to provide sustainable and fully integrated maternity services. It could be argued that sustainability is the antithesis of neoliberalism, and it has been suggested that a midwifery philosophy of care transcends professional disciplines, and is effective in improving outcomes for women and babies (Renfrew et al, 2014). This chapter provides an exploration of the potential for alignment of the midwifery model of provision with the principles of sustainability, as a contribution to strengthening maternity care provision globally.

A rapidly changing world

The complex challenges that the world currently faces include climate change, population growth, loss of biodiversity and changing patterns of disease. These issues are unprecedented in scope. It is widely accepted that at least some of these effects are associated with anthropocentric (human-instigated) activity (Neumayer, 2013). For too long societies have maintained the myth that humans exist in a state of separation from the natural world. The ecosystems that sustain human life have been viewed primarily as a means of expanding economic growth. This assumption has shaped worldviews and influenced social establishments and political and economic practices. It has resulted in societal norms of behaviour that ignore or undervalue other life forms in order to maximise short-term human gain, at the risk of long-term system instability. The planet, and its components and processes, are viewed in mechanistic terms, ignoring the complexities of the ecological and social systems that all living beings are part of (Blewitt, 2014).

A framework of sustainability that promotes the protection of the natural environment, as well as the social considerations of intergenerational equity and social justice, offers a counterpoint to the existing hegemonic worldview.

The word 'sustainability' is trending

The word 'sustainability' is used extensively in the media, in politics, in corporate parlance and in public sector areas such as health and education. Yet in spite of its almost ubiquitous status, the concept is not easy to define. A relatively modern term that emerged from the environmental movement in the 1970s, sustainability means, in a literal sense, the 'capacity to endure' (Harper, 2018). It was the Brundtland Report, *Our Common Future*, which launched the concept of sustainability in a very broad and global sense, using ecological, economic and social dimensions as the 'three pillars' of sustainability (World Commission on Environment and Development (WCED), 1987).

These three pillars (or tenets) are commonly referred to as the Triple Bottom Line (3BL) (Elkington, 1998). The term was introduced to assimilate ecological, economic and social dimensions within a framework that could be effectively used by businesses and organisations. 3BL set out to measure the financial, social and environmental performance of companies and corporations, and it continues to be a pivotal concept that pervades business reporting, and business engagement with sustainability (Milne, Marcus and Gray, 2012). From an ethical perspective, the three tenets are seen to present a means of achieving a balance of ecological health, social equity and justice and economic welfare. However, much of the mainstream debate about what constitutes sustainability has paid little consideration to the worldviews of indigenous communities, such as the Māori philosophy of *whakapapa* (interconnection) and *mauri* (life-supporting capacity) (Morgan, 2004), or the African philosophy of *Ubunto* that incorporates a holistic view of the sharing of resources and spaces (Shumba, 2011). In recognition of this gap, the three tenets have been expanded to provide a more inclusive and holistic perspective of less tangible aspects such as ethical, spiritual and temporal. These additional perspectives may have special relevance with regard to the territory of childbirth. For example, the tenet of spirituality evokes inspiration, purpose and meaning, important features in the field of new life (Crowther and Hall, 2017). An ethical dimension incorporates an inclusive view of humanity as sharing resources and spaces with others (Shumba, 2011). A temporal perspective takes into account intergenerational interconnectedness across time and space and provides links to both the past and the future, engendering 'rootedness, connection and remembering' (Murphy-Lawless, 2006, p439).

Healthcare and sustainability

The economic growth-driven ideological approach of neoliberalism has been associated with significant effects on human health and wellbeing by some authors (Schroeder et al, 2012; Coburn, 2014). Such effects include the escalation of lifestyle-related non-communicable diseases and socially mediated mental health conditions (Sakellariou & Rotarou, 2017; MacNamarra, 2017). McMichael (2013) describes these changes as a syndrome

> *'that reflects the interrelated pressures, stresses, and tensions arising from an overly large world population, the pervasive and increasingly systemic environmental impact of many economic activities, urbanization, the spread of consumerism, and the widening gap between rich and poor.'* (p1335)

In recent years there has been a growing interest in the value of adopting more sustainable approaches within healthcare. Sustainable health organisations have proliferated in many countries, pledging to transform healthcare to achieve objectives relating to sustainability (Davies 2017). Journals such as the *BMJ* and the *Lancet* have published editions advancing the agenda of climate change in health (*Lancet* Planetary Health Series 2017; *BMJ* 2019). A number of midwifery research studies have explored the concept of sustainability in relation to models of care and resilience (Sandall et al, 2016; Hunter and Warren, 2014; McAra Couper et al, 2014; Crowther et al, 2017). The findings have provided some valuable insights into broader workforce needs, especially in relation to burnout and self-care. However, the studies do not specifically explore how a sustainability framework could inform maternity care, particularly in relation to the tenets model of sustainability (Davies, 2017). Similarly, in obstetrics, although the word 'sustainability' is more prevalent in articles and textbooks than a decade ago, the word is used in a very generic sense with the concept largely used as a driver for economic benefit (Davies, 2017). This might suggest the need for a more philosophical discourse around the integration and application of sustainability within maternity care.

Childbirth and sustainability

Since the evolutionary emergence of *Homo sapiens*, women have given birth. Vaginal birth has proved to be a sustainable mammalian act of reproduction and it has allowed for the propagation of the human population. It would also appear from archaeological evidence that birth attendants have been around to support the process of human childbirth for as long as women have been doing it. Over millennia, midwifery and childbirth practice has continuously adapted and transformed in order to meet the changing needs of women, society and more recently the maternity care professions. As Wickham (2016) states, knowledge of history allows understanding of what it is like to '*practice an ancient art in a modern world*' as a sustainable healthcare practice.

Midwifery: a sustainable healthcare practice

Sustainability is about learning from the past. It is also about being mindful of what lies ahead with regard to the future of humankind and the relationships between humans and all other living entities. Those who work within the context of maternity care with mothers and their babies are, by default, working with 'the future of humankind' in an intergenerational context.

The midwifery model defined by ICM (2014) is sited within a social model, in which pregnancy and birth are viewed as normal physiological life experiences rather than as medical events (Kirkham, 2010; Miller & Wilkes, 2015). This manifests as a primary care-based community service that works towards strengthening family relationships and promoting normality within the context of birth (ICM, 2014), integrated into effective collaborative obstetric, neonatal and wider medical care where this is needed, as well as into social support from family and others, such as TBAs and doulas (Renfrew et al, 2016). The model supports a 'low tech, high touch' approach, which should result in the minimising of unnecessary intervention, and rapid seamless access to such interventions when they are really needed (Davis, 2004). The provision of maternity care should require very little in terms of resources where pregnancy, labour, birth, and the postpartum periods are straightforward. Designing services on this basis would also ensure that minimal waste is generated (Martis, 2011).

Community-based care and continuity of care

Within a primary-care model, care may be provided in women's homes or community settings, where the focus is on enhancing and supporting pregnancy and childbirth as a normal life process. In this context, support of the physical, psychosocial, cultural and spiritual wellbeing of the woman is more likely to be sensitive to the particular, dynamic needs of the woman and her family (Hatem et al, 2008; RCM, 2014; Homer, 2016).

A holistic midwifery model depends on positive interpersonal relationships between the caregiver and the service user (Sandall, 2016). This is much more likely to be realised if maternity care is set up within a framework of continuity of care (Homer, 2016; Sandall et al, 2016). Indeed, many definitions of social sustainability are marked by their inclusion of the terms 'communities', 'relationships' and 'communication' (Barron & Gauntlett, 2002).

In providing continuity of carer, midwives and increasingly doulas are given the opportunity to foster relationships that enable them to educate, encourage, support and listen to women. Where they are able to do this, obstetricians and GPs and the women they work with are likely to benefit from an approach based around relational aspects of care (Barker et al, 2017). There is an abundance of evidence that demonstrates the benefits for both women and midwives when a continuity model is mindfully adopted. The relationship that the woman develops with her caregivers over the period of childbearing may have a significance that lies beyond the physical monitoring processes that are carried out during this time (Sandall 2014; Page 2014). In such a relational context, all care providers, and particularly midwives, are in a strong position to facilitate the connection between the woman and her baby. Early attachment in the mother/baby dyad is theorised to provide the individual with a greater ability to form relationships throughout life (Van der Horst, 2011; Viaux-Savelon, 2016). This is an important consideration in terms of social sustainability because it is theorised that the ability to forge relationships is a significant factor in achieving wellbeing (Helne and Hirvilammi, 2015). People who readily form relationships are said to be generally happier, healthier and more likely to make a positive contribution to society (Layard, 2011; Adler, Dolan and Kavetsos, 2017).

If social sustainability hinges on positive relationships, then all maternity care givers have an important role in promoting socially sustainable healthcare more generally. In midwife-led continuity of care models, the midwife is able to play a significant role in connecting women (and their significant family members) with others in their local community, by taking on the role of 'social connector' (Gladwell, 2000). This may be achieved in the form of childbirth and parenting education, or through other ventures that may promote relationships and assist women in establishing their own new network of friends and support. This model could also be adopted by other maternity care providers. An example of where this has been successful is the Centering Pregnancy Scheme, in which women attend their antenatal assessment within a group setting and then share experiences and discussion with the guidance and support of midwives (Gaudion et al, 2011; Thiellen, 2012). Midwives and doulas may also act as social connectors by encouraging the active involvement of partners or other family members, where, with skilful communication and interpersonal skills, existing relationships may be strengthened. Facilitation of social connection may also involve other members of the community, for example, by providing education about pregnancy and birth in the local community promoting the benefits of physiological birth, or organising tours of birthing facilities for grandmothers. In the role of social connector, carers have an opportunity to integrate information about issues relating to sustainability. Indeed, women's groups in low-income countries are associated with dramatic improvements in maternal and child survival, with minimal impact on resource use (Prost, 2013).

In high-income countries, birth at home or in a birth centre has significant cost advantages over hospital birth (Sandall et al, 2016; Rogers et al, 2016). Such birthing environments carry less risk of intervention with no additional risk for most healthy women and babies, and they therefore are more likely to result in lower resource use and less likelihood of the need for follow-on care.

Conclusion

In practice, the strategies that maternity care providers can draw upon to effect change are dependent on the extent of the control that they have over their immediate working conditions and environments. However, with time, trust and patience, even in difficult circumstances, it is possible to find new ways of thinking, doing and being that may facilitate change. Any adoption of a sustainable framework will require a paradigmatic shift in thinking. Capra (1986) describes paradigms as:

> 'A constellation of concepts, values, perceptions and practices shared by a community, which forms a particular vision of reality and a collective mood that is the basis of the way the community organises itself'. (p14)

It is important to remember that dominant social paradigms are only ever contingent on local cultural norms and values. These can shift over time. Consequently, windows of opportunity arise that can give way to discussion of new paradigms and a paradigm shift can even be enacted. What is needed are ways of working that encourage human connection and engagement and transcend systemic flaws and shortfalls. Midwives specifically, and maternity carers more widely, have adapted and provided agency for change across millennia. It may be time to rise to the challenge yet again if the care provided for women, their babies and their families is to be sustainable in the long term.

Key points for consideration

- Vow to become more politicised. It's too easy to become engrossed in our own day-to-day activities and to overlook the socio-economic and political occurrences that impact on our lives and practice.
- Consider how the tenets of sustainability align with any projects or developments such as guidelines or policies in your own workplace.
- Promote, protect and preserve physiological childbirth at every opportunity. It is the cornerstone of sustainable practice.
- Use every opportunity to be a 'social connector' in practice both with clients and colleagues.
- Join a sustainability and healthcare group or forum such as the Centre for Sustainable Healthcare (UK); Health Care without Harm (US); Ora Taiao (New Zealand Climate Change and Health Council) or Healthy Planet UK.

References

Adler, MD., Dolan, Kavetsos, G. (2017) Would you choose to be happy? Tradeoffs between happiness and the other dimensions of life in a large population survey, *Journal of Economic Behavior & Organization*. Vol. 139 Pages 60-73,

Avdic, D. Lundborg, P . Vikström J (2018) Mergers and Birth Outcomes: Evidence from Maternity Ward Closures IZA Institute of Labour Economics. Bonn http://ftp.iza.org/dp11772.pdf

Barker I, Steventon A, Deeny SR 2017 Association between continuity of care in general practice and hospital admissions for ambulatory care sensitive conditions: cross sectional study of routinely collected, person level data. BMJ. 1;356:j84. doi: 10.1136/bmj.j84.

Barron, L. and Gauntlett, E. (2002) "'Housing and Sustainable Communities Indicators Project',." In , 4. Adelaide. http://www.adelaide.sa.gov.au/soc/pdf/barron_gauntlett.pdf.

Bick, D (Findings from a UK feasibility study of the Centering Pregnancy model.British Journal of Midwifery. Vol. 19 N0.12 pp.796-802

Blewitt, J. (2014) *Understanding Sustainable Development*. 2nd ed. Milton Park, Didcot: Taylor and Francis.

BMJ (2019) Climate Change. https://www.bmj.com/campaign/climate-change

Capra, F. (1986) *The Concept of Paradigm and Paradigm Shift*. ReVision 9 (1): 14

Coburn, D. (2014). Neoliberalism and Health. *The Wiley Blackwell Encyclopedia of Health, Illness, Behavior, and Society*.

Crowther S, and Hall, J. (2017) *Spirituality and Childbirth*, Abingdon, Oxon, Routledge.

Crowther, S. (2017) Resilience and sustainability amongst maternity care providers. In Thomson G Schmied V, editors: *Psychosocial resilience and risk in the perinatal period: Implications and guidance for professionals*. Abingdon, Oxon, Routledge, pp.185-200.

Davis, E. (2004). *Heart & Hands: A Midwife's Guide to Pregnancy & Birth*. Celestial Arts.

Downe, S., Finlayson, K., Oladapo, O. T., Bonet, M., & Gülmezoglu, A. M. (2018). What matters to women during childbirth: A systematic qualitative review. *PloS one, 13*(4), e0194906. doi:10.1371/journal.pone.0194906

Elkington, J. (1998) *Cannibals with Forks: The Triple Bottom Line of 21st Century Business*. New Society Publishers.

Gaudion, A. Menka, Y. Demilew, J. Walton, C. Yiannouzis, K. Robbins, J. and Schindler- Rising,S. (2011) Centering Pregnancy: Moving from 'Traditional' Individual Antenatal Care to Group Care. British journal of Midwifery. Vol 19.No 7.433-438

Grace, N. (2018) Agnes Gereb sentenced to two years in prison for attending home births. ARM News. 18th January 2018 www.midwifery.org.uk/news/agnes-gereb-sentenced-to-two-years-in-prison-for-attending-home-births

Gladwell, M. *(2000). The Tipping Point: How Little Things Can Make a Big Difference. New York:* Little Brown.

Glynos, J. (2014) "Neoliberalism, Markets, Fantasy: The Case of Health and Social Care." *Psychoanalysis, Culture and Society,* 19 (1). 5 – 12

Harper, D. (2018) Online Etymology Dictionary. https://www.etymonline.com/

Helne, T and Hirvilammi T (2015) Wellbeing and Sustainability: A relational approach. *Sustainable Development*. 23: (3) 167-175 https://doi.org/10.1002/sd.1581

Homer, C.S.E. (2016) "Models of Maternity Care: Evidence for Midwifery Continuity of Care." *The Medical Journal of Australia* 205 (8): 370–74. doi:10.5694/mja16.00844.

Humpage, L. (2014) *Policy Change, Public Attitudes and Social Citizenship: Does Neoliberalism Matter?* Bristol: Policy Press.

Hunter, B. and Warren, L. (2014). "Midwives' Experiences of Workplace Resilience." Midwifery, Special Focus on Mental Health and Special Focus on Education, 30 (8): 926–34. doi:10.1016/j.midw.2014.03.010.

International Confederation Midwives (2014) Philosophy and Model of Midwifery Care. https://www. internationalmidwives.org/assets/files/definitions-files/2018/06/eng-philosophy-and-model-of-midwifery-care.pdf

Lancet Planetary Health Series 2017 https://doi.org/10.1016/S2542-5196(17)30013-X https://www.thelancet.com/journals/lanplh/article/PIIS2542-5196(17)30013-X/fulltext

McAra-Couper, J. Gilkison, A. Crowther,S. Hunter, M. Hotchin, C. and Gunn.J. (2014) "Partnership and Reciprocity with Women Sustain Lead Maternity Carer Midwives in Practice." *New Zealand College of Midwives Journal* 49 (June): 29–33. doi:10.12784/nzcomjnl49.2014.5.29-33.

McMichael, A.J. (2013) Globalisation, Climate Change and Human Health. N Engl J Med; 368:1335-1343April 4, 2013DOI: 10.1056/NEJMra1109341.

McNamara, C. (2017) Trade liberalization and social determinants of health: A state of the literature review, *Social Science & Medicine*, 176, (1): 1-13 doi: 10.1016/j.socscimed.2016.12.017

Martis, . (2011) "Good Housekeeping in Midwifery Practice." In *Sustainability, Midwifery and Birth*, edited by Davies,L. Daellenbach, R. and Kensington, M. 141–55. London: Routledge.

Miller, S. and Wilkes, L. (2015). "Working in Partnership." In *Preparation for Practice*, edited by Sally Pairman, Sally K Tracy, Jan Pincombe, and Carol Thorogood, 3rd ed., 412–26. Morrinsville: Elsevier Health Sciences.

Milne, M. J. and Gray, R. (2012). "W(h)Ither Ecology? The Triple Bottom Line, the Global Reporting Initiative, and Corporate Sustainability Reporting." *Journal of Business Ethics* 118 (1): 13–29. doi:10.1007/s10551-012-1543-8.

Morgan, B. (2004). "A Tangata Whenua Perspective on Sustainability Using the Mauri Model." In , 14. Auckland.

Murphy-Lawless, J. (2006). "Birth and Mothering in Today's Social Order: The Challenge of New Knowledge's." *MIDIRS Midwifery Digest* 16 (4): 439–44.

Murphy-Lawless, J. (2018) Confronting the state of emergency which is our maternity services in Murphy Lawless, J. Mander, R. and Edwards N (Eds) (2018) Untangling the Maternity Crisis, First, London, Routledge,

Neumayer, E. (2013). *Weak versus Strong Sustainability : Exploring the Limits of Two Opposing Paradigms*. Cheltenham:

Edward Elgar Publishing.

Page, L. (2014) "The known and trusted midwife." *British Journal of Midwifery*, 22(4), p. 234

Prost A, Colbourn T, Seward N, Azad K, Coomarasamy A, Copas A, Houweling TA, Fottrell E, Kuddus A, Lewycka S, MacArthur C, Manandhar D, Morrison J, Mwansambo C, Nair N, Nambiar B, Osrin D, Pagel C, Phiri T, Pulkki-Brännström AM, Rosato M, Skordis-Worrall J, Saville N, More NS, Shrestha B, Tripathy P, Wilson A, Costello A 2013 Women's groups practising participatory learning and action to improve maternal and newborn health in low-resource settings: a systematic review and meta-analysis. Lancet. 2013 May 18;381(9879):1736-46. doi: 10.1016/S0140-6736(13)60685-6.

Renfrew, M.J., McFadden, A., Bastos, M.H., Campbell, J., Channon, A.A., Cheung, N.F., Delage, D., Downe, S.M., Kennedy, H.P. Malata, A .McCormick, F. Wick,L. Declercq,E. (2014) *Midwifery* and *quality care*: *findings* from a *new evidence informed framework* for *maternal* and *newborn care*, The *Lancet 384(9948):11291145*, 2014

Rogers, A. J., Rogers, N. G., Kilgore, M. L., Subramaniam, A., & Harper, L. M. (2016). Economic Evaluations Comparing a Trial of Labor with an Elective Repeat Cesarean Delivery: A Systematic Review. *Value in health : the journal of the International Society for Pharmacoeconomics and Outcomes Research*, *20*(1), 163-173.

Sakellariou, D., & Rotarou, E. S. (2017). The effects of neoliberal policies on access to healthcare for people with disabilities. *International journal for equity in health*, *16*(1), 199. doi:10.1186/s12939-017-0699-3

Sandall, J. (2014) The contribution of continuity of midwifery care to high quality maternity care. Royal College of Midwives https://www.rcog.org.uk/globalassets/documents/guidelines/highqualitywomenshealth careproposalforchange.pdf.Accessed.

Sandall J, Soltani H, Gates S, Shennan A, Devane D.(2016) Midwife-led continuity models versus other models of care for childbearing women. *Cochrane Database of Systematic Reviews,* Issue 4. Art. No.: CD004667. DOI: 10.1002/14651858.CD004667.pub5.

Schroeder, K, Thompson, T. Frith, K. and Pencheon, D. (2012) *Sustainable Healthcare*. Chichester: John Wiley & Sons.

Shumba, Overson. 2011. "Commons Thinking, Ecological Intelligence and the Ethical and Moral Framework of Ubuntu : An Imperative for Sustainable Development." *Journal of Media and Communication Studies* 3 (3): 84–96.

Small, J. (2016) "Government in Mediation with Midwives over Gender Pay Discrimination." *Sunday Star Times*, August 10.

Thielen K. (2012). Exploring the group prenatal care model: a critical review of the literature. *The Journal of perinatal education*, *21*(4), 209-18.

Viaux-Savelon S. (2016) Establishing Parent-Infant Interactions. In: Sutter-Dallay AL., Glangeaud-Freudenthal NC., Guedeney A., Riecher-Rösler A. (eds) *Joint Care of Parents and Infants in Perinatal Psychiatry*. Springer Cham. Heidelberg New York Dordrecht London.

Wickham S (2016) Midwifery, resilience and sustainability. Dr Sarah Wickham. https://www.sarawickham.com/research-updates/midwives-resilience-and-sustainability/ accessed 5th January 2019.

World Commission on Environment and Development. (1987) *Our Common Future*. Oxford: Oxford University Press.

PART III

New thinking
in the field: the
interconnectivity
of psychological,
emotional,
and physiological
states

CHAPTER 13

Epigenetics in healthy women and babies: short and medium term maternal and neonatal outcomes

Soo Downe, Holly Powell Kennedy, Hannah Dahlen and Jeffrey Craig

Introduction

In a 1990 article in the *British Medical Journal* entitled 'The fetal and infant origins of adult disease; the womb may be more important than the home', British epidemiologist David Barker set out his hypothesis linking early life events with risk for chronic diseases.[1] He based it on studies linking birth weight and infant mortality with an elevated risk for cardiometabolic diseases in adults, and cited evidence that neurodevelopmental and neurodegenerative diseases also fitted his model. Barker also recommended that research should be directed towards the intrauterine environment rather than the environments in later childhood and adulthood. Although his advice has been largely unheeded, Barker's hypothesis has evolved into the phenomenon known as the developmental origins of health and disease (DOHaD) and has since gained mainstream acceptance. This chapter discusses the growing evidence on the epigenetic origins of disease, and then outlines the developing hypothesis that the processes of physiological labour and birth might be epigenetic triggers for positive health for the offspring, in the short, medium and longer term.

Exploring the epigenetic origins of disease

The DOHaD phenomenon has grown through evidence from studies of animals and humans which have shown that prenatal and early postnatal factors such as stress, nutrition and inflammation in mothers and infants can predispose offspring to chronic diseases, ranging from the cardiometabolic to the neurocognitive.[2] These include childhood onset disorders such as autism and obesity, adolescent onset disorders such as schizophrenia, and adult onset disorders such as Parkinson's Disease, cardiovascular disease, cerebrovascular disease and some cancers. No precise timing for this early developmental vulnerability has been pinned down, and is likely to depend on the different maturation times of developing tissues and organs, but a useful concept is the idea of the sensitive 'first 1,000 days' from conception to age two.[3] The main goals of DOHaD research are to identify biomarkers and mechanisms that link early-life environment with later health outcomes. This critical knowledge will lead to early detection of chronic disorders, leading to early interventions in childhood in place of treatment in adulthood.

There is accumulating evidence that epigenetics is one of the mechanisms mediating DOHaD.[4] Epigenetic state has strong ties to development: epigenetic control of gene expression guides cell specialisation. Epigenetic mechanisms involve chemical modification of the DNA molecule or the proteins that bind to DNA, and combinations of epigenetic modifications at each gene determine its activity. The most widely-studied epigenetic modification is the methylation of the cytosine base of the cytosine-phosphate-guanine (CpG) sequence. CpG methylation is associated with reduced gene expression when present at the promoter – the region of a gene from which transcription is initiated.

As epigenetic state is a likely mediator of the effects of early life environment on later health outcomes, epigenetic studies of DOHaD have been based on the broad question of whether we can detect the precise genetic locations at which early-life environment can 'program', in Barker's parlance, risk for later disease. This is being investigated through use of embedding epigenetic analysis within prospective cohort studies and randomised controlled trials, and such research has advanced in areas including nutrition,[3] stress and trauma,[5] physical exercise,[6] and environmental toxins.[7,8] In parallel to human studies, animal studies are providing essential information about the role of epigenetics in DOHaD, aided by shorter generation times and the ability to sample tissues such as brain that are not accessible from humans.[9]

A landmark human DOHaD study is that of the Dutch famine,[10,11] in which undernutrition in early gestation at the end of World War Two was linked, 60 years later, to an increased risk of a range of chronic diseases and epigenetic differences in a number of genes compared to unexposed siblings. A notable example in animals is a set of experiments in rats centred around the effects of neglect on stress response in later life.[12,13] Rats that were not licked and groomed in the first few days of postnatal life grew up to be more sensitive to stress as adults than cared-for controls, and had altered DNA methylation within a region of DNA that regulates the activity of the glucocorticoid receptor gene involved in stress response. This series of studies went further, to show that pharmaceutical and nutritional interventions reversed the phenotypic and epigenetic effects of perinatal neglect.

Most human studies on the role of epigenetics in DOHaD have focused on the relationship between early-life environment and epigenetic state; few have focused on epigenetic state as a potential predictor of chronic disease risk[14-16] and even fewer have put the two together to link early-life environment, epigenetic state in the first 1,000 days and risk for chronic disease.[17] There are even fewer studies on the impact of intrapartum or postnatal events, such as caesarean section[18] or breastfeeding[19] on the epigenetics of the neonate. As far as we are aware there are no studies to date looking at this issue through a health-promoting lens. Taking this approach opens up 'different questions' (Kennedy, 2018) about which factors during labour and birth could promote optimal epigenetic states for long-term wellbeing in offspring.

The next section of this chapter examines the epidemiological evidence relating to the impact of intrapartum interventions on longer term ill-health, and how epigenetics may explain these findings. The subsequent section takes up the issue of longer term wellbeing.

Studies of birth interventions and chronic non-communicable disease

Epidemiological studies have linked mode of birth (particularly caesarean section) to increasing rates of asthma, eczema, Type 1 diabetes, infant bronchiolitis and obesity.[20-30] There is epidemiological and biological evidence of an increase in short-term effects in babies from caesarean section such as impairments in lung function, reduced thermogenic response, altered metabolism, altered feeding, altered immune phenotype and altered blood pressure.[20] Caesarean section has been linked to asthma and allergies[20,24,27,28] gastroenteritis, Type 1 diabetes,[21] childhood leukaemia,[33,34] testicular cancer,[22] obesity,[23] multiple sclerosis[26] and potential brain development.[31,32] Some critics dispute these findings, since they are generally the result of either retrospective or prospective cohort studies that cannot rule out the influence of family history, or other factors. However, in general, the researchers in this area try to control for a wide range of pre-existing factors, and the consistency of the findings in many studies is increasingly convincing.

The biological plausibility of a real cause/effect relationship is strengthened by epigenetic data in this area. The impact of mode of birth on DNA methylation has been previously reported.[18,35] In 2009, Schlinzig and colleagues[18] studied 37 healthy term infants who were born by caesarean section without labour (n=16) or by vaginal birth (n=21). They extracted DNA from the babies' cord blood at birth and again at 3–5 days post-birth when the newborn screening heel-prick was done. They found that a global measure of DNA methylation in white blood cells demonstrated higher methylation at birth if the baby was born by caesarean section compared to vaginal birth (p<0.001). At 3–5 days, while DNA methylation patterns did not alter in the vaginal group, they significantly decreased in the caesarean group. Five years later, Almgren and colleagues also examined neonatal cord blood following caesarean section with no labour and vaginal birth.[35] They found DNA from CD34+ cells from babies delivered by caesarean section were globally more methylated than DNA from babies born vaginally (p=0.02). They also found a relationship between the length of labour and DNA methylation. The researchers hypothesised that altered methylation may have implications for disease in later life.

Much of the emphasis in this area has been on mode of birth. However, more recently scientists have begun to consider the impact of other intrapartum interventions, specifically induction and augmentation of labour. The complex differences between the biological and neurohormonal effects of endogenous compared to exogenous oxytocin have been explored in detail in Chapter 2. A recent study has looked at both mode of birth and labour induction (separately and together) in a large Australian cohort of almost half a million healthy mothers and babies.[36] The data show impacts of childbirth interventions on chronic non-communicable conditions up to the age of at least five years old. Further analysis up to the age of 10 for the children is currently in progress.

If the mediating effect of mode of birth is stress, this could be a similar pathway for labour induction/augmentation. The use of exogenous oxytocin could impact on stress response and maternal-paternal-infant bonding in the first few days of life.[37] With the rapid rise of induction and augmentation in some high and middle-income countries this needs to be examined urgently. Based on the 2013 EPIIC (Epigenetic Impact of Childbirth) hypothesis, the timing of both a-stress and dys-stress events may be important for development, with compensatory mechanisms becoming overwhelmed over time. Positive maternal mood and sensitive mothering, which are modulated by endogenous oxytocin, are critical to normal child development.[38,39] Given the evidence that intrapartum factors can predict postpartum mood disturbance[40] and successful or unsuccessful breastfeeding[41,42] and that perinatal manipulation of the oxytocin system can predict dysfunctional maternal care in animals[43,44] the oxytocin receptor gene (OXTR) is a potential candidate for epigenetic modulation.

From chronic disease to wellbeing

As can be seen from the brief overview above, the field of intrapartum epigenetics is now growing. However, few researchers have hypothesised that labour itself may be an important salutogenic phenomenon that is an essential, priming agent in the dynamic process of labour and birth. This concept of labour as a dynamic salutogenic phenomenon was first proposed by Downe and McCourt in 2004[46] (reprinted in this volume). In 2013, the EPIIC hypothesis proposed that, when physiological labour and birth occurs (primarily without intervention), a healthy, positive form of stress (eustress) is exerted on the mother and baby.[47] The argument was made that eustress might be an important mediator of physiological epigenomic effects on specific genes, such as those that program immune responses, or weight regulation. Excessively high levels of stress during labour and birth (dys-tress) and excessively low levels (a-stress) were hypothesised to be associated with pathological priming, principally through the epigenetic pathway. The EPIIC hypothesis suggests that eustress during labour is physiologically desirable, and that it may enable optimal epigenetic priming in the neonate. In later publications[48] the EPIIC team have suggested that the EPIIC hypothesis and so-called Extended Hygiene Hypothesis[49] could both be working together to establish the optimal environment for long-term wellbeing for the offspring. The former appears to operate through epigenetic priming and the latter through seeding of the neonatal gut microbiome through ingestion of vaginal flora during birth. The hygiene hypothesis is explored in more detail in Chapter 14. Working from the perspective of both these theories may help generate a more effective synergistic analysis of the situation.

What does this mean? The complex and cascading events of labour

The context in which this new knowledge is sited is one in which technological interventions in labour and birth are increasing exponentially, with very little understanding of the potential longer-term consequences for the mother, or for her baby. For example, induction of labour is increasing worldwide. Rates doubled in the United States between 1990 and 2012, despite no change in pregnancy complications.[50] The 2015 'Listening to Mothers' study[51] found that 41% of 2,400 women reported that their providers tried to start their labour. Of those that were induced, 44% were because the baby was due or overdue, and not for any actual pathology. An Australian study found that rates ranged from 9.7% to 41.2% between hospitals between 2010 and 2011,[52] which is a rate that is very unlikely to be explained by clinical need. In the UK the most recent data show that induction of labour rates have increased from 29.4% in 2016–17 to 31.6% in 2017–18.[53] In the north of England region, this rate was almost 50%.

It is biologically implausible that one-third, or even one-half, of pregnant women need to have their labour induced for their health, or for the health of their baby. It is arguably reckless to expose so many women and babies to such an intervention without knowing the long-term consequences. Indeed, the World Health Organization (WHO) has cautioned against unnecessary interventions in childbirth.[54] Every intervention (or non-intervention) will have a 'knock on' effect on the consequent neurohormonal and/ or physiological state of the labouring mother and her baby. Clinicians are 'instruments' of care.[55] Clinical beliefs and values translate into decisions and actions and ultimately contribute to what happens to a woman during her labour and birth. In other words, intrapartum care is socialised, and reflects the setting in which it occurs, and the ethos of the caregivers within that setting. This socialisation probably contributes directly to the mother's capacity to effectively produce endogenous oxytocin and modulate the sensitive interacting catecholamine, beta-endorphin, and hormonal demands of labour and birth. These, in turn, may influence epigenetic priming in the offspring, with very long term, or even transgenerational, effects.

Conclusion

The philosophical premise of healthcare is to 'first, do no harm'. There is no question that some women will need intervention in order to have an optimal outcome. However, as discussed throughout this book, in a global society that increasingly values technology and algorithms over human touch and wisdom, it is probably unsurprising that funding for technical solutions is prioritised over resources for personal presence and watchful waiting, even though the neurohormonal and biological benefits of the latter are well known. Not only can unnecessary interventions cause harms, many of which may not yet be apparent, they can also strip a woman of her confidence in the physiological capacity of her body, her ability to birth, and, potentially, her ability to mother. The onset and progression of spontaneous labour and subsequent birth is exquisitely timed through evolutionary processes to be most beneficial to the mother and infant,[56] and should therefore be trusted on an individual basis, until shown to be actually veering into pathology. To do otherwise leads to situations in which many healthy women will receive 'too much too soon', with opportunity costs for healthcare systems that will mean there are limited resources when women and babies really do need interventions, meaning that some who are desperately in need of intervention receive 'too little too late'.[57] In the light of the emerging evidence associated with epigenetic processes, a re-evaluation of the value of physiological labour and birth is particularly important and urgent.

Future implications for exploring this critical balance are twofold. Reversing the trend in which women, clinicians, and society do not trust birth will require examining models of care that are successful in achieving the optimal balance, and listening to women themselves. This process needs to be underpinned by research that identifies and describes aspects of care that optimise, and those that disturb, the biological/physiological processes for healthy childbearing women and foetus/newborn infants and those who experience complications.[58] This includes research into the epigenetic consequences of labour and birth in the short, medium and longer term.

Key points for consideration

- Evidence is growing that what happens during labour and birth may have epigenetic consequences that could have profound impacts on the neonatal immune system.

- The long-term effects of this on non-communicable autoimmune disease are still at an early stage of investigation.

- New questions arise about the positive value of physiological labour and birth on neonatal, child and adult priming for health and wellbeing, that could even be transgenerational.

- Health professionals, service designers, policy-makers, service users and civil society should be informed about what is known (and what is currently not known) in this area.

- Until the evidence is more substantial, it is incumbent on those designing and delivering maternity care to pay attention to the precautionary principle, and to design services to minimise childbirth interventions unless they are highly likely to bring more harm than benefit, on the basis of the moral obligation to 'first, do no harm'.

References

1   Barker DJ. The fetal and infant origins of adult disease. Bmj. 1990;301(6761):1111.
2   Gluckman PD, Hanson MA, Buklijas T. A conceptual framework for the developmental origins of health and disease. Journal of Developmental Origins of Health and Disease. 2010;1(1):6-18.
3   Koletzko B, Brands B, Chourdakis M, Cramer S, Grote V, Hellmuth C, et al. The Power of Programming and the EarlyNutrition project: opportunities for health promotion by nutrition during the first thousand days of life and beyond. Ann Nutr Metab. 2014;64(3-4):187-96.
4   Gluckman PD. Epigenetics and metabolism in 2011: Epigenetics, the life-course and metabolic disease. Nat Rev Endocrinol. 2012;8(2):74-6.
5   Ryan J, Chaudieu I, Ancelin ML, Saffery R. Biological underpinnings of trauma and post-traumatic stress disorder: focusing on genetics and epigenetics. Epigenomics. 2016;8(11):1553-69.
6   Denham J. Exercise and epigenetic inheritance of disease risk. Acta Physiol (Oxf). 2017.
7   Ji H, Biagini Myers JM, Brandt EB, Brokamp C, Ryan PH, Khurana Hershey GK. Air pollution, epigenetics, and asthma. Allergy Asthma Clin Immunol. 2016;12:51.
8   Manikkam M, Haque MM, Guerrero-Bosagna C, Nilsson EE, Skinner MK. Pesticide methoxychlor promotes the epigenetic transgenerational inheritance of adult-onset disease through the female germline. PLoS One.

2014;9(7):e102091.

9   Dickinson H, Moss TJ, Gatford KL, Moritz KM, Akison L, Fullston T, et al. A review of fundamental principles for animal models of DOHaD research: an Australian perspective. J Dev Orig Health Dis. 2016;7(5):449-72.

10 Heijmans BT, Tobi EW, Stein AD, Putter H, Blauw GJ, Susser ES, et al. Persistent epigenetic differences associated with prenatal exposure to famine in humans. Proceedings of the National Academy of Sciences of the United States of America. 2008;105(44):17046-9.

11 Portrait F, Teeuwiszen E, Deeg D. Early life undernutrition and chronic diseases at older ages: the effects of the Dutch famine on cardiovascular diseases and diabetes. Soc Sci Med. 2011;73(5):711-8.

12 McGowan PO, Meaney MJ, Szyf M. Diet and the epigenetic (re)programming of phenotypic differences in behavior. Brain Res. 2008;1237:12-24.

13 Weaver IC, Champagne FA, Brown SE, Dymov S, Sharma S, Meaney MJ, et al. Reversal of maternal programming of stress responses in adult offspring through methyl supplementation: altering epigenetic marking later in life. J Neurosci. 2005;25(47):11045-54.

14 Relton CL, Groom A, St Pourcain B, Sayers AE, Swan DC, Embleton ND, et al. DNA methylation patterns in cord blood DNA and body size in childhood. PloS one. 2012;7(3):e31821.

15 Clarke-Harris R, Wilkin TJ, Hosking J, Pinkney J, Jeffery AN, Metcalf BS, et al. Peroxisomal proliferator activated receptor-gamma-co-activator-1alpha promoter methylation in blood at 5-7 years predicts adiposity from 9 to 14 years (EarlyBird 50). Diabetes. 2014.

16 Lillycrop KA, Costello PM, Teh AL, Murray RJ, Clarke-Harris R, Barton SJ, et al. Association between perinatal methylation of the neuronal differentiation regulator HES1 and later childhood neurocognitive function and behaviour. Int J Epidemiol. 2015;44(4):1263-76.

17 Godfrey KM, Sheppard A, Gluckman PD, Lillycrop KA, Burdge GC, McLean C, et al. Epigenetic gene promoter methylation at birth is associated with child's later adiposity. Diabetes. 2011;60(5):1528-34.

18 Schlinzig T, Johansson S, Gunnar A, Ekstrom TJ, Norman M. Epigenetic modulation at birth - altered DNA-methylation in white blood cells after Caesarean section. Acta Paediatr. 2009;98(7):1096-9.

19 McInerny TK. Breastfeeding, early brain development, and epigenetics--getting children off to their best start. Breastfeed Med. 2014;9(7):333-4.

20 Hyde MJ, Mostyn A, Modi N, Kemp PR. The health implications of birth by cesarean section. Biol Rev Camb Philos Soc. 2012;87:229–43. [PubMed]

21 Cardwell CR, Stene LC, Joner G, et al. Cesarean section is associated with an increased risk of childhood-onset type 1 diabetes mellitus: a meta-analysis of observational studies. Diabetologia. 2008;51:726–35. [PubMed]

22 Cook MB, Graubard BI, Rubertone MV, Erickson RL, McGlynn KA. Perinatal factors and the risk of testicular germ cell tumors. Int J Cancer. 2008;122:2600–6. [PubMed]

23 Goldani HA, Bettiol H, Barbieri MA, et al. Cesarean delivery is associated with an increased risk of obesity in adulthood in a Brazilian birth cohort study. Am J Clin Nutr. 2011;93:1344–7. [PubMed]

24 Hakansson S, Kallen K. Cesarean section increases the risk of hospital care in childhood for asthma and gastroenteritis. Clin Exp Allergy. 2003;33:757–64. [PubMed]

25 Joffe TH, Simpson NA. Cesarean section and risk of asthma. The role of intrapartum antibiotics: a missing piece? J Pediatr. 2009;154:154. [PubMed]

26 Maghzi AH, Etemadifar M, Heshmat-Ghahdarijani K, Nonahal S, Minagar A, Moradi V. Cesarean delivery may increase the risk of multiple sclerosis. Mult Scler. 2012;18:468–71. [PubMed]

27 Pistiner M, Gold DR, Abdulkerim H, Hoffman E, Celedon JC. Birth by cesarean section, allergic rhinitis, and allergic sensitization among children with a parental history of atopy. J Allergy Clin Immunol. 2008;122:274–9. [PMC free article] [PubMed]

28 Thavagnanam S, Fleming J, Bromley A, Shields MD, Cardwell CR. A meta-analysis of the association between cesarean section and childhood asthma. Clin Exp Allergy. 2008;38:629–33. [PubMed]

29 McKay JA, Groom A, Potter C, et al. Genetic and non-genetic influences during pregnancy on infant global and site specific DNA methylation: role for folate gene variants and vitamin B12. PLoS One. 2012;7:e33290. [PMC free article] [PubMed]

30 Huh SY, Rifas-Shiman SL, Zera CA, et al. Delivery by cesarean section and risk of obesity in preschool age children: a prospective cohort study. Arch Dis Child. 2012;97:610–6. [PMC free article] [PubMed]

31 MacKay DF, Smith GC, Dobbie R, Pell JP. Gestational age at delivery and special educational need: retrospective cohort study of 407,503 school children. PLoS Med. 2010;7:e1000289. [PMC free article] [PubMed]

32 Polidano C, Zhu A, Bornstein JC. The relation between caesarean birth and child cognitive development. Scientific Reports. 2017. 7:11483. DOI:10.1038/s41598-017-10831-y

33 Kaye SA, Robison LL, Smithson WA, Gunderson P, King FL, Neglia JP. Maternal reproductive history and birth characteristics in childhood acute lymphoblastic leukemia. Cancer. 1991;68:1351–5. [PubMed]

34 Cnattingius S, Zack M, Ekbom A, Gunnarskog J, Linet M, Adami HO. Prenatal and neonatal risk factors for childhood myeloid leukemia. Cancer Epidemiol Biomarkers Prev. 1995;4:441–5. [PubMed]

35 Almgren M, Schlinzig T, Gomez-Cabrero D, Gunnar A, Sundin M, Johansson S, Norman

M2, Ekström TJ 2014 Cesarean delivery and hematopoietic stem cell epigenetics in the newborn infant: implications for future health? Am J Obstet Gynecol. 211(5):502.e1-8. doi: 10.1016/j.ajog.2014.05.014. Epub 2014 Jul 1.

36 Peters LL, Thornton C, de Jonge A, Khashan A, Tracy M, Downe S, Feijen-de Jong EI, Dahlen HG. 2018 The effect of medical and operative birth interventions on child health outcomes in the first 28 days and up to 5 years of age: A linked data population-based cohort study. Birth 45(4):347-357. doi: 10.1111/birt.12348. Epub 2018 Mar 25.

37 Neumann ID 2008. Brain oxytocin: a key regulator of emotional and social behaviours in both females and males. J Neuroendocrinol, 20 858-65.

38 Tronick E, Reck C. Infants of depressed mothers. Harv Rev Psychiatry. 2009;17:147–56. [PubMed]

39 Carter CS, Grippo AJ, Pournajafi-Nazarloo H, Ruscio MG, Porges SW. Oxytocin, vasopressin, and sociality. Prog Brain Res. 2008;170:331–6. [PubMed]

40 Blom EA, Jansen PW, Verhulst FC, et al. Perinatal complications increase the risk of postpartum depression, the generation R study. BJOG. 2010;117:1390–8. [PubMed]

41 Gonzales ME. Hard data about the side effects of synthetic oxytocin. Mid-pacific conference on birth and primal health research; Honolulu, HI. 2012.

42 Olza Fernandez I, Marin Gabriel M, Malalana Martinez A, Fernandez-Canadas Morillo A, Lopez Sanchez F, Costarelli V. Newborn feeding behaviour depressed by intrapartum oxytocin: a pilot study. Acta Paediatr. 2012;101:749–54. [PubMed]

43 Poindron P. Mechanisms of activation of maternal behaviour in mammals. Reprod Nutr Dev. 2005;45:341–51. [PubMed]

44 Leng G, Meddle SL, Douglas AJ. Oxytocin and the maternal brain. Curr Opin Pharmacol. 2008;8:731–4. [PubMed]

45 Downe S, McCourt C 2004. From Being to Becoming: Reconstructing childbirth knowledges. In: Downe S (ed.) Normal Birth, evidence and debate. Oxford: Elsevier.

46 Dahlen H, Kennedy H, Anderson CM, Bell AF, Clark A, Foureur M, Ohm JE, Shearman AM, Taylor JY, Wright ML, Downe S 2013. The EPIIC hypothesis: Intrapartum effects on the neonatal epigenome and consequent health outcomes. Medical Hypothesis, 8, 656-62.

47 Dahlen HG, Downe S, Wright ML, Kennedy HP, Taylor JY 2016 Childbirth and consequent atopic disease: emerging evidence on epigenetic effects based on the hygiene and EPIIC hypotheses. (BMC Pregnancy Childbirth. 13;16:4. doi: 10.1186/s12884-015-0768-9.

48 Rautava S, Ruuskanen O, Ouwehand A, Salminen S, Isolauri E 2004 The hygiene hypothesis of atopic disease - an extended version. J Pediatr Gastroenterol Nutr. 38(4):378-88.

50 Osterman MJ, Martin JA. Recent declines in induction of labor by gestational age. NCHS Data Brief 2014:1–8.

51 Declercq ER, Sakala C, Corry MP, Applebaum S, Herrlich A. Listening to Mothers SM III: Pregnancy and Childbirth. New York: Childbirth Connection, May 2013.

52 Nippita TA, Trevena JA, Patterson JA, Ford JB, Morris JM, Roberts CL 2015 Variation in hospital rates of induction of labour: a population-based record linkage study. BMJ Open 2;5(9):e008755. doi: 10.1136/bmjopen-2015-008755.

53 UK Hospital Episode Statistics (HES) NHS Maternity Statistics 2017-18 report. Available from: https://digital.nhs.uk/news-and-events/latest-news/nhs-maternity-statistics-2017-18. Accessed 11th Jan 2019

54 World Health Organization 2018. Intrapartum care for a positive childbirth experience. Available from: https://www.who.int/reproductivehealth/publications/intrapartum-care-guidelines/en/. Accessed 11th Jan 2019

55 Kennedy HP. 2002 The midwife as an "Instrument" of care. Am J Public Health. 2002 Nov;92(11):1759-60.

56 Buckley, Sarah J. Hormonal Physiology of Childbearing: Evidence and Implications for Women, Babies, and Maternity Care. Washington, D.C.: Childbirth Connection Programs, National Partnership for Women & Families, January 2015.

57 Miller, S., Abalos, E., Chamillard, ... Althabe, F. (2016). Beyond too little, too late and too much, too soon: a pathway towards evidence-based, respectful maternity care worldwide. Lancet, 388, 2176-2192.

58 Kennedy, H. P., Yoshida, S., Costello, A., Declercq, E., Dias, M. A., Duff, E., ... Renfrew, M. J. 2016. Asking different questions: research priorities to improve the quality of care for every woman, every child. Lancet Glob Health, 4 (11), e777-e779.

CHAPTER 14

The microbiome relating to labour and birth

Holly Jenkins and *Matthew Hyde*

Introduction

The human microbiome, a term given to represent the population of microorganisms that inhabit the human body, has long been associated with health and disease.[1] The largest and most researched of the human microbiomes is the gut microbiome. The gut microbiome is a complex microbial community that has co-evolved symbiosis with the host, to perform essential protective, structural, metabolic and immunological functions.[2] Alterations to the microbiome can be pathological, and understanding how a healthy gut microbiome is developed and maintained is important.

This chapter will focus on what is known about the development of the gut microbiota (the microorganisms present in a defined environment) in early life, and especially the impact of birth and the labour process.[3]

The origins of the gut microbiota

How and when bacterial colonisation begins is still debated. Earlier studies provided evidence for a bacterial presence in amniotic fluid, umbilical cord blood, placental tissue, foetal membranes and meconium.[4-8] For example, a study by Aagard et al (2014) reported that the placenta harbours unique non-pathogenic bacterial species.[9] However, these findings have been heavily criticised by other groups who fail to separate placental samples from negative controls.[10,11] Similarly, Lim et al (2018) have shown that amniotic fluid from healthy term pregnancies does not harbour detectable bacterial species.[12] In contrast, meconium has been shown to be characterised by *Bacilli* and *Firmicutes* species.[3,7,9] Although it remains unknown whether detected bacteria are live (functional) or remnant bacterial DNA,[14] these meconium findings challenge the assumption of a sterile *in utero* environment and indicate prenatal establishment of the gut microbiota.

During vaginal delivery, the baby passes through the birth canal and over the perineum, receiving inoculation with bacteria from the mother's gut microbiota. Intake of breastmilk (rich in bacteria) further populates the infant gut.[15] Infants typically acquire a mixture of aerobes and anaerobes including *Lactobacillus, Bifidobacterium* and *Enterobacteriaceae* spp.,[14] establishing a microbiota that has low diversity and a dominance of the *Proteobacteria* and *Actinobacteria* phyla. Diversity increases with time as *Firmicutes* and *Bacteroidetes* spp. Proliferate.[16] Early colonization with facultative anaerobes creates an environment that promotes the later proliferation of strict anaerobes such as *Bacteroides, Clostridium* and *Bifidobacterium* genera,[8,17] and with increasing time postpartum the gut microbiota becomes largely anaerobic.[7] Establishment of the gut microbiota is facilitated by the low pH of the neonatal gut.[18] As time after birth increases, the bacterial diversity increases and converges towards an adult-like microbiota by 3–5 years of age.[8] Once established, the gut microbiota remains relatively stable, though subject to dysbiotic shifts throughout life.

Perinatal influences on gut colonisation

Many perinatal factors influence colonisation, including mode of delivery, diet, antibiotic exposure and gestational age. These will be reviewed in greater detail.

Mode of birth

Mode of birth is thought to significantly influence colonisation.[8] Caesarean section delivery disrupts the vaginal-faecal-foetal bacterial transmission, resulting in lower bacterial diversity compared to vaginally delivered infants.[13] Exposure to the skin microbiota results in colonisation with organisms such as *Staphylococcus* and *Actinetobacter*.[8,19] High levels of bacteria from the skin microbiota have been reported in obstetric operating theatres, which may contribute to the pattern of colonisation in caesarean section babies.[20] Postnatal colonisation of *Bifidobacterium* and *Bacteroides* spp. is often delayed and there is an increased presence of *Clostridium* genera in caesarean section-born infants.[21,22] Similar findings have been reported in a number of other studies with caesarean section-associated differences in the gut microbiota persisting for anything between six months and two years post-birth.[4,19,20] The clinical relevance of the differential establishment of the microbiota between caesarean section and vaginally-born infants remains unclear. Several studies have reported that caesarean section delivery is associated with long-term health complications for the infant.[25,26] In particular, caesarean section delivery is associated with an increased risk of obesity, allergies and immune deficiencies.[27-30] Aberrant establishment of the microbiota has been implicated as a potential mechanism underlying these associations, but this remains unproven.[5]

However, a small study carried out by Dominguez-Bello et al, (2010) compared the bacterial communities of vaginally and caesarean section-delivered neonates across several body sites (skin, oral mucosa, nasopharyngeal aspirates and meconium) within the first 24 hours postpartum. They found that the neonates harboured homogenous communities that did not change across body sites regardless of delivery mode.[19] More recently Chu et al (2017) reported that infants undergo rapid bacterial expansion between

4 and 6 weeks of age, but this was not influenced by mode of birth (when controlled for confounding factors).[31] Similarly Stewart and colleagues (2017) found that mode of birth did not influence the longitudinal development of the microbiota in preterm infants.[32] It is possible that the previously reported differences between birth mode and colonisation are related to laboratory methods, e.g. sequencing techniques.

Infant diet

Diet has a strong influence on bacterial colonisation. Infant diet may include breastmilk (mother's own, at the breast or expressed and bottle/tube fed), donor human milk or infant formula. Breastmilk provides antimicrobial and immunomodulatory benefits that promote growth and provide protection against infections and inflammation.[33]

Breastfeeding provides live bacteria for ingestion by the infant, producing healthy bacterial colonisation. Initially it was thought that the bacterial cells found in human milk were skin contaminants, but given some of the bacteria found in milk are strict anaerobes, this theory has been largely discredited.[34] The most commonly isolated genera in breastmilk include *Bifidobacterium, Staphylococcus, Streptococcus,* and *Lactobacillus.*[35]

Breastmilk also contains many bioactive molecules and complex proteins, lipids and carbohydrates. These provide nutrition, but many also have prebiotic functions.[36] Human milk oligosaccharides (HMO; the third largest carbohydrate component) are indigestible and act as prebiotics – encouraging colonisation with beneficial bacteria (e.g. *Bifidobacterium infantis*) while preventing pathogenic colonisation.[36]

If breastmilk is unavailable, infant formula may be used. Formula is designed to mimic human breastmilk composition, although it has much lower bacterial counts than breastmilk. Sterilised infant formula and pasteurised human donor milk do not provide a beneficial bacterial source.[37]

Studies have shown marked differences in the gut microbiota of breast and formula-fed term infants.[38] Regardless of diet, the most represented bacterial species belong to the *Bifidobacterium* genus, although the species present and their relative abundance may differ. Formula-fed infants tend to have higher numbers of *Bacteroides, Clostridium, Enterobacteriaceae* and *Enterococcus* spp.[21,39] In general, breastfed infants have a more stable and uniform gut microbiota.[21] Supplementing breastmilk with formula leads to a shift in bacterial patterns, with noted increases of *Clostridium, Streptococcus, Bacillus, Escherichia coli* and *Enterococcus faecalis.*[17,40]

Mode of birth and diet interact. We have shown that, worldwide, caesarean section is associated with reduced breastfeeding initiation.[41] This complicates separating the individual impacts of mode of birth and infant nutrition on the development of the infant microbiota.

Antibiotics

Antibiotic exposure around birth is recognised as impacting the gut microbiota. Antibiotic usage varies across the world. Following UK NICE guidelines, all UK mothers delivering by caesarean section are given prophylactic antibiotics before skin incision (intra-operatively).[42]

In some regions, intrapartum antibiotic prophylaxis (IAP) is administered to prevent early-onset infections in the infant (particularly Group B *Streptococcus* infections), and following pre-labour rupture of membranes. Several studies report bacterial gut dysbiosis in infants born to mothers exposed to IAP. Most commonly, antibiotics reduce the species richness, with underrepresentation of *Bacteroides*, over-representation of *Enterococcus* and *Clostridium* organisms and lower *Bifidobacteria* counts.[43] IAP has a profound impact one month postpartum, with unexposed infants exhibiting higher *Staphylococcaceae, Bacilli* and *Bifidobacteriaceae*. By 90 days of age these differences had largely disappeared.[44] In contrast, Jaureguy et al, (2004) found that short-term IAP did not have a major effect on the infant microbiota, nor did it favour colonisation with antibiotic-resistant species.[45]

Approaches to the prevention of early-onset neonatal infection differ internationally. The UK applies a risk-factor based approach in giving prophylactic antibiotics, but a minority of term infants receive antibiotics.[46] In contrast, most infants admitted to neonatal intensive care units (NICU) are administered antibiotics.[5] Antibiotic administration typically occurs just as acquisition of the microbiota enters its crucial phase, and thus impacts its development.[47]

In preterm neonates, exposure to ampicillin and gentamicin during the first week post-birth reduces the bacterial diversity,[48] increases the abundance of pathogenic *Enterobacteriaceae* and reduces beneficial microbes including *Bifidobacterium, Lactobacillus* and *Bacilli* spp., when compared to unexposed neonates.[48] Broad-spectrum antibiotic use can alter gastrointestinal gene expression and influence functionality and development of the intestinal barrier.[49] In very low birth weight neonates administration of a 10-day course of antibiotics increased the likelihood of developing necrotising enterocolitis, with each additional day increasing the risk.[50]

Premature birth

The development of the microbiota in preterm infants differs from that of the healthy term infant. The gut of the preterm infant is under-developed at birth. A high caesarean section rate, reduced skin-to-skin contact, the NICU environment, less feeding at the breast, use of human donor milk and parenteral feeding, among other factors, all affect establishment of the gut microbiota.[51-54]

Broadly, development of the preterm infant's gut microbiota is characterised by delayed *Bifidobacterium* colonisation, underrepresentation of anaerobes and over-representation of *Staphylococci, Streptococcus, Enterococci* and *Enterobacteriaceae*.[8,40,55] Aujoulat et al (2014) explored the temporal bacterial dynamics and report similar patterns including an under-representation of *Bacteroidetes* and a dominance of gram-positive bacteria (*Staphylococci, Enterococci* and *Clostridia*).[56]

Other factors

The areas reviewed here represent only a few of the many aspects of labour, birth and perinatal care practices which impact the establishment of the gut microbiota. Wider environmental factors must not be forgotten. Within the family environment, studies show that having siblings impacts on the infant's microbiota.[21] Place of birth, in terms of hospital vs home, can determine the predominant bacterial species present in the gut.[21] For example, Combellick et al (2018) recently found that infants born in a hospital had lower levels of *Bacteroides, Bifidobacterium, Lactococcus* and *Streptococcus,* but higher *Clostridium* and *Enterobacteriaceae* members when compared to those born at home.[57] A pan-European study has also shown that the geographical region of birth was a more significant determinant of intestinal colonisation than mode of birth.[39]

This is an emerging area of research and further studies are required. For example, as yet there is little information regarding the impact of birthing in water or being born in the caul, on the infant microbiota.[58]

Impact of early-life disruption on the life course of the microbiota

The gut microbiota is inherently dynamic and fluctuates over time. This is partly attributable to dietary patterns, illness and medical treatment. It is not yet fully known how 'permanent' the gut microbiota is, and whether the signature of the gut microbiota established in early infancy persists throughout life, or if it has an impact on neonatal neurohormonal programming in the early days of life, independent of later changes in gut microbiota composition, as discussed below.

In a study of preterm infants neither post-discharge antibiotic exposure nor significant illness had a detectable impact on the microbiota, although a decline in organisms commonly associated with a NICU environment was observed after discharge.[59] Overall, the preterm infants showed the capacity to develop a complex microbiota that was comparable to a healthy term infant, regardless of the time spent in NICU.

The effect of caesarean birth on the adult microbiota has not been extensively described, but Goedert et al, (2014) report distinct faecal bacterial communities in adults born by caesarean section, although confounding factors could not be eliminated.[60]

The early microbiota and programming of later-life health

It is known that bacterial colonisation influences maturation of the immune system,[61] particularly the gut immune system,[62] and aberrant bacterial growth in the gut may have long-term health consequences.

Differences in the gut microbiota of children with food allergies and those without have been described.[63] Allergic infants had lower bacterial diversity and elevated *En terobacteriaceae:Bacteroidaceae* ratio. Differences in the microbiota may modulate T-cell regulation.[64] It has been postulated that the gut microbiota modifies the risk of developing Type 1 and Type 2 diabetes,[65,66] incidence of obesity and metabolic syndrome[67] and intestinal diseases (e.g. inflammatory bowel disease).[68]

Restoring the aberrant microbiota

In adults, evidence suggests that the microbiota may be reset or restored.[69] For example, faecal microbiota transplants are being increasingly used to treat patients with *Clostridium difficile*. Results from these studies are promising and have shown partial restoration of a 'healthy' microbiota.[70-72]

More recently, there has been much interest in the potential for restoring the aberrant microbiota in caesarean section babies at birth by seeding them with bacteria from the mother's vagina. Seeding is not necessarily confined to oral and nasal cavities, but to the entire baby. Dominguez-Bello et al conducted a pilot study in which caesarean section infants were exposed to maternal vaginal fluids at birth.[73] The composition of the infants' microbiota was longitudinally assessed, and it was found that caesarean section infants exposed to vaginal fluids had bacterial communities resembling those of vaginally delivered infants. Further studies are needed to determine whether the effects persist into later life.

Major concerns about the safety of seeding with vaginal bacteria have been raised, with suggestions that it may increase risk of sepsis.[74,75] As with all new interventions caution must be exercised, and long-term monitoring of the seeded infants is required to confirm safety and efficacy. Several interventions have received wide clinical usage before retrospective analysis has demonstrated harm. *Caveat emptor*!

Conclusions

It seems likely that the perinatal establishment of the infant microbiota has significant impact on the infant's short and long-term health and development. Evidence suggests that several factors can significantly disrupt normal colonisation. These include routine clinical practices which have generally been recognised as being 'safe'. Only now, when very high percentages of babies are being born abdominally around the world, is the lasting impact of caesarean section on the gut microbiota being discovered. It remains to be proven what later life sequelae follow disruption of the developing gut microbiota. As a minimum, these findings suggest caution in the overuse of surgical delivery. Where a caesarean section is really necessary, preliminary data suggests that the bacterial effects may not be long-standing, though it is not clear if this will reverse any early neurohormonal impacts of bacterial disruption. The neonatal microbiota is an emerging field of research. This chapter reports an interim understanding of the field.

Points for consideration

- Learn to identify babies born preterm, by caesarean section, or who have received antibiotics as 'high risk' for development of an aberrant gut microbiome.
- Review and regularly audit unit policies aimed at reducing the number of 'high risk' babies.
- Encourage and support breastfeeding (not just breastmilk, but actually feeding at the breast), but especially in 'high risk' babies.
- Audit and minimise the use of antibiotics in the peripartum period.
- Outside of participation in clinical trials, wait patiently for further confirmatory data supporting novel microbiome interventions before adopting them on your unit.

References

1   Manor O, Borenstein E. Systematic Characterization and Analysis of the Taxonomic Drivers of Functional Shifts in the Human Microbiome. *Cell Host Microbe*. 2017;21(2): 254–267.

2   Kinross JM, Darzi AW, Nicholson JK. Gut microbiome-host interactions in health and disease. *Gen Med*. 2011;3(3): 14.

3   Marchesi JR, Ravel J. The vocabulary of microbiome research: a proposal. *Microbiome*. 2015;3(1): 31.

4   Ardissone AN, de la Cruz DM, Davis-Richardson AG, Rechcigl KT, Li N, Drew JC, et al. Meconium Microbiome Analysis Identifies Bacteria Correlated with Premature Birth. *PLoS ONE*. 2014;9(3): e90784.

5   Neu J, Rushing J. Cesarean versus Vaginal Delivery: Long term infant outcomes and the Hygiene Hypothesis. *Clin Perinatol*. 2011;38(2): 321–331.

6   Watts DH, Krohn MA, Hillier SL, Eschenbach DA. The association of occult amniotic fluid infection with gestational age and neonatal outcome among women in preterm labor. *Obstet Gynecol*. 1992;79(3): 351–357.

7   Gritz EC, Bhandari V. The Human Neonatal Gut Microbiome: A Brief Review. *Front Pediatr*. 2015;3.

8   Rodriguez JM, Murphy K, Stanton C, Ross RP, Kober OI, Juge N, et al. The composition of the gut microbiota throughout life, with an emphasis on early life. *Microb Ecol Health Dis*. 2015;26: 26050.

9   Aagaard K, Ma J, Antony KM, Ganu R, Petrosino J, Versalovic J. The placenta harbors a unique microbiome. *Sci Transl Med*. 2014;6(237): 237ra65.

10   Lauder AP, Roche AM, Sherrill-Mix S, Bailey A, Laughlin AL, Bittinger K, et al. Comparison of placenta samples with contamination controls does not provide evidence for a distinct placenta microbiota. *Microbiome*. 2016;4(1): 29.

11   Leiby JS, McCormick K, Sherrill-Mix S, Clarke EL, Kessler LR, Taylor LJ, et al. Lack of detection of a human placenta microbiome in samples from preterm and term deliveries. *Microbiome*. 2018;6(1): 196.

12   Lim ES, Rodriguez C, Holtz LR. Amniotic fluid from healthy term pregnancies does not harbor a detectable microbial community. *Microbiome*. 2018;6(1): 87.

13   Romano-Keeler J, Weitkamp J-H. Maternal influences on fetal microbial colonization and immune development. *Pediatr Res*. 2015;77(1–2): 189–195.

14   Mueller NT, Bakacs E, Combellick J, Grigoryan Z, Dominguez-Bello MG. The infant microbiome development: mom matters. *Trends Mol Med*. 2015;21(2): 109–117.

15   Jost T, Lacroix C, Braegger CP, Chassard C. New Insights in Gut Microbiota Establishment in Healthy Breast Fed Neonates. *PLoS ONE*. 2012;7(8): e44595.

16   Fujimura KE, Slusher NA, Cabana MD, Lynch S V. Role of the gut microbiota in defining human health. *Expert Rev Anti Infect Ther*. 2010;8(4): 435–454.

17   Guaraldi F, Salvatori G. Effect of Breast and Formula Feeding on Gut Microbiota Shaping in Newborns. *Frontiers in Cellular and Infection Microbiology*. 2012;2: 94.

18   Miclat NN, Hodgkinson R, Marx GF. Neonatal gastric pH. *Anesth Analg*. 1978;57(1): 98–101.

19   Dominguez-Bello MG, Costello EK, Contreras M, Magris M, Hidalgo G, Fierer N, et al. Delivery mode shapes the acquisition and structure of the initial microbiota across multiple body habitats in newborns. *Proc Natl Acad Sci USA*. 2010;107(26): 11971–11975.

20   Shin H, Pei Z, Martinez KA, Rivera-Vinas JI, Mendez K, Cavallin H, et al. The first microbial environment of infants born by C-section: the operating room microbes. *Microbiome*. 2015;3(1): 59.

21   Penders J, Thijs C, Vink C, Stelma FF, Snijders B, Kummeling I, et al. Factors Influencing the Composition of the Intestinal Microbiota in Early Infancy. *Pediatrics*. 2006;118(2): 511–521.

22   Biasucci G, Rubini M, Riboni S, Morelli L, Bessi E, Retetangos C. Mode of delivery affects the bacterial community in the newborn gut. *Early Hum Dev*. 2010;86(1): 13–15.

23   Fanaro S, Chierici R, Guerrini P, Vigi V. Intestinal microflora in early infancy: composition and development. *Acta Paediatr Suppl*. 2003;91(441): 48–55.

24   Madan J, Hoen A, Lundgren S, Al E. Association of cesarean delivery and formula supplementation with the intestinal microbiome of 6-week-old infants. *JAMA Pediatr*. 2016;170(3): 212–219.

25   Hyde MJ, Mostyn A, Modi N, Kemp PR. The health implications of birth by Caesarean section. *Biol Rev Camb Philos Soc*. 2012;87(1): 229–243.

26   Hyde MJ, Griffin JL, Herrera E, Byrne CD, Clarke L, Kemp PR. Delivery by Caesarean section, rather than vaginal delivery, promotes hepatic steatosis in piglets. *Clin Sci (Lond)*. 2009;118(1): 47–59.

27   Pistiner M, Gold DR, Abdulkerim H, Hoffman E, Celedon JC. Birth by cesarean section, allergic rhinitis, and allergic sensitization among children with a parental history of atopy. *J Allergy Clin Immunol*. 2008;122(2): 274–279.

28   Huh SY, Rifas-Shiman SL, Zera CA, Edwards JWR, Oken E, Weiss ST, et al. Delivery by caesarean section and risk of obesity in preschool age children: a prospective cohort study. *Arch Dis Child*. 2012;97(7): 610–616.

29   Thavagnanam S, Fleming J, Bromley A, Shields MD, Cardwell CR. A meta-analysis of the association between Caesarean section and childhood asthma.*Clin Exp Allergy*. 2008;38(4): 629–633.

30   Riiser A. The human microbiome, asthma, and allergy. *Allergy Asthma Clin Immunol*. 2015;11: 35.

31 Chu DM, Ma J, Prince AL, Antony KM, Seferovic MD, Aagaard KM. Maturation of the infant microbiome community structure and function across multiple body sites and in relation to mode of delivery. *Nat Med*. 2017;23(3): 314-326.

32 Stewart CJ, Embleton ND, Clements E, Luna PN, Smith DP, Fofanova TY, et al. Cesarean or Vaginal Birth Does Not Impact the Longitudinal Development of the Gut Microbiome in a Cohort of Exclusively Preterm Infants. *Front Microbiol*. 2017;8: 1008.

33 Gregory KE, Samuel BS, Houghteling P, Shan G, Ausubel FM, Sadreyev RI, et al. Influence of maternal breast milk ingestion on acquisition of the intestinal microbiome in preterm infants. *Microbiome*. 2016;4(1): 68.

34 Rodriguez JM. The Origin of Human Milk Bacteria: Is There a Bacterial Entero-Mammary Pathway during Late Pregnancy and Lactation? *Adv Nutr*. 2014;5(6): 779–784.

35 Rodriguez JM. The Origin of Human Milk Bacteria: Is There a Bacterial Entero-Mammary Pathway during Late Pregnancy and Lactation? *Adv Nutr*. 2014;5(6): 779–784.

36 Andreas NJ, Kampmann B, Mehring Le-Doare K. Human breast milk: A review on its composition and bioactivity. *Early Hum Dev*. 2015;91(11): 629–635.

37 Meier P, Patel A, Esquerra-Zwiers A. Donor Human Milk Update: Evidence, Mechanisms and Priorities for Research and Practice. *J Pediatr*. 2017;180: 15–21.

38 Gale C, Logan KM, Santhakumaran S, Parkinson JR, Hyde MJ, Modi N. Effect of breastfeeding compared with formula feeding on infant body composition: a systematic review and meta-analysis. *Am J Clin Nutr*. 2012;95(3): 656–669.

39 Fallani M, Young D, Scott J, Norin E, Amarri S, Adam R, et al. Intestinal microbiota of 6-week-old infants across Europe: geographic influence beyond delivery mode, breast-feeding, and antibiotics. *J Pediatr Gastroenterol Nutr*. 2010;51(1): 77–84.

40 Groer MW, Luciano AA, Dishaw LJ, Ashmeade TL, Miller E, Gilbert JA. Development of the preterm infant gut microbiome: a research priority. *Microbiome*. 2014;2: 38.

41 Prior E, Santhakumaran S, Gale C, Philipps LH, Modi N, Hyde MJ. Breastfeeding after cesarean delivery: a systematic review and meta-analysis of world literature. *Am J Clin Nutr*. 2012;95(5): 1113–1135.

42 NICE Guidelines. *Caesarean Section* (update). 2012. Available from https://www.nice.org.uk/guidance/cg132 [Accessed Feb 2017].

43 Azad M, Konya T, Persaud R, Guttman D, Chari R, Field C, et al. Impact of maternal intrapartum antibiotics, method of birth and breastfeeding on gut microbiota during the first year of life: a prospective cohort study. *BJOG*. 2015;123(6): 983-93.

44 Arboleya S, Sánchez B, Milani C, Duranti S, Solís G, Fernández N, et al. Intestinal microbiota development in preterm neonates and effect of perinatal antibiotics. *J Pediatr*. 2015;166(3): 538–544.

45 Jauréguy F, Carton M, Panel P, Foucaud P, Butel M-J, Doucet-Populaire F. Effects of Intrapartum Penicillin Prophylaxis on Intestinal Bacterial Colonization in Infants. *J Clin Microbiol*. 2004;42(11): 5184–5188.

46 NICE Guidelines (2012) *Neonatal infection : antibiotics for prevention and treatment*. Available from https://www.nice.org.uk/guidance/cg149 [Accessed Feb 2017].

47 Munyaka PM, Eissa N, Bernstein CN, Khafipour E, Ghia J-E. Antepartum Antibiotic Treatment Increases Offspring Susceptibility to Experimental Colitis: A Role of the Gut Microbiota. *PLoS ONE*. 2015;10(11): e0142536.

48 Gibson MK, Crofts TS, Dantas G. Antibiotics and the developing infant gut microbiota and resistome. *Curr Opin Microbiol*. 2015;27: 51–56.

49 Westerbeek EAM, van den Berg A, Lafeber HN, Knol J, Fetter WPF, van Elburg RM. The intestinal bacterial colonisation in preterm infants: A review of the literature. *ClinI Nutr*. 2006;25(3): 361–368.

50 Alexander VN, Northrup V, Bizzarro MJ. Antibiotic Exposure in the Newborn Intensive Care Unit and the Risk of Necrotizing Enterocolitis. *J Pediatr*. 2011;159(3): 392–397.

51 Brooks B, Firek BA, Miller CS, Sharon I, Thomas BC, Baker R, et al. Microbes in the neonatal intensive care unit resemble those found in the gut of premature infants. *Microbiome*. 2014;2(1): 1.

52 Schwiertz A, Gruhl B, Lobnitz M, Michel P, Radke M, Blaut M. Development of the intestinal bacterial composition in hospitalized preterm infants in comparison with breast-fed, full-term infants. *Pediatr Res*. 2003;54(3): 393–399.

53 Unger S, Stintzi A, Shah P, Mack D, O'Connor DL. Gut microbiota of the very-low-birth-weight infant. *Pediatr Res*. 2015;77(1–2): 205–213.

54 Delnord M, Blondel B, Drewniak N, Klungsøyr K, Bolumar F, Mohangoo A, et al. Varying gestational age patterns in cesarean delivery: an international comparison. *BMC Preg Childbirth*. 2014;14(1): 321.

55 Magne F, Abely M, Boyer F, Morville P, Pochart P, Suau A. Low species diversity and high interindividual variability in faeces of preterm infants as revealed by sequences of 16S rRNA genes and PCR-temporal temperature gradient gel electrophoresis profiles. *FEMS Microbiol Ecol*. 2006;57(1): 128–138.

56 Aujoulat F, Roudière L, Picaud J-C, Jacquot A, Filleron A, Neveu D, et al. Temporal dynamics of the very premature infant gut dominant microbiota. *BMC Microbiol*. 2014;14(1): 325.

57 Combellick JL, Shin H, Shin D, Cai Y, Hagan H, Lacher C, et al. Differences in the fecal microbiota of neonates

born at home or in the hospital. *Sci Rep*. 2018;8(1): 15660.

58 Fehervary P, Lauinger-Lorsch E, Hof H, Melchert F, Bauer L, Zieger W. Water birth: microbiological colonisation of the newborn, neonatal and maternal infection rate in comparison to conventional bed deliveries. *Arch Gynecol Obstet*. 2004;270(1): 6–9.

59 Stewart CJ, Skeath T, Nelson A, Fernstad SJ, Marrs ECL, Perry JD, et al. Preterm gut microbiota and metabolome following discharge from intensive care. *Sci Rep*. 2015;5: 17141.

60 Goedert JJ, Hua X, Yu G, Shi J. Diversity and Composition of the Adult Fecal Microbiome Associated with History of Cesarean Birth or Appendectomy: Analysis of the American Gut Project. *EBioMedicine*. 2014;1(2–3): 167–172.

61 Round JL, Mazmanian SK. The gut microbiota shapes intestinal immune responses during health and disease. *Nat Rev Immunol*. 2009;9(5): 313–323.

62 Belkaid Y, Hand T. Role of the Microbiota in Immunity and inflammation. *Cell*. 2014;157(1): 121–141.

63 Ngoc PL, Gold DR, Tzianabos AO, Weiss ST, Celedon JC. Cytokines, allergy, and asthma. *Curr Opin Allergy Clin Immunol*. 2005;5(2): 161–166.

64 Fujimura KE, Sitarik AR, Havstad S, Lin DL, Levan S, Fadrosh D, et al. Neonatal gut microbiota associates with childhood multisensitized atopy and T cell differentiation. *Nat Med*. 2016;22(10): 1187–1191.

65 Paun A, Danska JS. Modulation of type 1 and type 2 diabetes risk by the intestinal microbiome. *Pediatr Diabetes*. 2016;17(7): 469–477.

66 Needell JC, Zipris D. The Role of the Intestinal Microbiome in Type 1 Diabetes Pathogenesis. *Curr Diab Rep*. 2016;16(10): 89.

67 Garcia-Mantrana I, Collado MC. Obesity and overweight: Impact on maternal and milk microbiome and their role for infant health and nutrition. *Mol Nutr Food Res*. 2016;60(8): 1865–1875.

68 Knoll RL, Forslund K, Kultima JR, Meyer CU, Kullmer U, Sunagawa S, et al. Gut microbiota differs between children with Inflammatory Bowel Disease and healthy siblings in taxonomic and functional composition - a metagenomic analysis. *Am J Physiol Gastro Liver Physiol*. 2016; ajpgi.00293.2016.

69 Van den Abbeele P, Verstraete W, El Aidy S, Geirnaert A, Van de Wiele T. Prebiotics, faecal transplants and microbial network units to stimulate biodiversity of the human gut microbiome. *Microbl Biotech*. 2013;6(4): 335–340.

70 Rohlke F, Stollman N. Fecal microbiota transplantation in relapsing Clostridium difficile infection. *Therap Adv Gastroenterol*. 2012;5(6): 403–420.

71 Mullish BH, Marchesi JR, Thursz MR, Williams HRT. Microbiome manipulation with faecal microbiome transplantation as a therapeutic strategy in Clostridium difficile infection. *QJM*. 2015;108(5): 355–359.

72 Juul FE, Garborg K, Bretthauer M, Skudal H, Øines MN, Wiig H, et al. Fecal Microbiota Transplantation for Primary Clostridium difficile Infection. *NEJM*. 2018;378(26): 2535–2536.

73 Dominguez-Bello MG, De Jesus-Laboy KM, Shen N, Cox LM, Amir A, Gonzalez A, et al. Partial restoration of the microbiota of cesarean-born infants via vaginal microbial transfer. *Nat Med*. 2016;22(3): 250–253.

74 Cunnington AJ, Sim K, Deierl A, Kroll JS, Brannigan E, Darby J. 'Vaginal Seeding' of infants born by caesarean section. *BMJ*. 2016;352.

75 Stinson LF, Payne MS, Keelan JA. A Critical Review of the Bacterial Baptism Hypothesis and the Impact of Cesarean Delivery on the Infant Microbiome. *Front Med*. 2018;5: 135.

CHAPTER 15

Interconnectivity in the birth room

Athena Hammond and Maralyn Foureur

Introduction

Internationally, there is an increasing focus on improving the quality of maternity services provided in facilities (Kennedy et al, 2016; Renfrew, 2014; Koblinsky et al, 2016). In particular, there is concern about the reducing rates of physiological labour and birth occurring in these settings and the associated implications for quality and health outcomes (Tracy et al, 2007; Peters et al, 2018). Change is required to improve the quality of experiences and clinical outcomes of childbearing women, increase the wellbeing and efficacy of maternity care providers, and to shift the attitudes, behaviours and organisational culture of maternity services towards authentically person-centred care (Deery and Fisher, 2017; Moncrieff, 2018; Vedam, 2017). Despite significant effort and many anecdotal reports of individual, team or unit success, at a systems level change of this type remains elusive in all country settings.

Factors including the physical environment (Foureur et al, 2010; Hammond et al, 2017), staff stress and wellbeing (Pezaro et al, 2018), activities and behaviour of staff (MacLellan, 2011), socio-cultural discourse (Davis and Walker, 2010a), model of care (Homer, 2016; Sandall et al, 2013) and organisational culture (Frith et al, 2014; Catling et al, 2017) have been identified as playing a role in the provision of quality maternity care and the construction of the birth environment. Such factors tend to be considered individually, or even compared to one another, but in this chapter we explore the idea that these factors are interconnected and therefore can be distilled and considered *as a mutually influencing system*, rather than as separate constructs. To do this we propose a model of interconnectivity based on four evidence-based domains that provide a basis for the design and delivery of effective, good-quality maternity services, including an increase in the rate of normal, physiological births occurring in facility settings.

In the next section we present a brief explanation of the concept of interconnectivity in general terms and subsequently present our model of interconnected domains of influence in the birth room. Information and evidence relating to the domains and their influence on quality, and on each other, are then described in detail.

The concept of interconnectivity

Interconnectivity, or the state of interconnectedness, describes the way in which a group of things (such as people, objects, constructs or places) interact with each other to create a complex whole that operates as a system (Western Washington University, 2019). Interconnectivity is seen in the ecosystems of the natural world, as well as in human physiology, social networks, global technology and in many other complex and changeable systems. Emerging research exploring issues as diverse as justice (Nygren, 2018), workplace stress (McCraty et al, 2009), hypertension treatment (Alabdulgader, 2012) and cancer immunology (Walker et al, 2018) suggest that interconnectivity is far more pervasive and nuanced than we might have once imagined and may therefore affect all of us in ways that we are only just starting to understand.

In this chapter we interpret interconnectivity as:

'an event or state that can occur when two or more people, places or constructs exhibit a mutual exchange or influence over one another – these exchanges or influences may or may not be visible but the effects of the exchange or influence are generally observable.'

Domains of interconnectivity

There are implied relationships in any kind of interconnectedness. As illustrated in Figure 1, we propose relationships exist between four domains that influence quality in maternity services and contribute to construction of the birth environment. The domains are spatial, neurobiological, behavioural and cultural. The four domains have arisen from our own and others' research investigating the physical, physiological, neurobiological and psychosocial factors that play a significant part in shaping the experiences and outcomes of childbearing women, healthcare staff and organisations engaged in providing maternity care.

When considered and addressed as a mutually influencing system, we believe the four domains have significant potential to promote change and support good-quality maternity care services, including increasing the rate of normal, physiological birth in facilities. Our rationale for these beliefs is explained in the next sections of this chapter, which explore each domain.

Figure 1.
Four interconnected domains of influence in the birth room (Hammond & Foureur 2018).

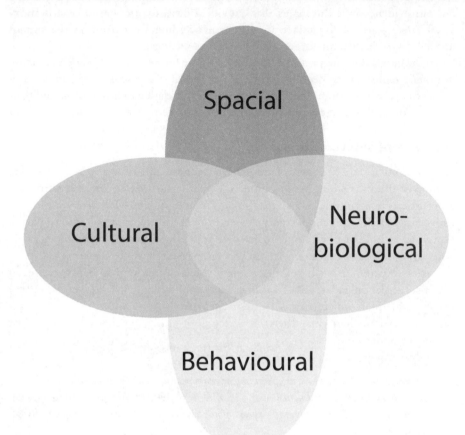

The spatial domain

Across hundreds of years, architects and philosophers have explored the concept of interconnectivity between space, place and people (Day, 2014; Tuan, 1977; Lounsbury, 2010). Thus, the idea that the design of places we inhabit can influence the way we feel and behave is neither controversial nor experimental. There is good evidence from diverse fields such as sociology, psychology, evidence-based design, architecture, neuroscience, salutogenics and human geography that we affect places and places affect us (Caan, 2011; Ulrich et al, 2010; Lawson, 2010; Gieryn, 2000; Golembiewski, 2016). Knowing this, we can seek to design spaces that shape human experiences and behaviours at both functional and emotional levels (Chan et al, 2007; Nanda et al, 2013).

While the spatial domain affects all users of a space, much of the evidence in maternity services comes from research with midwives and with childbearing women. The next section summarises the main findings of this body of research.

The influence of the spatial domain has been described by midwives working in homes, hospitals and birth centres (Davis and Walker, 2010a; Bourgeault et al, 2012; Keating and Fleming, 2009; Blix, 2011; Walsh, 2006). Midwives are deeply affected at both personal and professional levels by the design and aesthetics of the birth environment and have reported that the designed environment influences the way they practice, including by making the facilitation of normal birth more or less difficult to achieve (Hammond et al, 2013; Coddington et al, 2017; Hammond et al, 2014). This may be one reason why some facility spaces, particularly those described as ambient or alternately designed, are associated with higher rates of normal, physiological birth than other standard clinical facility spaces (Hodnett et al, 2012).

Ambient or alternative spaces are more likely to display the three design characteristics identified as supporting midwife wellbeing and quality midwifery practice: friendliness, functionality and freedom (Hammond et al, 2017). Friendliness relates to design and aesthetic features that are warm, relaxing and non-threatening and is associated with environments that midwives perceive as authentic. Functionality relates to spaces that are practical and adaptable, and provide uncluttered, easy-to-use spaces with plenty of storage and surfaces. Freedom relates to midwives' sense of being able to provide person-centred care in a space that is comfortable, safe, well resourced and flexible enough to cater to the diverse and changeable needs of childbearing women and families. It is suggested that spaces that provide these characteristics reduce midwife stress and support the provision of quality care (Hammond, 2017), one indicator of which is facilitation of physiological birth (Escuriet et al, 2015).

Unfortunately, practitioners working in high-income countries report with remarkable consistency that the design and aesthetics of standard facility birth environments do not support them to do their jobs easily or to provide what they consider optimal care to women (Keating and Fleming, 2009; O'Connell and Downe, 2009; Davis, 2010). This is important as spaces that do not support the functional, social and psychological needs of staff are likely to increase stress and decrease wellbeing, morale, efficacy and quality (Vischer, 2008; Ruohomäki et al., 2015).

The effects of the spatial domain on midwives are further highlighted in research from New Zealand which suggests that the same midwives – working within the same model of continuity of midwifery care – practise differently in home, birth centre and hospital spaces, thereby facilitating different experiences and different clinical outcomes for women (Miller and Skinner, 2012; Davis et al, 2011; Davis and Walker, 2010b; Hunter, 2003; Freeman et al, 2006). We acknowledge that these differences result from complex influences and are about more than just space, but the spatial domain undoubtedly has an influence and is a good place to begin unpacking the concept of interconnectedness given how spaces shape our lives. Certainly, a growing body of evidence attests to the influence of place of birth on clinical outcomes (Scarf et al, 2018; Birthplace in England Collaborative Group, 2011) and a recent ground-breaking report – while acknowledging the interconnected roles of cultural and contextual factors – suggests an association between facility design and caesarean section rates (Ariadne Labs and MASS Design Group, 2017). All of this work points towards the significance of the spatial domain in maternity care as one part of an interconnected model of influences.

For women, the spatial qualities of birth rooms have a significant impact upon how easy or hard it is to give birth (Singh and Newburn, 2006; Dagustan, 2009). Spatial factors that make a difference include the architectural design, which is usually replete with well lit, highly reflective, hard-edged, right-angled structures and contains fixtures, fittings and signage which convey unconscious meanings about whether birth is regarded as safe or dangerous in this space (Fannin, 2003; Davis and Walker, 2010a; Foureur et al, 2010). Studies have identified parts of the brain that respond to spatial factors such as curved or straight-edged surfaces, enclosed or open spaces with high ceilings, stimulating the release of stress-related neurohormones (Stenglin, 2009). Other spatial factors identified include sufficient room within the space to enable the labouring woman to move about freely and assume a range of positions (Lepori, 1994); the presence or absence of clutter (Hammond et al, 2013) and noise (Oliviera et al, 2011).

Other major spatial issues are the dominant and powerfully persuasive position of the bed within the space (Mondy et al, 2016); the position of the neonatal resuscitaire within the woman's line of sight (Duncan, 2011) and the lack of privacy afforded by a door into the room that opens directly from an outer public space. A recent study identified that accommodation for the woman's chosen birth companions provided within the space is also a factor that influences the quality of her experience (Harte, 2016). Interviews with Australian women have highlighted their desire for an environment that was softer, more home-like and more comfortable than a standard facility birth room (Watson, 2009). Women wanted an environment that felt welcoming and private and looked recognisably different from the usual hospital setting. The design and aesthetic cues inherent in such a differentiated space are arguably valuable for childbearing women of all risk, including those who require complex medical care. Whether birth is straightforward or complex, a carefully considered space can act to mediate the anxiety and fear frequently associated with childbirth, and its associated neurohormonal consequences.

Women tend to prefer an environment that supports their physical needs in labour: for flexibility, privacy, capacity to get low to the ground, objects to lean on, space to move freely and access to an ensuite bathroom with a deep bath (Jenkinson et al, Lepori, 1994; Forbes et al, 2008). These features may enhance women's autonomy and help make active labour and physiological birth more achievable when appropriate (Walsh and Gutteridge, 2011; Romano and Lothian, 2008). As well as being functionally supportive, there is evidence that such spaces may have neurobiological effects on the brain and body (Stark et al, 2016; Foureur, 2008) as discussed in the next section.

The neurobiological domain

The brain controls the way the world is experienced and interpreted by people, how they perceive themselves, and how meaning is made of life (Berkmann, 2014; Pulvermüller, 2013). It is constantly receiving and organising information that is gathered by the senses, as information about the environments people move through every day. One of the most important tasks of the brain is to constantly monitor these environments for threats, making decisions about the safety of any given space, place, action or interaction

(Öhman, 2005). This applies to things that are actually happening as well as events or interactions that our brain thinks *might* happen. The brain is interpreting the complex and constantly changing world around us, and determining the likelihood of something weird, uncomfortable, dangerous or life-threatening happening in each space or situation. Essentially, the brain is asking over and over again, 'Am I safe here?'

At a pre-cognitive or unconscious level, the answer to this question determines whether individuals should *approach* or *avoid* any given place or situation (Nanda et al, 2013). When the brain decides a threat is present that should be *avoided*, the hypothalamus initiates a sequence of chemical changes including the release of adrenaline, noradrenaline and cortisol into the bloodstream. This is often referred to as the 'fight or flight' response. Fight or flight is an innate, primal response that prepares for either confrontation or running away from a place or situation that threatens safety or survival. The heart rate increases, breathing becomes faster, blood rushes to the muscles and reflexes sharpen. Importantly, once fight or flight has been triggered there is a tendency to see *everything* in the near environment as a potential threat (Nanda et al, 2013; Schmidt et al, 2017).

To avoid triggering the fight or flight response in labour, birth rooms need to trigger the complementary, but less well known, psychophysiological response of 'calm and connect'. First described by Swedish researchers, the calm and connect response is mediated not by adrenaline, but by oxytocin (Uvnäs Moberg et al, 2005). Oxytocin is a neurohormone that is known to increase calm, buffer stress and facilitate positive human relationships (IsHak et al, 2011; Feldman, 2012). It is also critical to the normal progress of labour and birth, and to bonding and breastfeeding (Buckley, 2015). Brains synthesise and release oxytocin in response to environmental and social cues.

Environments that are perceived as warm, friendly, calm and non-threatening stimulate oxytocin release, which facilitates the physiological process of labour and can increase feelings of trust, empathy and connection between people. Thus, we think consideration of the interconnectivity between the spatial and neurobiological domains has been vastly underestimated as a tool to support the neurobiology of straightforward, normal birth and to promote trusting relationships between women and maternity care providers.

Social cues are also an important mediator of the effects of oxytocin (Averbeck, 2010; Groppe et al, 2013). Social cues are the verbal and non-verbal signals received from each other about how to behave and interact; we use them to interpret how others are feeling. A disconnect between environmental and social cues can occur when, for example, the physical space is perceived as safe, but people present *in* the space are perceived as unsafe. This kind of disconnect can actually negate the effects of oxytocin and *reduce or reverse* feelings of trust and social bonding (Olff et al, 2013; Bartz et al, 2011). The corollary of this effect is that the provision of a safe and relaxing space is necessary but not sufficient. In order to ensure neurobiological responses in the woman that optimise physiological labour and birth, caregivers within the birth environment must also promote a safe psychological and emotional space for women through their attitudes and behaviours.

The behavioural domain

Most people are familiar with the way in which spaces can trigger memories, feelings or expectations about what may be about to happen. Less familiar is the concept that the spatial environment can actually alter the structure and function of our brains, thus influencing the way we feel and behave in any given place. At a 2003 conference of the Academy of Neuroscience for Architecture, American neuroscientist Professor Rusty Gage, President of the Salk Institute and leading specialist in neuroplasticity, famously explained this concept as simply, 'Change the environment, change the brain, change the behaviour,' (The Salk Institute, 2012). Gage and others have demonstrated that how we feel and behave, the decisions we make and the ways in which we relate to others are all directly influenced by our perceptions of the spaces in which we live and work (Techau et al, 2016; Gage, 2004; Uvnäs Moberg et al, 2005).

Architects have long known that certain types of spatial qualities can be used to shape the behaviour of individuals and groups in buildings and public spaces (Alexander et al, 1977). This is because we receive *messages* about how to behave from cues embedded in our near environment and because the way we *feel* about where we are can have effects on our brain that influence behaviour (Caan, 2011; Nanda et al, 2013; Gage, 2004). For example, experiments have shown that looking at curved spaces and objects makes us happier and more relaxed than looking at sharp edged places and things (Vartanian et al, 2017; Dazkir and Read, 2011) and contact with nature increases our psychological wellbeing and sense of humour (Herzog and Strevey, 2008). The interconnectivity between spatial, neurobiological and behavioural domains has provided an evidence-based foundation for the rise of what is now called neuroarchitecture – architecture that explicitly designs with the brain and behaviour in mind (Metzger, 2018).

In our research, midwives have told us that they believe the design and aesthetics of facility birth rooms influence the way they feel and behave (Hammond et al, 2014). Midwives have shown they can view a photo of their own or another facility birth room and then describe in detail how they behave, or predict they would behave, in response to that space. Often, descriptions of behaviour are linked to midwives' perceptions of how much stress they experience, or anticipate they will experience, in a particular space (Hammond et al, 2017; Bourgeault et al, 2012; Davis, 2010). In spaces where stress is reduced, maternity care staff may be more able to behave in a way congruent with quality, human-centred care, regardless of whether birth is straightforward or medically complex (Foureur et al, 2010; Stenglin and Foureur, 2013; Sleutel et al, 2007; Dilani, 2009).

The influence of space on behaviour has also been observed in labouring women. In rooms described as domestic, as opposed to conventional, women have been observed to take more ownership of the space and behave in a more creative, uninhibited and active way (Mondy et al, 2016). This could be because the arrangement and aesthetics of conventional birth rooms send a 'bed-centric' message to women about the role – and the position – they are expected to assume during labour and birth (Townsend et al, 2016; Bowden et al, 2016). Writing more than 30 years ago, the French obstetrician Michel Odent (1984) described how, although he and his team had transformed what we would nowadays call their philosophy and model of care, it was not until the bed was removed from the centre of the birth room that women felt they had permission to behave instinctively during labour. Odent also reported that removing the labour room bed resulted in more sensitive staff responses to women. Worldwide, the challenge is to provide a safe birth space, which supports women to behave instinctively, and labour room staff to behave sensitively in response to women's clinical and psychosocial needs.

The cultural domain

In facility birth rooms, the domain of culture has enormous influence over what happens, to whom, why and how (Coast et al, 2014; Kirkham and Stapleton, 2004). This is partly because, at a societal level, culture contributes to the construction of what is often called the 'dominant discourse'. That is, the accepted way of thinking, understanding and talking about a particular issue or event. Worldwide, the dominant discourse positions childbirth primarily as a medical-technological event that is controlled by managerially driven healthcare institutions (Perez-Botella et al, 2015). The nature of this 'risk discourse', and the atmosphere of fear that tends to accompany it, is examined in more detail in Chapter 7. In response, most birth rooms in facilities in high-income countries, and in tertiary maternity centres around the world, include an array of medical technology that is intended to ensure safety, and that signals this intent to those using such spaces. Ironically, some researchers have demonstrated that it is this very medical technology that contributes to perceptions of the birth room as a dangerous and stressful place for healthcare staff and women, thus creating non-optimal neurobiological and behavioural responses that may interrupt facilitation of straightforward, normal birth (Watson, 2009; Hammond et al, 2014; Stenglin and Foureur, 2013; Fahy, 2008; Copeland et al, 2014; Duncan, 2011; Foureur, 2008).

Organisational culture is both constructed and reflected by modern birth rooms and the activities and behaviours that occur within them. Highly technocratic rooms represent a culture of childbirth that is replete with new myths, ideologies and values about the benefits of machines and monitoring that may undermine women's beliefs about their capacity to labour and give birth unaided (Scamell and Alaszewski, 2012). New rituals and customs have arisen around the use of symbolic artefacts, such as the CTG monitor, IV stand, syringe pump, blood pressure cuff and neonatal resuscitation equipment. This happens in environments that emphasise the need for continuous surveillance and ease of access to the woman's body. However, it must also be acknowledged that for some women such highly technocratic birth spaces are reassuring. This may be particularly important for women or babies whose health is compromised, or for women who have experienced previous trauma and for whom an apparently technologically controlled environment inspires feelings of safety.

In all birth environments, organisational culture can be physically 'seen' through artefacts and spatial arrangements that provide cues about the permissible or preferred behaviour of childbearing women, midwives and other staff in any given setting. Unfortunately, many midwives (and other health professionals) and childbearing women report that their personal values and beliefs about what could or should be happening in the birth room are overridden by organisational and institutional culture (Freemantle, 2013; O'Connell and Downe, 2009; Catling et al, 2017; Davies and Hodnett, 2002). In contrast, some researchers have demonstrated what can happen when alignment is achieved between personal, organisational and institutional culture – a flexible environment that improves experiences and outcomes for women and increases wellbeing and efficacy for staff can result (Misago et al, 2001; Guteridge and Giles, 2013; Walsh, 2006).

Conclusion

Taking an interconnected approach to the birth environment and quality of care is one way to approach the challenge of shifting maternity care towards a more authentically person-centred practice that supports childbearing women and the staff who care for them. We argue that the design and aesthetics of any space have direct neurobiological effects on the users of the space, which in turn shape behaviour and thus contribute to the construction and expression of culture in both the physical and discursive environment. We believe that the four domains of influence – spatial, neurobiological, behavioural and cultural – are always present and interacting, and can therefore always be considered, regardless of differences in facility location, models of care or childbearing populations. Acknowledging the need to address all four interconnected domains of influence in the birth room will allow us to ask important new questions about how birth environments can be constructed to facilitate optimal neurobiological and behavioural conditions in which safe, satisfying birth can take place.

Key points for consideration

- Make a list of the visible artefacts and spatial arrangements in your birth spaces and consider what message is conveyed about birth here.
- Describe where and how the woman's chosen birth companions are supported within your birth spaces.
- Discuss the design and aesthetics of your birth spaces with your colleagues and with childbearing women to explore where changes could be made.
- Source photos of other birth spaces and compare them with yours to determine what messages they convey and which you prefer.
- Create spaces that consider and address the interconnected influence of the spatial, neurobiological, behavioural and cultural domains.

References

ALABDULGADER, A. A. 2012. Coherence: A Novel Nonpharmacological Modality for Lowering Blood Pressure in Hypertensive Patients. *Global Advances in Health and Medicine* 1, 54-62.

ALEXANDER, C., ISHIKAWA, S. & SILVERSTEIN, M. 1977. *A Pattern Language,* Oxford, United Kingdom, Oxford University Press.

ARIADNE LABS AND MASS DESIGN GROUP 2017. Designing Capacity for High Value Healthcare: The Impact of Design on Clinical Care in Childbirth.

AVERBECK, B. B. 2010. Oxytocin and the salience of social cues. *Proceedings of the National Academy of Sciences,* 107, 9033-9034.

BARTZ, J. A., ZAKI, J., BOLGER, N. & OCHSNER, K. N. 2011. Social effects of oxytocin in humans: context and person matter. *Trends in Cognitive Sciences,* 15, 301-309.

BERKMANN, E. 2014. *Me, My Brain and I* [Online]. Psychology Today. [Accessed 08.04.2018 2018].

BIRTHPLACE IN ENGLAND COLLABORATIVE GROUP 2011. Perinatal and maternal outcomes by planned place of birth for healthy women with low risk pregnancies: The birthplace in England national prospective cohort study. *British medical Journal (Open Access).*

BLIX, E. 2011. Avoiding disturbance: Midwifery practice in home birth settings in Norway. *Midwifery,* 27, 687-692.

BOURGEAULT, I. L., SUTHERNS, R., MACDONALD, M. & LUCE, J. 2012. Problematising public and private work spaces: Midwives' work in hospitals and in homes. *Midwifery,* 28, 582-590.

BOWDEN, C., SHEEHAN, A. & FOUREUR, M. 2016. Birth room images: What they tell us about childbirth. A discourse analysis of birth rooms in developed countries. *Midwifery,* 35, 71-77.

BUCKLEY, S. 2015. Hormonal Physiology of Childbearing: Evidence and Implications for Women, Babies and Maternity Care. Washington: National Partnership for Women and Families.

CAAN, S. 2011. *Rethinking Design and Interiors: Human Beings in the Built Environment,* London, Laurence King Publishing.

CATLING, C. J., REID, F. & HUNTER, B. 2017. Australian midwives' experiences of their workplace culture. *Women and Birth,* 30, 137-145.

CHAN, J., BECKMAN, S. & LAWRENCE, P. 2007. Workplace design: A new managerial imperative. *California Management Review,* 49, 6-22.

COAST, E., JONES, E., PORTELA, A. & LATTOF, S. 2014. Maternity Care Services and Culture: A Systematic Global Mapping of Interventions. *PLoS ONE.*

CODDINGTON, R., CATLING, C. & HOMER, C. S. E. 2017. From hospital to home: Australian midwives' experiences of transitioning into publicly-funded homebirth programs. *Women and Birth,* 30, 70-76.

COPELAND, F., DAHLEN, H. G. & HOMER, C. S. E. 2014. Conflicting contexts: Midwives' interpretation of childbirth through photo elicitation. *Women and Birth,* 27, 126-131.

DAGUSTAN, J. 2009. Why do so few women give birth at home? Interpreting place in childbirth discourse. *School of Geography Working Paper Series* [Online].

DAVIES, B. L. & HODNETT, E. 2002. Labor Support: Nurses' Self-Efficacy and Views About Factors Influencing Implementation. *Journal of Obstetric, Gynecologic, & Neonatal Nursing,* 31, 48-56.

DAVIS, D., BADDOCK, S., PAIRMAN, S., HUNTER, M., BENN, C., WILSON, D., DIXON, L. & HERBISON, P. 2011. Planned Place of Birth in New Zealand: Does it Affect Mode of Birth and Intervention Rates Among Low-Risk Women? *Birth: issues in Perinatal Care,* 38, 111-119.

DAVIS, D. & WALKER, K. 2010a. The corporeal, the social and space/place: Exploring intersections from a miidwifery perspective in New Zealand. *Gender, Place & Culture: A Journal of Feminist Geography,* 17, 377-391.

DAVIS, D. L. & WALKER, K. 2010b. Case-loading midwifery in New Zealand: making space for childbirth. *Midwifery,* 26, 603-608.

DAVIS, J. A. P. 2010. Midwives and Normalcy in Childbirth: A Phenomenologic Concept Development Study. *Journal of Midwifery & Women's Health,* 55, 206-215.

DAY, C. 2014. *Places Of The Soul,* New York, Routledge.

DAZKIR, S. & READ, M. 2011. Furniture forms and their influence on our emotional responses toward interior environments. *Environment and Behaviour,* 10, 1-13.

DEERY, R. & FISHER, P. 2017. Professionalism and person-centredness: developing a practice-based approach to leadership within NHS maternity services in the UK. *Health Sociology Review,* 26, 143-159.

DILANI, A. Psychosocially supportive design: A salutogenic approach to the design of the physial environment. 1st International Conference on Sustainable Healthy Buildings, 2009 Seoul, Korea.

DUNCAN, J. 2011. The effect of colour and design in labour and delivery: A scientific approach. *Optics and Laser Technology,* 43, 420-424.

ESCURIET, R., WHITE, J., BEECKMAN, K., FRITH, L., LEON-LARIOS, F., LOYTVED, C., LUYBEN, A., SINCLAIR, M., VAN TEIJLINGEN, E., AND EU COST ACTION IS. 'CHILDBIRTH CULTURES, C. & CONSEQUENCES' 2015. Assessing the performance of maternity care in Europe: a critical exploration of tools and indicators. *BMC Health Services Research,* 15, 491.

FAHY, K. 2008. Power and the Social Construction of the Birth Territory. *In:* FAHY, K., FOUREUR, M. & HASTIE, C. (eds.) *Birth Territory and Midwifery Guardianship: Theory for Practice, Education and Research.* London: Butterworth Heinemann.

FANNIN, M. 2003. Domesticating birth in the hospital: 'family-centered' birth and the emergence of 'homelike' birthing rooms. *Antipode,* 35, 513-534.

FELDMAN, R. 2012. Oxytocin and social affiliation in humans. *Hormones and Behavior,* 61, 380-391.

FORBES, I., HOMER, C., FOUREUR, M. & LEAP, N. 2008. Birthing unit design: Researching new principles. *World Health Design,* Oct 2008, 47-53.

FOUREUR, M. 2008. Creating Space to Enable Undisturbed Birth. *In:* FAHY, K., FOUREUR, M. & HASTIE, C. (eds.) *Birth Territory and Midwifery Guardianship: Theory for Practice, Education and Research.* Sydney: Butterworth Heinemann Elsevier.

FOUREUR, M., DAVIS, D., FENWICK, J., LEAP, N., IEDEMA, R., FORBES, I. & HOMER, C. S. 2010. The relationship between birth unit design and safe, satisfying birth: Developing a hypothetical model. *Midwifery,* 26, 520-525.

FREEMANTLE, D. 2013. Part 1: The cultural web -- A model for change in maternity services. *British Journal of Midwifery,* 21, 648-653.

FRITH, L., SINCLAIR, M., VEHVILÄINEN-JULKUNEN, K., BEECKMAN, K., LOYTVED, C. & LUYBEN, A. 2014. Organisational culture in maternity care: a scoping review. *Evidence Based Midwifery,* 12, 16-22.

GAGE, F. 2004. Structural plasticity of the adult brain. *Dialogues in Clinical Neuroscience,* 6, 135-141.

GIERYN, T. F. 2000. A space for place in sociology. *Annual Review of Sociology,* 26, 463.

GOLEMBIEWSKI, J. 2016. Saultogenic Architecture in Healthcare Settings. *In:* MITTLELMARK, M., SAGY, S., ERIKSSON, M., BAUER, G., PELIKAN, J., LINDSTROM, B. & ESPNES, G. (eds.) *The Handbook of Salutogenesis.* New York: Springer.

GROPPE, S. E., GOSSEN, A., RADEMACHER, L., HAHN, A., WESTPHAL, L., GRÜNDER, G. & SPRECKELMEYER, K. N. 2013. Oxytocin Influences Processing of Socially Relevant Cues in the Ventral Tegmental Area of the Human Brain. *Biological Psychiatry,* 74, 172-179.

GUTERIDGE, K. & GILES, H. 2013. Setting the standard. *Midwives.* Redactive Publishing.

HAMMOND, A. 2017. *Oxytocin and Adrenaline Spaces.* PhD, University of Technology Sydney.

HAMMOND, A., FOUREUR, M. & HOMER, C. 2013. The hardware and software implications of birth unit design: A midwifery perspective. *Midwifery,* In Press.

HAMMOND, A., HOMER, C. & FOUREUR, M. 2014. Messages from space: An exploration of the relationship between hospital birth environments and midwifery practice. *Health Environments Research & Design Journal (HERD),* 7, 81-95.

HAMMOND, A., HOMER, C. S. E. & FOUREUR, M. 2017. Friendliness, functionality and freedom: Design characteristics that support midwifery practice in the hospital setting. *Midwifery,* 50, 133-138.

HARTE, J. D. 2016. Childbirth Supporters 19 Experiences in a Built Hospital Birth Environment. *HERD,* 9, 135-161.

HERZOG, T. & STREVEY, S. 2008. Contact with nature, sense of humour and psychological wellbeing. *Environment and Behaviour,* 40, 747-776.

HODNETT, E., WALSH, D. & DOWNE, S. 2012. Alternative versus conventional institutional settings for birth. *Cochrane Database of Systematic Reviews.*

HOMER, C. 2016. Models of maternity care: evidence for midwifery continuity of care. *Medical Journal of Australia,* 205, 370-374.

HUNTER, M. 2003. Autonomy, clinical freedom and responsibility. *In:* KIRKHAM, M. (ed.) *Birth Centres: A Social Model for Maternity Care.* London: Elsevier Science.

INSTITUTE, S. 2012. Do Changes in the Environment Affect the Brain? YouTube.

ISHAK, W. W., KAHLOON, M. & FAKHRY, H. 2011. Oxytocin role in enhancing well-being: A literature review. *Journal of Affective Disorders,* 130, 1-9.

JENKINSON, B., JOSEY, N. & KRUSKE, S. BirthSpace: An evidence-based guide to birth environment design. Queensland: Queensland Centre for Mothers and Babies, The University of Queensland.

KEATING, A. & FLEMING, V. E. M. 2009. Midwives' experiences of facilitating normal birth in an obstetric-led unit: a feminist perspective. *Midwifery,* 25, 518-527.

KENNEDY, H. P., YOSHIDA, S., COSTELLO, A., DECLERCQ, E., DIAS, M. A., DUFF, E., GHERISSI, A., KAUFMAN, K., MCCONVILLE, F., MCFADDEN, A., MICHEL-SCHULDT, M., MOYO, N. T., SCHUILING, K., SPECIALE, A. M. & RENFREW, M. J. 2016. Asking different questions: research priorities to improve the quality of care for every woman, every child. *The Lancet Global Health,* 4, e777-e779.

KIRKHAM, M. & STAPLETON, H. 2004. The Culture of the Maternity Services in Wales and England as a Barrier to Informed Choice. *In:* KIRKHAM, M. (ed.) *Informed Choice in Maternity Care.* Basingstoke; Hampshire UK: Palgrave Macmillan.

KOBLINSKY, M., MOYER, C. A., CALVERT, C., CAMPBELL, J., CAMPBELL, O. M. R., FEIGL, A. B., GRAHAM, W. J., HATT, L., HODGINS, S., MATTHEWS, Z., MCDOUGALL, L., MORAN, A. C., NANDAKUMAR, A. K. & LANGER, A. 2016. Quality maternity care for every woman, everywhere: a call to action. *The Lancet,* 388, 2307-2320.

LAWSON, B. 2010. Healing Architecture. *Arts and Health: An International Journal for Research, Policy and Practice,* 2, 95-108.

LEPORI, B. 1994. Freedom of movement in birth places. *Children's Environments,* 11, 1-12.

LOUNSBURY, C. 2010. Architecture and Cultural History. *In:* HICKS, D. & BEAUDRY, M. (eds.) *the Oxford Handbook of Material Culture Studies.* Oxford: Oxford University Press.

MACLELLAN, J. 2011. The art of midwifery practice: A discourse analysis. *MIDIRS Midwifery Digest,* 21, 25-31.

MCCRATY, R., ATKINSON, M., LIPSENTHAL, L. & ARGUELLES, L. 2009. New Hope for Correctional Officers: An Innovative Program for Reducing Stress and Health Risks. *Applied Psychophysiological Biofeedback,* 34, 251-272.

METZGER, C. 2018. *Neuroarchitecture,* Berlin, Jovis.

MILLER, S. & SKINNER, J. 2012. Are first time mothers who plan home birth more likely to receive evidence-based care? A comparative study of home and hospital care provided by the same midwives. *Birth,* 39, 135-144.

MISAGO, C., KENDALL, C., FREITAS, P., HANEDA, K., SILVEIRA, D., ONUKI, D., MORI, T., SADAMORI, T. & UMENAI, T. 2001. From 'culture of dehumanization of childbirth' to 'childbirth as a transformative experience': changes in five municipalities in north-east Brazil. *International Journal of Gynecology & Obstetrics,* 75, S67-S72.

MONCRIEFF, G. 2018. Can continuity bring birth back to women and normality back to midwives? *British Journal of Midwifery,* 26, 642-650.

MONDY, T., FENWICK, J., LEAP, N. & FOUREUR, M. 2016. How domesticity dictates behaviour in the birth space: Lessons for designing birth environments in institutions wanting to promote a positive experience of birth. *Midwifery,* 43, 37-47.

NANDA, U., PATI, D., GHAMARI, H. & BAJEMA, R. 2013. Lessons from neuroscience: form follows function, emotions follow form. *Intelligent Buildings International,* 5, 61-78.

NYGREN, A. 2018. Inequality and interconnectivity: Urban spaces of justice in Mexico. *Geoforum,* 89, 145-154.

O'CONNELL, R. & DOWNE, S. 2009. A metasynthesis of midwive's experience of hospital practice in publicly funded settings: Compliance, resistance and authenticity. *Health: An Interdisciplinary Journal for the Social Study of Health, Illness and Medicine,* 13, 589-609.

ODENT, M. 1984. *Birth Reborn,* London, Random House.

ÖHMAN, A. 2005. The role of the amygdala in human fear: Automatic detection of threat. *Psychoneuroendocrinology,* 30, 953-958.

OLFF, M., FRIJLING, J. L., KUBZANSKY, L. D., BRADLEY, B., ELLENBOGEN, M. A., CARDOSO, C., BARTZ, J. A., YEE, J. R. & VAN ZUIDEN, M. 2013. The role of oxytocin in social bonding, stress regulation and mental health: An update on the moderating effects of context and interindividual differences. *Psychoneuroendocrinology,* 38, 1883-1894.

OLIVIERA, F., KAKEHASHI, T., TSUNEMI, M. & PINHEIRO, E. 2011. Noise levels in the delivery room. *Text and Context Nursing,* 20, 287-293.

PEREZ-BOTELLA, M., DOWNE, S., MAGISTRETTI, M., LINDSTROM, B. & BERG, M. 2015. The use of salutogenesis theory in empirical studies of maternity care for healthy mothers and babies. *Sexual & Reproductive Healthcare,* 6, 33-39.

PETERS, L. L., THORNTON, C., DE JONGE, A., KHASHAN, A., TRACY, M., DOWNE, S., FEIJEN-DE JONG, E. I. & DAHLEN, H. G. 2018. The effect of medical and operative birth interventions on child health outcomes in the first 28 days and up to 5 years of age: A linked data population-based cohort study. *Birth-Issues in Perinatal Care,* 45, 347-357.

PEZARO, S., PEARCE, G. & BAILEY, E. 2018. Childbearing women's experiences of midwives' workplace distress: Patient and public involvement. *British Journal of Midwifery,* 26, 659-669.

PULVERMÜLLER, F. 2013. How neurons make meaning: brain mechanisms for embodied and abstract-symbolic semantics. *Trends in Cognitive Sciences,* 17, 458-470.

RENFREW, M. J. 2014. Midwifery and quality care: findings from a new evidence-informed framework for maternal and newborn care. *The Lancet (British edition),* 384, 1129-1145.

ROMANO, A. M. & LOTHIAN, J. A. 2008. Promoting, Protecting, and Supporting Normal Birth: A Look at the Evidence. *JOGNN: Journal of Obstetric, Gynecologic & Neonatal Nursing,* 37, 94-105.

RUOHOMÄKI, V., LAHTINEN, M. & REIJULA, K. 2015. Salutogenic and user-centred approach for workplace design. *Intelligent Buildings International,* 7, 184-197.

SANDALL, J., SOLTANI, H., GATES, S., SHENNAN, A. & DEVANE, D. 2013. Midwife-led continuity models versus other models of care for childbearing women. *The Cochrane Database of Systematic Reviews,* 8, CD004667.

SCAMELL, M. & ALASZEWSKI, A. 2012. Fateful moments and the catergorisation of risk: Midwifery practice and the ever-narrowing window of normality during childbirth. *Health, Risk and Society,* 14, 207-221.

SCARF, V. L., ROSSITER, C., VEDAM, S., DAHLEN, H. G., ELLWOOD, D., FORSTER, D., FOUREUR, M. J., MCLACHLAN, H., OATS, J., SIBBRITT, D., THORNTON, C. & HOMER, C. S. E. 2018. Maternal and perinatal outcomes by planned place of birth among women with low-risk pregnancies in high-income countries: A systematic review and meta-analysis. *Midwifery,* 62, 240-255.

SCHMIDT, L. J., BELOPOLSKY, A. V. & THEEUWES, J. 2017. The time course of attentional bias to cues of threat and safety. *Cognition and Emotion,* 31, 845-857.

SINGH, D. & NEWBURN, M. 2006. Feathering the nest: what women want from the birth environment. *RCM Midwives,* 9, 266-269.

SLEUTEL, M., SCHULTZ, S. & WYBLE, K. 2007. Nurses' Views of Factors That Help and Hinder Their Intrapartum Care. *Journal of Obstetric, Gynecologic, & Neonatal Nursing,* 36, 203-211.

STARK, M. A., REMYNSE, M. & ZWELLING, E. 2016. Importance of the Birth Environment to Support Physiologic Birth. *Journal of Obstetric, Gynecologic & Neonatal Nursing,* 45, 285-294.

STENGLIN, M. & FOUREUR, M. 2013. Designing out the Fear Cascade to increase the likelihood of normal birth. *Midwifery,* 29, 819-825.

STENGLIN, M. K. 2009. Space odyssey: towards a social semiotic model of three-dimensional space. *Visual Communication,* 8, 35-64.

TECHAU, D., OWEN, C., PATON, D. & FAY, R. 2016. Buildings, Brains and Behaviour: Towards an affective neuroscience of architecture. *Design and Health Scientifc Review,* 24-37.

TOWNSEND, B., FENWICK, J., THOMSON, V. & FOUREUR, M. 2016. The birth bed: A qualitative study on the views of midwives regarding the use of the bed in the birth space. *Women and Birth,* 29, 80-84.

TRACY, S., SULLIVAN, E., WANG, Y., BLACK, D. & TRACY, M. 2007. Birth outcomes associated with interventions in labour amongst low risk women: A population based study. *Women & Birth,* 20, 41-48.

TUAN, Y. 1977. *Space and Place,* Minneapolis, University of Minnesota Press.

ULRICH, R., BERRY, L., XIAOBO, Q. & TURNER PARISH, J. 2010. A Conceptual Framework for the Domain of Evidence-Based Design. *Health Environments Research & Design Journal (HERD),* 4, 95-114.

UVNÄS MOBERG, K., ARN, I. & MAGNUSSON, D. 2005. The Psychobiology of Emotion: The Role of the Oxytocinergic System. *International Journal of Behavioral Medicine,* 12, 59-65.

VARTANIAN, O., NAVARRETE, G., CHATTERJEE, A., FICH, L., LEDER, H., MODROÑO, C., ROSTRUP, N., SKOV, M., CORRAD, G. & NADAL, M. 2017. *Preference for Curvilinear Contour in Interior Architectural Spaces: Evidence From Experts and Nonexperts.*

VEDAM, S. 2017. The Mothers on Respect (MOR) index: measuring quality, safety, and human rights in childbirth. *SSM - population health,* 3, 201-210.

VISCHER, J. 2008. Towards an environmental psychology of workspace: How people are affected by environments for work. *Architectural Science Review,* 51, 97-108.

WALKER, R., POLESZCZUK, J., PILON-THOMAS, S., KIM, S., ANDERSON, A., CZERNIECKI, B. J., HARRISON, L. B., MOROS, E. G. & ENDERLIN, H. 2018. Immune interconnectivity of anatomically distant tumors as a potential mediator of systemic responses to local therapy. *Scientific Reports,* 8.

WALSH, D. 2006. Subverting the assembly-line: childbirth in a free-standing birth centre. *Social Science & Medicine,* 62, 1330-1340.

WALSH, D. & GUTTERIDGE, K. 2011. Using the birth environment to increase women's potential in labour. *MIDIRS Midwifery Digest,* 21, 143-147.

WATSON, A. 2009. *Examining the Content Validity of the BUDSET Instrument Within a Woman-Centred Framework.* Bachelor of Midwifery (Honours), University of Technology, Sydney.

WESTERN WASHINGTON UNIVERSITY. 2019. *Interconnectedness* [Online]. : Western Washington University. Available: https://www.facingthefuture.org/pages/interconnectedness [Accessed 04/01/2019 2019].

CHAPTER 16

Approaches to pain in labour: implications for practice

Nicky Leap, Elizabeth Newnham and *Sigfridur Inga Karlsdottir*

Introduction

'Pain is never the sole creation of our anatomy and physiology; it emerges only at the intersection of bodies, minds and culture' (Morris, 1991, p1).

This statement reminds us to consider the influences of 'bodies, minds and culture' when thinking about the complexity of how a person approaches the subject of pain in labour. When translated into values and beliefs, these influences can have a profound effect on how practitioners engage with women around pain in labour and ultimately, on women's experiences of birth. Indeed, as Ellen Hodnett has noted:

'The influences of pain, pain relief, and intrapartum medical interventions on subsequent satisfaction are neither as obvious, as direct, nor as powerful as the influences of the attitudes and behaviors of the caregivers'. (Hodnett, 2002 S160).

With these considerations in mind, in this chapter we explore perspectives on pain in labour drawing on work describing three paradigms. (When we use the word 'paradigm' we mean ways of thinking and being in the world that affect how we behave and interact with others and contribute to an identifiable culture.) We provide an overview of the paradigms of 'pain relief' and 'working with pain in labour' (Leap and Anderson, 2008), drawing on literature identifying how these discordant perspectives can affect women's experiences, particularly in hospital institutions where the dominant culture encourages the use of epidural analgesia (Newnham, McKellar et al, 2016, 2018).

Women's perspectives on pain in labour have been described as 'the third paradigm in labour preparation and management' (Karlsdottir, Halldorsdottir et al, 2014).

Arguably, however, women's perspectives should be seen as the central paradigm in terms of maternity care, since understandings of women's different approaches to pain management in labour are essential if maternity care providers are to adapt care to the needs of individual women (Escott, Spiby et al, 2004; Klomp, Maniën et al, 2014). We therefore summarise evidence from studies that have explored women's experiences of pain in labour.

A full discussion about the opposing paradigms of 'pain relief 'and 'working with pain' can be accessed elsewhere (Leap and Anderson 2008; Leap and Hunter 2016). Although it is tempting to conceptualise the 'pain relief' paradigm as 'medical' and the 'working with pain' paradigm as belonging to 'midwifery', we suggest that this can limit understandings of the pervasive influence of the technocratic culture on institutionalised birth and caregivers (Davis-Floyd 2001; Reiger and Dempsey 2006; Newnham 2014). We want to avoid generalisations that undermine individual midwives', doctors', and others' attempts to support women with healthy pregnancies who want to avoid interventions in the way they manage pain.

The 'pain relief' paradigm

The International Association for the Study of Pain defines pain as '*an unpleasant sensory and emotional experience associated with actual or potential tissue damage or described in terms of such damage.*' (IASP, 2014). This definition explains why the pursuit of 'adequate pain relief' is an important feature of nursing and medical practice in the context of pathology. When transferred into the arena of childbirth, the definition translates into the biomedical discourse that labour pain is problematic and should be avoided or relieved through pharmacological methods, in particular the use of epidural anaesthesia (Newnham, McKellar et al, 2016). This approach has been described as 'the pain relief paradigm' (Leap and Anderson, 2008) and has become the dominant philosophy of technocratic birth (Davis-Floyd, 2001), embraced by practitioners as well as the general public (See Table 1).

Table 1.
Potential attitudes associated with the 'pain relief paradigm'

No woman should have to suffer pain in labour in this day and age.
Women have unrealistic expectations about how they will cope with labour; most will end up using drugs or an epidural, including those who say they want to manage without.
A paternalistic 'rescuing' approach underestimates women's own ability to work with pain in normal labour.
Discomfort with the noise that women make in response to contractions.
A belief that some midwives withhold pain relief because of their normal birth agenda, causing women to suffer.
Pharmacological pain relief gives women a sense of control.

The 'pain relief menu'

Central to the 'pain relief paradigm' is the notion of 'choice'. Practitioners working within this frame of reference tend to present women with a list of all the things that are on offer to help women manage pain (See Table 2). In the name of informed choice, those working this way will usually draw on formal RCT evidence to describe the 'pros and cons' of each method. This has been described as offering the 'pain relief menu' (Leap and Anderson, 2008). The (often unintentional) message can be that the woman will need pharmacological pain relief even when labour is uncomplicated; it is just a question of her choosing the right thing for her. Although the menu might start with things the woman can do for herself or with her birth supporters, this can be undermined by an inference that many women have unrealistic expectations of how they will cope using their own resources and will end up needing pharmacological pain relief when in labour (Lally, Murtagh et al, 2008). There is therefore a need for sensitivity about the messages women are receiving when practitioners are discussing the 'pros and cons' of different ways of managing pain in labour.

Table 2.
The pain relief 'menu' (examples)

Methods controlled by the woman: water, changing positions, moving around, vocalising, breathing techniques, relaxation, psychoprophylaxis, music.
Methods with chosen attendant/support person: heat packs, massage, breathing techniques, counting, chanting, labour coaching, hiring a doula.
Complementary therapies: herbs, homeopathy, acupuncture, acupressure, reflexology, hypnotism, biofeedback machines.
TENS machine (transcutaneous electrical nerve stimulation).
Entonox/nitrous oxide.
Sterile water injections in the lower back.
Pethidine/morphine (or equivalent parenteral opioid).
Epidural anaesthesia.

The 'working with pain' paradigm

In response to understanding the potential for women to experience birth as transformational (Van der Gucht and Lewis, 2015), many practitioners adopt an approach to supporting women in normal labour using what has been described as 'working with pain' (Leap, 1997). In this approach, pain is seen as part of a productive, physiological process aided by the intricate, interwoven hormonal physiology of pregnancy, labour and birth, breastfeeding and mother-baby bonding (Buckley, 2015). Labour is acknowledged as challenging, with women's coping strategies emphasised, all with a view to building women's confidence in their abilities to find ways to manage pain with appropriate support (Leap, Sandall et al, 2010; Karlsdottir, Halldorsdottir et al, 2014).

A 'working with pain' approach highlights the essential role of supportive birth companions and acknowledges that women are likely to need encouragement when they experience crises of confidence during both pregnancy and labour (Dempsey, 2013). The rationale for this approach is discussed in terms of reducing the potential for intervention and the benefits of physiological birth. This includes articulating the sense of triumph and pride women often describe after surmounting the challenges they experience during labour and birth: feelings that contribute to a positive start to new motherhood (Leap and Anderson 2008; Karlsdottir, Halldorsdottir et al, 2014).

The central features of the 'working with pain' approach are summarised in Table 3:

Table 3.
The 'working with pain' approach

Uterine activity is explained as something that women can work with during the normal physiology of labour with the help of endogenous hormones.
'Normal pain' is part of 'normal labour' and has a different quality to the pain of injury or ill health. It has an important role in the physiology of labour and most women will be able to cope with 'normal' levels of pain.
'Abnormal pain' is associated with complicated labour, stimulation of contractions with intravenous oxytocin, poor support and usually the need for pharmacological pain relief.
The wave-type nature of contractions and the rests in between are emphasised in order to construct contractions as manageable, one at a time.
Pain is a stimulator of endogenous opioids and part of the hormonal cascades that promote uninterrupted birth physiology.
Continuous support and encouragement are essential features of supporting women to face the challenges associated with labour and birth.
The unsolicited offering of pharmacological pain relief to a woman during labour can undermine her confidence, reducing the chances of a normal labour and birth.

The third paradigm: women's approaches to pain in labour

In Western society pain is generally looked at as a very negative phenomenon. Many women, however, describe childbirth pain in a positive way, psychologically and emotionally, even though they often experience it objectively as the most painful event of their lives (Lundgren and Dahlberg, 1998; Karlsdottir, Halldorsdottir et al, 2014). Labour pain is remembered as being different from any other pain, a unique kind of pain that brings pleasure and excitement as well as anxiety and fear of the unknown (Callister, Khalaf et al, 2003; Lundgren, Karlsdottir et al, 2009; Karlsdottir, Halldorsdottir et al, 2014).

In studies across the world, women have identified the meaning they attach to managing pain in terms of a sense of control and a positive experience of giving birth (Lowe 2002; Larkin, Begley et al, 2009). They have described pain as an important component of a rite of passage that brings human growth and a sense of pride and accomplishment (Lundgren and Dahlberg, 1998; Kennedy, Shannon et al, 2004;

Karlsdottir, Halldorsdottir et al, 2014).

In contrast, there are women who describe the pain of labour as too much for them, leaving them with a feeling of exhaustion and fear (Lundgren, Karlsdottir et al, 2009). Memories of poor support, inadequate pain relief and feeling a lack of control can contribute to post-traumatic stress, harming their relationships and severely affecting their physical and mental health (Waldenström, Hildingsson et al, 2004; Birth Trauma Association, 2017). Many years after giving birth, these memories can still affect women negatively (Lundgren, Karlsdottir et al, 2009). These feelings can be affected by unexpected events that happen during labour and birth and a sense of lack of support and control as labour progresses.

Women's expectations of pain in labour

Women's expectations about the intensity of pain in labour vary considerably. It is therefore important that, early and throughout pregnancy, midwives and healthcare professionals address these expectations in order to assist women to prepare themselves for the pain of labour (Karlsdottir, Sveinsdottir et al, 2015). Midwives, childbirth educators and birth supporters can help pregnant women to develop their own unique set of practical and cognitive coping strategies for labour through reflection on their individual coping styles and awareness of any unhelpful patterns of pain catastrophising (Whitburn, Jones et al, 2014). This is particularly effective where there are opportunities to reinforce and practise these coping strategies with birth partners (Escott, Slade et al, 2009).

A woman's life experiences and personal attitudes will affect how she prepares for labour (Larkin, Begley et al, 2009; Mander 2010). The approaches of caregivers, however, can have a profound effect on how women actually experience their labour pain (Hodnett, 2002; Gibson, 2014). Several authors have suggested that most women do not come into maternity units with polarised views about pain in labour and that there is value in understanding a spectrum of approaches (Haines, Rubertsson et al, 2012; Dempsey, 2013; Klomp, Maniën et al, 2014; Karlsdottir, Sveinsdottir et al, 2015; Newnham, McKellar et al, 2018). At one end of the spectrum are women who are completely clear that they do not want to have any pain and at the other end are those who will embrace pain as part of normal labour. Between these two ends of the spectrum are the majority of women, most of whom will adopt a 'wait and see approach'. Many will rely on the advice of 'experts', unaware that their pain tolerance can be affected by the type of support they receive (Dempsey, 2013) and that they are in a particularly vulnerable group for operative birth if they choose to 'take it as it comes' (Haines, Rubertsson et al, 2012, p12).

Where women are able to build a trusting relationship with a midwife, they identify their midwife as the most useful source of information in preparing for labour and birth (Grimes, Forster et al, 2014). This relational continuity of care can play a major role in building a woman's confidence in her ability to manage pain in labour (Leap, Sandall et al, 2010); particularly if she is fearful of birth (Nilsson and Lundgren, 2009) or considered to be 'high-risk' (Berg, 2005). Discussions during pregnancy about labour can take into consideration the complexity of individual women's opinions, feelings, values, expectations and preferences as well as social, cultural and political influences

(Haines, Rubertsson et al, 2012; Noseworthy, Phibbs et al, 2013). This approach is potentially more valuable than one-off discussions in which women are expected to make decisions about which methods of 'pain relief' they are going to want to use during labour (Lally, Thomson et al, 2014).

Engaging with pregnant women about managing pain in labour

Increasingly, pregnant women are relying on information sources that are readily accessible through the Internet and television in order to prepare for labour and birth (Lagan, Sinclair et al, 2010). Portrayals of normal birth tend to be missing in the dramatic presentations of labour and birth in the televisual media (see Chapter 10) and this appears to influence how women engage with childbirth (Morris and McInerney, 201; Luce, Cash et al, 2016). The overwhelming messages from reality television tend to perpetuate fear and the idea that obstetric interventions and technology make labour pain more manageable (Stoll and Hall 2013a; Stoll and Hall, 2013b; D'Cruz and Lee, 2014; Sanders 2015).

It has been suggested that all birth attendants should watch reality TV shows such as *One Born Every Minute* so that they understand the potential messages women are getting, can provide alternative sources of information, and can attempt to build or restore women's confidence in their abilities to manage pain in labour (Garrod, 2012; Leap and Hunter, 2016). For the same reasons, midwives have been encouraged to critique how pain is portrayed in the books that many women are turning to in order to get information about labour (Kennedy, Nardini et al, 2009; Grimes, Forster et al, 2014).

Conversations during antenatal care about what women have recently viewed on television about labour and birth or have read in books or magazines open up the possibility for women to discuss anxieties about how they will manage pain in labour (Talbot, 2012). Women and their partners also value having such discussions in small-group learning environments where they can learn from each other as well as the facilitator (Nolan 2009; Schrader, McMillan, Barlow et al, 2009).

Discussing evidence about managing pain in labour

Reporting on non-pharmacological measures for managing pain in labour is relatively neglected in the health and medical literature (Caton, Corry et al, 2002; Simkin and Bolding, 2004). This often results in discussions about evidence and risk occurring in ways that minimise the potential side effects of epidurals, while emphasising the lack of strong evidence for non-pharmacological measures. Such an approach perpetuates a dominant culture that privileges technology over normal physiology (Newnham, McKellar et al, 2015, 2016, 2018).

Overall, non-pharmacological approaches to pain management in labour are associated with a reduction in epidural rates and women using these methods report a higher satisfaction with their experiences of labour and birth (Chaillet, Belaid et al, 2014). This is reflected in Cochrane systematic reviews reporting on the following:

- Midwifery-led continuity of care (Sandall, Soltani et al, 2016)
- Continuous support for women during labour (Bohren, Hofmeyer et al, 2017)
- Acupuncture and hypnotherapy (Smith, Collins et al, 2006)
- Immersion in water (Cluett, Burns et al, 2018)
- Upright positions and moving around spontaneously (Lawrence, Lewis et al, 2013)
- Alternative birth settings (Hodnett, Downe et al, 2012)

Conversely, effective pharmacological pain relief in the form of epidural analgesia is one of the factors associated with less positive experiences of birth, affecting short and long-term mental health (Carvalho and Cohen, 2013; Lindholm and Hildingsson, 2015). It appears that many women who have epidural analgesia continue to have worrying memories of labour pain, particularly those who perceive their labours to have been traumatic (Waldenström, 2006; Waldenström and Schytt, 2009). Epidural analgesia is acknowledged as the most effective form of pain relief, but it is also associated with an increase in interventions and instrumental birth (Anim-Somuah, Smyth et al, 2018; Jones, Othman et al, 2013). It thus can dramatically change birth outcomes for a woman who is considered to be low risk (Tracy and Tracy, 2003; Tracy, Sullivan et al, 2007; Newnham, McKellar et al, 2016, 2018).

Continuous support for women during labour

The importance of continuous support in labour has been a central feature of women's responses in studies conducted across geographical and cultural boundaries over the last 50 years (Bohren, Hoffmeyer et al, 2017). High-quality support not only reduces medical interventions, including the use of epidurals, but also improves women's perceptions of their birth experience, promoting a positive adaptation to motherhood and reducing the risk of post-traumatic stress disorder and other perinatal mental health problems (Ross-Davie and Cheyne, 2014).

In many studies, women have identified the importance of support from midwives who have a positive approach to helping them manage labour through drawing on their own resources and coping strategies (Haines, Rubertsson et al, 2012; Karlsdottir, Halldorsdottir et al, 2014; Van der Gucht and Lewis, 2015). In high-income countries, though, there is often a dissonance between what women want in order to cope with pain and the realities of clinical practice (Van der Gucht and Lewis, 2015). Most women will be cared for in labour by a midwife they are unlikely to have met before whose philosophy of care around pain may or may not be congruent with theirs. Care from a known midwife in labour can considerably reduce women's decisions to use pharmacological pain relief (Homer, Leap et al, 2017) while promoting positive experiences of labour (Leap, Sandall et al, 2010); however, it would benefit women if all midwives (and other healthcare providers) who work with women in labour are open to adopting a 'working with pain' approach, providing a caring presence and continuous support (Kennedy, Anderson et al, 2010; Ross-Davie and Cheyne, 2014; Ross-Davie, McElligott et al, 2014).

Conclusion

There is a wealth of evidence identifying that women want continuous support in labour and that many would like this to be provided by midwives or other caregivers who accept pain as part of the process of promoting normal birth and an empowering transition to motherhood. There is therefore an imperative for health professionals to take seriously this evidence and the NICE guideline that they should: 'consider how their own values and beliefs inform their attitude to coping with pain in labour and ensure their care supports the woman's choice' (National Collaborating Centre for Women's and Children's Health, 2014, p329). Pain management in labour is not, however, a simple matter of providing information about the 'pain relief menu' and asking women to make choices. Maternity services tend to be dominated by approaches that privilege a culture of 'pain relief' as opposed to one where the value of 'working with pain' is discussed and promoted between practitioners, and in turn, with women. The attitudes of maternity care providers will affect the conversations that take place with pregnant women and their labour supporters and the level of support they receive during labour. This can have both a positive and negative effect on the choices women make and how they manage and remember pain in labour. The long-term consequences of these experiences can be profound in terms of the wellbeing of women and their families.

Key points for consideration

- Incorporate a 'working with pain' paradigm into your practice.
- Most women want to 'go with the flow' in labour and women who are well-supported in labour have fewer pain-relief requirements.
- The approach of the caregivers can have a profound effect on how women actually experience the pain of labour.
- Non-pharmacological approaches to pain management in labour are associated with a reduction in epidural rates.
- Women using non-pharmacological methods have less intervention and report a higher satisfaction with their experiences of labour and birth.

References

Anim-Somuah, M., R.M.D. Smyth, A.M. Cyna and A. Cuthbert. Epidural versus non-epidural or no analgesia for pain management in labour. Cochrane Database of Systematic Reviews 2018, Issue 5. Art. No.: CD000331. DOI: 10.1002/14651858.CD000331.pub4.

Berg, M. (2005). "A midwifery model of care for childbearing women at high risk: genuine caring in caring for the genuine." *Journal of Perinatal Education* **14**(1): 9-21.

Bohren MA, Hofmeyr G, Sakala C, Fukuzawa RK, Cuthbert A. Continuous support for women during childbirth. Cochrane Database of Systematic Reviews 2017, Issue 7. Art. No.: CD003766. DOI: 10.1002/14651858.CD003766. pub6

Birth Trauma Association. (2017). "What is Birth Trauma? http://www.birthtraumaassociation.org.uk/index.php/help-support/what-is-birth-trauma. Accessed 25/4/2017." Retrieved 25th April 2017.

Buckley, S. J. (2015). Hormonal Physiology of Childbearing: Evidence and Implications for Women, Babies, and Maternity Care. Washington, D.C, Childbirth Connection Programs, National Partnership for Women & Families.

Callister, L. C., I. Khalaf, S. Semenic, R. Kartchner and K. Vehvilainen-Julkunen (2003). "The pain of childbirth: perceptions of culturally diverse women." *Pain Management in Nursing* **4**(4): 145-154.

Carvalho, B. and S. E. Cohen (2013). " Measuring the labor pain experience: delivery still far off. Editorial." *International Journal of Obstetric Anesthesia* **22**: 6-9.

Caton, D., M. P. Corry, F. Frigoletto, D,, D. P. Hopkins, E. Lieberman, L. J. Mayberry, J. P. Rooks, A. Rosenfield, C. Sakala, P. Simkin and D. Young (2002). "The nature and management of labor pain: Executive Summary." *American Journal of Obstetrics and Gynecology* **186**(5, Supplement 1): S1-S15.

Chaillet, N., L. Belaid, C. Crochetière, L. Roy, G.-P. Gagné, J. M. Moutquin, M. Rossignol, M. Dugas, M. Wassef J. Bonapace (2014). "Nonpharmacologic approaches for pain management during labor compared with usual care: A Meta-Analysis " *Birth* **41**(2): 122-137.

Cluett ER, Burns E, Cuthbert A. Immersion in water during labour and birth. Cochrane Database of Systematic Reviews 2018, Issue 5. Art. No.: CD000111. DOI: 10.1002/14651858.CD000111.pub4.

D'Cruz, L. and C. Lee (2014). "Childbirth Expectations: an Australian study of young childless women." *Journal of Reproductive and Infant Psychology* **32**(2): 196-208.

Davis-Floyd, R. (2001). "The technocratic, humanistic and holistic paradigms of childbirth." *International Journal of Gynaecology & Obstetrics* **75**: S5-S23.

Dempsey, R. (2013). *Birth with Confidence. Savvy Choices for Normal Birth*. Fairfield, Australia, Boathouse Press.

Escott, D., P. Slade and H. Spiby (2009). "Preparation for pain management during childbirth: The psychological aspects of coping strategy development in antenatal education." *Clinical Pschology Review* **29**: 617-622.

Escott, D., H. Spiby, P. Slade and R. B. Fraser (2004). "The range of coping strategies women use to manage pain and anxiety prior to and during first experience of labour." *Midwifery* **20**(2): 144-156.

Garrod, D. (2012). "Birth as entertainment: What are the wider effects?" *British Journal of Midwifery* **20**(2): 81.

Gibson, E. (2014). "Women's expectations and experiences with labour pain in medical and midwifery models of birth in the United States." *Women and Birth* **27**(3): 185-189.

Grimes, H. A., D. A. Forster and M. S. Newton (2014). "Sources of information used by women during pregnancy to meet their information needs." *Midwifery* **30**: e26-e33.

Haines, H. M., C. Rubertsson, J. F. Pallant and I. Hildingsson (2012). "The influence of women's fear, attitudes and beliefs of childbirth on mode and experience of birth." *BMC Pregnancy and Childbirth* **12**: 55.

Hodnett, E. D. (2002). "Pain and women's satisfaction with the experience of childbirth: a systematic review." *American Journal of Obstetrics and Gynaecology* **186**(5): S160-S172.

Hodnett, E. D., S. Downe and D. Walsh (2012). "Alternative versus conventional institutional settings for birth." *Cochrane Database of Systematic Reviews*: Issue 8. Art. No.: CD000012.

Homer, C. S. E., N. Leap, N. Edwards and J. Sandall (2017). "Midwifery continuity of carer in an area of high socio-economic disadvantage in London: a retrospective analysis of Albany Midwifery Practice outcomes using routine data (1997–2009)." *Midwifery* **48**: 1-10.

IASP (2014). "International Association for the Study of Pain Definition of Pain. www.iasp-pain.org/Taxonomy."

Jones, L., M. Othman, T. Dowswell, Z. Alfirevic, Gates S, M. Newburn, S. Jordan, T. Lavender and J. P. Neilson (2013). "Pain management for women in labour: an overview of systematic reviews. Cochrane Database of Systematic Reviews 2013, Issue 6. Art. No.: CD009234."

Karlsdottir, S. I., S. Halldorsdottir and I. Lundgren (2014). "The third paradigm in labour pain preaparation and management: the childbearing woman's paradigm." *Scandinavian Journal of Caring Sciences* **28**: 315-327.

Karlsdottir, S. I., H. Sveinsdottir, O. A. Olafsdottir and H. Kristjansdottir (2015). "Pregnant women's expectations about pain intensity during childbirth and their attitudes towards pain management: Findings from an Icelandic national study." *Sexual & Reproductive Healthcare* **6**: 211-218.

Kennedy, H. P., T. Anderson and N. Leap (2010). Midwifery Presence: Philosophy, Science and Art. Chapter 7. *Essential Midwifery Practice: Intrapartum Care*. D. Walsh and S. Downe. Chichester, West Sussex, UK, Wiley-Blackwell: 105-124.

Kennedy, H. P., K. Nardini, R. McLeod-Waldo and L. Ennis (2009). "Top-Selling Childbirth Advice Books: A Discourse Analysis." *Birth* **36**(4): 318-324.

Kennedy, H. P., M. T. Shannon, U. Chuahorm and M. K. Kravetz (2004). "The Landscape of Caring for Women: A Narrative Study of Midwifery Practice." *Journal of Midwifery and Women's Health* **49**(1): 14-23.

Klomp, T., J. Maniën, A. de Jong, E. K. Hutton and A. L. M. Lagro-Janssen (2014). "What do midwives need to know about approaches of women towards labour pain management? A qualitative interview study into expectations of management of labour pain for pregnant women receiving midwife-led care in the Netherlands." *Midwifery* **30**: 432-438.

Lagan, B. M., M. Sinclair and W. Kernohan (2010). "Internet use in pregnancy informs women's decision making: a webbased survey." *Birth* **37**(2): 106-115.

Lally, J. E., M. J. Murtagh and S. Macphail (2008). "More in hope than expectation: women's experience and expectations of pain relief in labour. A review." *BMC Med* **6**(7): doi:10.1186/1741-7015-1186-1187.

Lally, J. E., R. G. Thomson, S. MacPhail and C. Exley (2014). "Pain relief in labour: a qualitative study to determine how to support women to make decisions about pain relief in labour." *BMC Pregnancy and Childbirth* **14**: 6.

http://www.biomedcentral.com/1471-2393/1414/1476.

Larkin, P., C. M. Begley and D. Devane (2009). "Women's experiences of labour and birth: an evolutionary concept analysis." *Midwifery* **25**: e49-e59.

Lawrence, A., L. Lewis, G. J. Hofmeyr and C. Styles (2013). "Maternal positions and mobility during first stage labour (Review)." *Cochrane Database of Systematic Reviews*: Issue 10. Art. No.: CD003934. DOI: 003910.001002/14651858. CD14003934.pub14651854.

Leap, N. (1997). "Being with women in pain - do midwives need to re-think their role?" *British Journal of Midwifery* **5**(5): 263.

Leap, N. and T. Anderson (2008). The role of pain in normal birth and the empowerment of women. Chapter 2. *Normal Childbirth: Evidence and Debate 2nd Edition*. S. Downe. Edinburgh, Churchill Livingstone/Elsevier: 29-46.

Leap, N. and B. Hunter (2016). *Supporting Women for Labour and Birth: a thoughtful guide*. London, Routledge.

Leap, N., J. Sandall, S. Buckland and U. Huber (2010). "Journey to Confidence: Women's Experiences of Pain in Labour and Relational Continuity of Care." *Journal of Midwifery and Women's Health* **55**(3): 235-242.

Lindholm, A. and I. Hildingsson (2015). "Women's preferences and received pain relief in childbirth – A prospective longitudinal study in a northern region of Sweden." *Sexual & Reproductive Healthcare* **6**: 74-81.

Lowe, N. K. (2002). "The nature of labor pain." *American Journal of Obstetrics and Gynecology* **186**(5): S16-S24.

Luce, A., M. Cash, V. Hundley, H. Cheyne, E. van Teijlingen and C. Angell (2016). ""Is it realistic?" the portrayal of pregnancy and childbirth in the media." *BMC Pregnancy and Childbirth* 16:40.

Lundgren, I. and K. Dahlberg (1998). "Women's experience of pain during childbirth." *Midwifery* **14**(2): 105-110.

Lundgren, I. S. I. Karlsdottir and T. Bondas (2009). "Long-term memories and experiences of childbirth in a Nordic context - a secondary analysis." *International Journal of Qualitative Studies on Health and Well-being* **4**: 115-128.

Mander, R. (2010). Skills for Working with (the Woman in) Pain. Chapter 8. *Essential Midwifery Practice: Intrapartum Care*. D. Walsh and S. downe. Chichester, West Sussex, UK, Wiley-Blackwell: 125-140.

Morris, D. (1991). *The Culture of Pain*. Berkeley, University of California Press.

Morris, T. and K. McInerney (2010). "Media representation and childbirth: An analysis of reality television programs in the United States." *Birth* **37**(134-140).

National Collaborating Centre for Women's and Children's Health (2014). Intrapartum Care. Care of healthy women and their babies during childbirth. Version 2. Clinical Guideline 190. Methods, evidence and recommendations. Commissioned by the National Institute for Health and Care Excellence (NICE). N. I. f. H. a. C. Excellence, National Collaborating Centre for Women's and Children's Health.

Newnham, E. (2014). "Birth control: Power/knowledge in the politics of birth." *Health Sociology Review* **23**(3): 254-268.

Newnham, E., L. McKellar and J. Pincombe (2015). "Documenting risk: A comparison of policy and information pamphlets for using epidural or water in labour." *Women and Birth* **28**: 221-227.

Newnham, E., L. McKellar and J. Pincombe (2016). "A critical literature review of epidural analgesia." *Evidence Based Midwifery* (14.1): 22-28.

Newnham, E., L. McKellar and J. Pincombe (2018). *Towards the humanisation of birth: A study of epidural analgesia and hospital birth culture*. Basingstoke, UK, Palgrave MacMillan.

Nilsson, C. and I. Lundgren (2009). "Women's lived experience of fear of childbirth." *Midwifery* **25**: e1-e9.

Nolan, M. (2009). "Information Giving and Education in Pregnancy: A Review of Qualitative Studies." *The Journal of Perinatal Education* **18**(4): 21-30.

Noseworthy, D. A., S. R. Phibbs and C. A. Benn (2013). "Towards a relational model of decision-making in midwifery care." *Midwifery* **29**: e42–e48.

Reiger, K. and R. Dempsey (2006). "Performing birth in a culture of fear: an embodied crisis of late modernity " *Health Sociology Review* **15**(4): 364-373.

Ross-Davie, M. C. and H. Cheyne (2014). "Intrapartum support: what do women want? A Literature review to identify how far the nature of labour support shapes women's assessment of their birth experiences." *Evidence Based Midwifery* **12**(2): 52-58.

Ross-Davie, M. C., M. McElligott, M. Little and K. King (2014). "Midwifery support in labour: how important is it to stay in the room?" *The Practising Midwife* **17**(6): 19-22(14).

Sandall, J., H. Soltani, S. Gates, A. Shennan and D. Devane (2016). "Midwife-led continuity models versus other models of care for childbearing women." *Cochrane Database of Systematic Reviews*_: Issue 4. Art. No.: CD004667.

Sanders, R. (2015). "Midwifery Facilitation: Exploring the Functionality of Labor Discomfort. Commentary." *Birth* **42**(3): 202-205.

Schrader McMillan, A., J. Barlow and M. Redshaw (2009). Birth and Beyond: A Review of the Evidence about Antenatal Education. Warwick, UK, University of Warwick.

Simkin, P. and A. Bolding (2004). "Update on nonpharmacologic approaches to relieve labor pain and prevent suffering." *Journal of Midwifery and Women's Health* **49**(6): 489-504.

Smith, C. A., C. T. Collins, A. M. Cyna and C. A. Crowther (2006). Complementary and alternative therapies for pain management in labour (Cochrane Review), Cochrane Database of Systematic Reviews Issue 4. Art. No.: CD003521. DOI: 10.1002/14651858.CD003521.pub2.

Stoll, K. and W. Hall (2013a). "Vicarious Birth Experiences and Childbirth Fear: Does It Matter How Young Canadian Women Learn About Birth?" *The Journal of Perinatal Education* **22**(4): 226-233.

Stoll, K. and W. Hall (2013b). "Attitudes and Preferences of Young Women With Low and High Fear of Childbirth." *Qualitative Health Research* **23**(11): 1495-1505.

Talbot, R. (2012). "Self-efficacy: women's experiences of pain in labour." *British Journal of Midwifery* **20**(5): 317-321.

Tracy, S., E. Sullivan, Y. Wang, D. Black and M. Tracy (2007). "Birth outcomes associated with interventions in labour amongst low-risk women: a population-based study " *Women and Birth* **20**(2): 41-48.

Tracy, S. and M. Tracy (2003). "Costing the cascade: estimating the costs of increased intervention in childbirth using population data." *British Journal of Obstetrics and Gynaecology* **110**(August): 717-224.

Van der Gucht, N. and K. Lewis (2015). "Women's experiences of coping with pain during childbirth: A critical review of qualitative research." *Midwifery* **31**: 349-358.

Waldenström, U., I. Hildingsson, C. Rubertsson and I. Radestad (2004). "A Negative Birth Experience: Prevalence and Risk Factors in a National Sample." *Birth* **31**(1): 17-27.

Waldenström, U., and E. Schytt (2009). "A longitudinal study of women's memory of labour pain – from 2 months to 5 years after the birth." *BJOG* March **116**(4): 577-583. doi:10.1111/j.1471-0528.2008.02020.x. Epub: 2008 Dec 9.

Waldenström, U. (2006). Obstetric pain relief and its association with remembrance of labor pain at two months and one year after birth. *Journal of Psychosomatic Obstetrics and Gynecology*, **27**(3), 147-156.

Whitburn, L. Y., L. E. Jones, M.-A. Davy and R. Small (2014). "Women's experiences of labour pain and the role of the mind: An exploratory study." *Midwifery* **30**: 1029-1035.

CHAPTER 17

Precision maternity care: using big data to understand trends and to make change happen

Melissa Cheyney and *Lilian Peters*

Introduction

In 2009, a new flu strain combining elements of bird and swine flu viruses called H1N1 was discovered, and global public health agencies feared the worst. In the United States, the Centers for Disease Control and Prevention (CDC, 2010) tracked the virus in hopes of developing strategies to slow its spread. However, a combination of the time it took for people to seek care, for physicians to detect and report cases and for the CDC to tabulate numbers resulted in a two-week lag time in tracking (Mayer-Schönberger and Cukier, 2013). Then, a few weeks before H1N1 hit the global media, Google published a landmark paper in the journal *Nature* (Ginsberg et al, 2009). The authors, Ginsburg and colleagues, described a methodology that used correlations between frequencies of specific Internet search queries and the spread of influenza-like illnesses (ILI) over time. This project, called Google Flu Trends (GFT), was heralded as an exemplary use of big data (Goel et al, 2010; McAfee et al, 2012) as it allowed researchers to 'nowcast' the spread of flu down to regional and even state levels, essentially removing the two-week lag time in tracking that traditional CDC methods entailed (Mayer-Schönberger and Cukier 2013).[*]

---

[*] Interestingly, a similar attempt is underway to use Google search trends to predict Zika virus outbreaks (See Teng et al, 2017).

Unfortunately, GFT successes were short lived. In February 2013, an article in *Nature* reported that GFT was predicting more than double the number of doctor visits for ILI than the CDC, despite the fact that GFT was built to predict CDC reports (Butler 2013; Lazer et al, 2014; Olson et al, 2013). Because millions of search terms were being fitted to the CDC's data, some terms ended up being strongly correlated to ILI simply by chance. Among other issues, GFT researchers had essentially created an algorithm that was highly vulnerable to overfitting to seasonal terms unrelated to H1N1 (like 'high school basketball', for example).* This story, now commonly referred to as the 'Parable of Google Flu' (Lazer et al, 2014), is widely regarded as a cautionary tale for the evangelists of the big data revolution. The purpose of this chapter is to provide an overview of the growth of big data as a field, and to begin to examine some of the ways that big data, when applied within a critical '*all data* revolution' framework (Lazer et al, 2014:1205), may be used to study physiological labour and birth. The ultimate goal is to reduce preventable maternal and newborn mortality and morbidity, as well as unnecessary clinical interventions globally.

What is 'big data'? More, messy and what, not why

There is no consistently accepted definition for big data. However, a review of the field suggests that while, initially, file size alone defined data as 'big' – e.g. the volume of information was so large that the data no longer fit within the memory used for processing – over time, size-based definitions have given way to more complex, characteristic-driven definitions (Ristevski and Chen, 2018). The term 'big data' is now commonly used to refer to large data sets created by merging several traditional and new sources of health-related information. Traditional sources include biomedical research and healthcare data (e.g. data from patient registries, clinical trials, bio banks) (Mittelstadt and Floridi, 2016; Mathaiyan, Chandrasekaran and Davis, 2013), national statistics data (e.g. death certificates), socioeconomic data (e.g. census bureau), and environmental data (e.g. air pollution monitors). New sources include: data generated from social media (e.g. reflecting individual preferences, behaviour and interests) (Lupton, 2014; Costa, 2014), personal health monitoring technologies including wearable devices (e.g. personal fitness services), smartphone applications (e.g. lifestyle apps) (Boye, 2012) and others. 'Big data' may also refer to any data set with huge numbers of participants with multiple data collection points within a longitudinal timeframe (Azmak et al, 2015).

One approach to synthesising this vast field is to think about 'big data' as data that are: more, messy, and focused on *what*, not *why* (Mayer-Schönberger and Cukier, 2013). Mayer-Schönberger and Cukier (2013), in particular, have argued that the main advantage of big data is that it allows research to move beyond the primary historical limitation of smaller data sets – that is, the need for sampling. Big data advocates argue that quantitative changes in data acquisition have produced a qualitative change in research potential that is not so much like moving from a photograph to a high-resolution digital image, but

---

* See Lazer et all (2014) for a detailed analysis of why GFT algorithms began to perform less well over time.

more like moving from a still image to film (Mayer-Schönberger and Cukier, 2013). Expectations for big data are high.

However, both lovers and critics of big data acknowledge that, as scale increases, so do the number of inaccuracies – that is, data become messier. Advocates of big data call on people to let go of their love affair with precision – not to give up exactitude entirely, but to contemplate how there can be beneficial tradeoffs between accuracy and size, especially for some research questions (Mayer-Schönberger and Cukier, 2013). What is lost in accuracy at the micro level, may be more than compensated for in insights gained at the macro level. To this way of thinking, imprecision is an accepted feature, not necessarily a shortcoming. By relaxing standards, more data are available for analysis. Others, in contrast, stress that data quality still matters, and that size does not always trump quality (Boyd and Crawford, 2012; Lazer et al, 2014). Traditional 'small data' can offer information that is 'not contained (or containable) in big data', and the know-ability of the nuances and contextual determinants of small data can mean that researchers are clearer on the reliability and validity of specific variables and the presence and potential effects of systematic bias (Lazer et al, 2014:1205).

More and messier data also require a move away from the search for causality towards contentment in discovering correlations and patterns in data that may lead to new insights – what some have called 'letting the data speak' (Mayer-Schönberger and Cukier, 2013:8). Big data often cannot explain why something is happening, just that it does appear to be happening. Big data is thus said to be more about the *what*, and less about the *why*. If big data means embracing messy to get more, letting the data speak, and finding contentment with the *what*, not *why*, then the issue is raised about applications to maternity care and physiological labour and birth research. How might big data, with all its caveats and cautions, be used to understand the nature and consequences of physiological labour and birth on a global scale?

Precision maternity care: moving beyond too much too soon and too little too late to the right amount at the right time in the right way

Miller and colleagues (2016) have described a continuum of global maternity care in which two extremes exist. They refer to this as 'too little, too late' (TLTL) and 'too much, too soon' (TMTS). TLTL is used to describe care where a push towards facility birth combines with inadequate staff, training, infrastructure, supplies and medications (Austin et al, 2014) and often results in care that is below an evidence-based standard, withheld, or simply unavailable until it is too late. The converse, too much, too soon (TMTS), is characterised by routine overuse of interventions and hyper-medicalisation of normal pregnancy and birth. Miller and colleagues (2016) argue that TMTS systems often include the unnecessary use of non-evidence-based interventions (e.g. continuous electronic foetal monitoring), as well as overuse of interventions that can be life-saving, but that are potentially harmful when applied routinely (e.g. caesarean section). As facility births have increased globally, so has the recognition that TMTS systems can produce harm, increase costs and concentrate disrespect, abuse and violations of human rights in childbirth (Freedman and Kruk, 2014; Miller and Lalonde, 2015; WHO, 2014; International Federation of Gynecology and Obstetrics, International Confederation of Midwives, White Ribbon Alliance et al, 2016). While TMTS systems are typically associated with high-resource nations and TLTL with low- and middle-resource ones, due to inequality these extremes often coexist in a given nation.

Big data could be used to help ensure that within particular cultural settings, the right amounts of care were offered at the right time, and delivered in a manner that respects, protects, and promotes human rights. We refer to this goal here as *precision maternity care,* and we see it as closely tied both to birth setting and to provider type. It is currently an absolute impossibility that all women everywhere will be able to give birth to every baby in a facility attended by a physician or skilled midwife, and recent work on TMTS systems calls us to question whether this should be a primary goal at all (Kruk et al, 2016). The push for facility birth for all overlooks the fact that the resources, quality of care and occupational cultures of those institutions are often more important predictors of outcomes than is access to the facility itself. Indeed, home and birth centre midwives in high-resource countries often have more reliable access to essential equipment and medications than do physicians in some hospitals in low-resource nations. Access to a facility alone cannot be the central aim in global maternity care reform. Knowing which births are likely to be successful in community settings (homes, birth centres, local clinics outside of a hospital), where first-line interventions for complications and mechanisms for transfer are available and managed by midwives, and which births would benefit from closer proximity to a facility or even a higher level of care with a specialist, would allow limited resources to be allocated more efficiently. By merging existing and new data sets that contain data on planned place of birth, maternal risk profiles, provider type, clinical interventions provided during pregnancy and birth and outcomes of care, including transfer to higher level facilities, for which something is also known about midwifery/practitioner education, models of care and systems integration, might enable researchers to use big data to build statistical models with portable applications that optimise the use of limited clinical resources. Table 1 lists a sample of selected, existing data sets that could be merged to contribute to such an agenda. A more comprehensive list with global representation is a critical first step.

As a note of caution, any such endeavour would have to be premised on the primary principle that macro-level trends and patterns should not supplant the autonomy and decision-making of individual women, nor the processes of shared decision-making between women, partners, families and care providers. However, robust predictive models could inform systems and population-level allocation of resources and provider-patient level decision-making around place of birth and level of care in a way that brings services closer to a model of *precision maternity.* This would allow for the right amount of care at the right time in the right way – that is, in a way that explicitly respects the rights of all childbearing people.

Table 1.

Examples of existing and emerging data sets that may be used to study precision maternity care.

Data Set	Nation/s
UK Place of Birth Data Set	United Kingdom
Dutch Perinatal Registry (Perined)	Netherlands
Swedish Birth Registry	Sweden
Danish Birth Registry	Denmark
Nordic Medical Birth Registry	Norway
MANA Statistics Project	USA
Perinatal Data Registry	USA
New Zealand Ministry of Health	New Zealand
Million Moms Study	Australia
New South Wales linkage data	Australia
Euro Peristat Project	Europe-wide
British Columbia Reproductive Care Program Perinatal Registry	Canada

Towards a critical, precision maternity care, all-data framework

Enormous progress has been made in the last decade around developing tools to capture and merge big data collected from diverse data sets (Jumbe, Murray and Kern, 2016). One such project, the Healthy Birth Growth and Development *knowledge integration* (HBGD*ki*) project funded by the Bill and Melinda Gates Foundation was launched in 2013 with the goal of generating predictive models from existing data that could be used to promote healthy birth, and prevent growth faltering and impaired neurocognitive development in children globally (Jumbe, 2016). The HBGD*ki* group has successfully merged data from 130 studies representing nearly 10 million children, enabling researchers to explore how to provide the right intervention(s), to the right child, at the right time, and at the right price. This process has enabled data scientists to develop and troubleshoot a data curation process for diverse data sets that involves intake, harmonisation to common data standards and preparation for analysis. However, to date, HBGD*ki* has focused almost exclusively on growth and development (rather than birth *per se*) using big data. There is, therefore, an opportunity to bring together the innovations in big data sharing and data set aggregation with a *precision maternity care* research agenda.

Mittelstadt and Floridi (2016:303) have argued that: '*As is often the case with the cutting edge of scientific and technological processes, understanding the ethical implications of big data lags behind.*' Indeed, a review of the literature on big data reveals numerous ethical concerns, many of which are in their intellectual infancy. To address these issues in maternity care, a *critical, precision maternity care, all data framework* could be used, to enable a systematic examination of the role big data may play in global midwifery and physiologic labour and birth research.

By *critical*, we mean that explicit attention should be paid to a series of ethical considerations (see Table 2 for summary of the 'Big Five'). The approach must not fall prey to what might be called 'big data hubris' or the 'often-implicit assumption that big data are a substitute for, rather than a supplement to, traditional data collection and analysis' (Lazer et al, 2014:1203). Nor should it lead to a widening of the data gap between 'data haves' and 'data have-nots'. This critical lens also needs to 'trouble' (Haraway, 2016) the n=all assumption and work to create data sets that are more inclusive cross-culturally and that capture multiple levels of care. This entails attention to whose data are currently included and whose are missing.

By *all data* we mean that an explicit recognition of the need to employ both traditional and new data sets, an approach Mayer-Schönberger and Cukier (2013) argue is analogous to recognising the need for both a microscope and a telescope in our work. National and facility-level data sets emerge from a particular socio-political milieu and a set of specific maternity care structures. As such, they will continue to be needed to address population-level quality assurance and improvement. Instead of focusing on a 'big data revolution', we see the need for an *'all data* revolution', which explicitly recognises that a critical change in the last two decades has been in innovative analytics that may be applied to both small and large data sets (Lazer et al, 2014). Using data from traditional (e.g. population-based reproductive health registries) and new sources (e.g. merged data sets, social media) together will provide a deeper, clearer, and more nuanced understanding of the global maternity care universe. There are enormous scientific possibilities in big data (Mayer-Schönberger and Cukier, 2013; Boyd and Crawford, 2012; Jumbe, Murray and Kern, 2016; Mittelstate and Floridi, 2016; Amzak et al, 2015), including exciting possibilities for producing evidence-informed systems of *precision maternity care* globally. However, it is important to ensure that excitement about data quantity does not result in glossing over foundational issues related to construct validity, measurement, reliability and dependencies among variables (Boyd and Crawford, 2012; Lazer et al, 2014). In response to the opportunities and limitations of big data, there is a need for an explicitly critical and inclusive stance focused on skilled midwifery care for all, tailored to specific cultural and maternity care settings and maternal risk profiles. This should encompass an approach to handling data that uses both traditional and new sources to refine and inform one another, while preventing de-contextualisation that may threaten the utility and efficacy of findings.

Table 2.
Summary of Mittelstadt and Floridi's (2016) 'big five' ethical concerns of big data, modified with permission.

Ethical Concern	Summary
1. Informed Consent	Consent has historically been solicited for a single study; broad, blanket consent mechanisms that pre-authorise for future studies limit autonomy of data subjects; relationships that may be revealed when data are linked cannot be accurately predicted, thus consent cannot be truly informed.
2. Privacy	Data subjects may not be aware of the extent to which data can be publicly 'scraped' and evaluated outside the context-sensitive spaces they were created in, especially data gathered from social media; often unclear whether the duties around confidentiality that accompany fiduciary, contractual and/or professional relationships are being honoured when big data are shared.
3. Ownership	Two forms of ownership must be considered – rights to control or manage data and rights to benefit from data; is data owned by the collector of data or the research participants who produce the data?; research participants need greater control over data when discrimination, surveillance or other undesired uses are likely.
4. Epistemology and Objectivity	The complexity of big data, the inherent difficulty of analysing vast data sets, and the complicated rationale of algorithms can limit significantly who can comment on the validity of relationships and supposed findings; the difficulty of questioning findings that emerge from the 'black box' of big data lead mass media, industry and thus, often the public as well, to assume that big data are objective or beyond the influence of human interpretation and researcher bias; the ideas of data-led objectives or 'letting the data speak' entirely discounts the role of interpretive frameworks.
5. Big Data Divides	There are inequalities between data subjects who provide information for big data analytics and those who do not, as well as differences between organisations who have the capacity, resources and infrastructures to engage in and understand outcomes from big data projects; this can create a divide in the kinds of knowing that are available; we must also question whether n=all is an accurate way to portray big data since some data subjects opt out, while others are systematically excluded by unequal systems of power.

How this might work in practice: big data, global midwifery, and physiologic labour and birth research

The *Lancet* series on Midwifery published in 2014 has provided a critical starting point for contemplating the potential role of big data in midwifery and physiologic labour and birth research. The four papers (Homer et al, 2014; Renfrew et al, 2014; ten Hoope-Bender et al, 2014; Van Lerberghe et al, 2014) in that series arguably represent the most comprehensive global examination to date of what women and newborns need to survive, thrive, and transform from preconception through to the early weeks of life (World Health Organization (WHO), 2016). Together, these *Lancet* papers highlight the need for a systems-level shift away from fragmented maternity care that is all too commonly consumed with the identification and treatment of pathology, towards what expert panellists call a 'whole-systems approach' that provides integrated, collaborative, holistic, and skilled care for all. Midwifery care and the support of normal physiologic labour and birth emerge as the core components of such a global shift.

Collectively, these works have compellingly answered the question: given resource limitations, where should research and policy endeavours be focused to have the broadest global impact on reducing preventable maternal and newborn death and suffering? The papers in the *Lancet* series and the vast body of work they draw upon make clear: the answer lies within a model of skilled midwifery care for all that promotes normal physiologic reproductive processes, first-line management of complications, family planning and access to emergency care when needed within healthcare systems, integrated across all birth settings.

The question as we see it now becomes: how can this skilled midwifery care for all framework be implemented in diverse cultural and political-economic settings characterised by unique and complex national healthcare systems with enormous variability and inequality in maternity care budgets? In another landmark paper, Kennedy and colleagues (2016) provide a strategic path forward that could use big data to help answer these core questions. Where past research funding has targeted the management of complications that contribute to high mortality (i.e. haemorrhage, hypertensive disorders, sepsis, obstructed labour, preterm birth etc.), Kennedy and colleagues have identified research priorities that restore balance between pathology and prevention.

An international research alliance committed to this end has formed (see Kennedy et al, 2018).[*] One working group within this alliance has begun cultivating collaborative relationships between midwifery researchers and big data scientists who can provide the technical support needed to merge existing and emerging data sets with the end goal of developing a *critical, all data framework* that may eventually help deliver evidence-informed, *precision maternity care* to all. Kennedy and colleagues have identified research priorities that restore balance between pathology and prevention (see Table 3).

---

*   See QMNC Alliance website: www.qmnc.org

Table 3.

Ranking of research topics by overall research priority score. Reprinted with permission from Kennedy et al. 2016.

	Research priorities	Research priority score
1	Evaluate the effectiveness of midwifery care across the continuum in increasing access to and acceptability of family planning for women	90.4
2	Evaluate the effectiveness of midwife-led care when compared to other models of care across various settings, particularly on rates of foetal and infant death, preterm birth and low birthweight	89.8
3	Determine which indicators are most valuable in assessing quality maternal and newborn care	89.7
4	Identify and describe aspects of care that optimise, and those that disturb, the biological/physiological processes for healthy childbearing women and foetus/newborn infants and those who experience complications	89.3
5	Evaluate the effectiveness of midwifery care in providing culturally appropriate information, education and health promotion (e.g. nutrition, substance use, domestic violence and mental health)	89.1
6	Identify and describe enabling factors from examples of success implementation of evidence-based maternal and newborn care across a variety of settings	89
7	Describe and evaluate the effectiveness of midwives working with others (such as health professionals, community health workers and traditional health attendants) in achieving quality maternal and newborn care including, but not limited to: • Timely transfer of women to appropriate level/site of care • Management of emergency situations • Maximal use of skills and competencies • Shared decision-making and accountability	89
8	Assess the views and preferences of women and families across a variety of settings about their experiences of maternal and newborn care including, but not limited to, care providers and sites of care (e.g. place of birth, antenatal care)	88.8
9	Develop setting-specific benchmarks to assess measurable progress on implementation of quality maternal and newborn care	88.3
10	Identify and describe aspects of maternal and newborn care that strengthen or weaken women's psychosocial wellbeing and mental health	88.0
11	Assess whether new measures of morbidity are needed to more effectively evaluate outcomes of maternal and newborn care	88.0

Conclusion

In summary, we are arguing for a merging of two critical conversations that we believe can inform global maternity care: big data science and research priority setting. Such a merger would combine existing and new data sets that contain information on planned place of birth, maternal wellbeing and risk profiles, provider type, key interventions and outcomes of care, maternity care provider education and models of care and systems integration. Knowledge arising from these analyses could enable researchers to use big data to build models with portable applications that optimise the use of limited clinical resources. Even the most robust predictive models must not be permitted to displace maternal choice, but, if used wisely, they may be able to inform systems-level allocation of resources and provider-service user-level decision-making around place of birth and level of care in a way that brings maternity care globally closer to a model of *precision maternity care*. This could be the basis for ensuring the right amount of care at the right time in the right way, in the right place, for every mother and baby, everywhere.

Key points for consideration

- Strive to collect data on: planned place of birth, maternal wellbeing and risk profiles, provider type, clinical interventions provided during pregnancy and birth, outcomes of care, transfers to higher level facilities, midwifery/practitioner education, models of care and systems integration.

- Ensure data collection that has been sensitised to ethical considerations that include at a minimum: informed consent, privacy, data ownership, questions of epistemology and objectivity and the mitigation of big data divides.

- Employ both traditional and new data sets to answer questions about what women and newborns need to survive, thrive and transform from preconception through to the early weeks of life.

- Always work on the notion that even the most robust predictive models cannot, and must not, be permitted to displace maternal choice.

- Promote a more equitable distribution of global maternity care resources premised on locally contextualised models of precision maternity care.

References

Austin A, Langer A, Salam RA, Lassi ZS, Das JK, Bhutta ZA. Approaches to improve the quality of maternal and newborn health care: an overview of the evidence. Reproductive Health. 2014;11(Suppl 2): S1. doi:10.1186/1742-4755-11-S2-S1. PubMed Central PMCID: PMC4160919.

Azmak O, Bayer H, Caplin A, Miyoung C, Glimcher P, Koonin S. Using Big Data to Understand the Human Condition. Big Data. 2015 Sept 1;3(3):173-188. doi: 10.1089/big.2015.001.

Boyd D, Crawford K. CRITICAL QUESTIONS FOR BIG DATA: Provocations for a cultural, technological, and scholarly phenomenon. Information, Communication & Society. 2012, May 10:15(5):662-679. doi: http://dx.doi.org/10.1080/1369118X.2012.678878.

Boye N. Co-production of Health enabled by next generation personal health systems. Studies in Health Technology Informatics. 2012;177:52-8. PubMed PMID: 22942030.

Butler D. When Google got flu wrong. Nature. 2013, Feb 14;494(7436):155-6.

Centers for Disease Control and Prevention (CDC). The 2009 H1N1 Pandemic: Summary Highlights, April 2009-April 2010. 2010 Jun 16:[17 pgs]. Available from: https://www.cdc.gov/h1n1flu/cdcresponse.htm.

Costa FF. Big data in biomedicine. Drug Discov Today. 2014 Apr;19(4):433-40. Epub 2013 Oct 29. doi: 10.1016/j. drudis.2013.10.012. PubMed PMID: 24183925.

Freedman LP, Kruk ME. Disrespect and abuse of women in childbirth: challenging the global quality and accountability agendas. The Lancet. 2014 Jun 22;384(9948):e42-4. doi: http://dx.doi.org/10.1016/S0140-6736(14)60859-X.

Ginsberg J, Mohebbi MH, Patel RS, Brammer L, Smolinski MS, Brilliant L. Detecting influenza epidemics using search engine query data. Nature. 2009 Feb 19;(457):1012-14. doi:10.1038/nature07634.

Goel S. Hofman JM, Lahaie S, Pennock DM, Watts DJ. Predicting consumer behavior with Web search. Levin SA, editor. Proceedings of the National Academy of Sciences. 2010;107(41):17486-90. doi: 10.1073/pnas.1005962107.

Haraway DJ. Staying with the trouble: Making kin in the Chthulucene. Duke University Press; 2016 Aug 19.

Homer CS, Friberg IK, Dias MAB, ten Hoope-Bender P, Sandall J, Speciale AM, et al. The projected effect of scaling up midwifery. The Lancet. 2014 Sept 20;384(9948):1146-57. doi: http://dx.doi.org/10.1016/S0140-6736(14)60790-X.

Jumbe S. Health Birth, Growth, and Development Knowledge Integration. Proceedings of the 2016 American Association for the Advancement of Science (AAAS) Annual Meeting; 2016 Feb 11-15; Washington D.C.

Jumbe NLN, Murray JC, Kern S. Data Sharing and Inductive Learning--Toward Healthy Birth, Growth, and Development. New England Journal of Medicine. 2016 Jun 23;374(25):2415-7. Epub 2016 May 11. doi: 10.1056/NEJMp1605441.

Kennedy HP, Yoshida S, Costello A, Declercq E, Dias MA, Duff E, et al. Asking different questions: research priorities to improve the quality of care for every woman, every child. The Lancet. 2016 Nov;4(11):e777-9. Epub 2016 Sept 20. doi: http://dx.doi.org/10.1016/S2214-109X(16)30183-8.

Kennedy HP, Cheyney M, Dahlen HG, Downe S, Foureur MJ, Homer CS, Jefford E, McFadden A, Michel-Schuldt M, Sandall J, Soltani H. Asking different questions: A call to action for research to improve the quality of care for every woman, every child. Birth. 2018 Jun 21.

Kruk ME, Leslie HH, Verguet S, Mbaruku GM, Adanu RM, Langer A. Quality of basic maternal care functions in health facilities of five African countries: an analysis of national health system surveys. The Lancet Global Health. 2016 Nov 1;4(11):e845-55.

Lazer D, Kennedy R, King G, Vespignani A. The Parable of Google Flu: Traps in Big Data Analysis. Science. 2014 Mar 14;343(6176):1203-5. doi: 10.1126/science.1248506.

Lupton D. The commodification of patient opinion: The digital patient experience economy in the age of big data. Sociology of Health and Illness. 2014 Jul;36(6):856-69. Epub 2014 Jan 21. doi: 10.1111/1467-9566.12109. PubMed PMID: 24443847.

Mathaiyan J, Chandrasekaran A, Davis S. Ethics of genomic research. Perspectives in Clinical Research. 2013 Jan-Mar;4(1):100-4. doi: 10.4103/2229-3485.106405. PubMed Central PMCID: PMC3601693.

Mayer-Schönberger V, Cukier K. Big Data: A Revolution That Will Transform How We Live, Work, and Think. Great Britain: John Murray An Hachette UK Company; 2013.

McAfee A, Brynjolfsson E. Big Data The Management Revolution. Harvard Business Review. 2012 Oct. Available from: https://hbr.org/2012/10/big-data-the-management-revolution.

Miller S, Abalos E, Chamillard M, Ciapponi A, Colaci D, Comandé D, et al. Beyond too little, too late and too much, too soon: a pathway towards evidence-based, respectful maternity care worldwide. The Lancet. 2016 Oct 29;388(10056):2176-2192. Epub 2016 Sep 16. doi: 10.1016/S0140-6736(16)31472-6. Pub Med PMID: 27642019.

Miller S, Lalonde A. The global epidemic of abuse and disrespect during childbirth: History, evidence, interventions, and FIGO's mother– baby friendly birthing facilities initiative. International Journal of Gynecology & Obstetrics. 2015;31:S49–52.

Mittelstadt BD, Floridi L. The Ethics of Big Data: Current and Foreseeable Issues in Biomedical Contexts. 2016 Apr;22(2):303-41. Epub 2015 May 23. doi: 10.1007/s11948-015-9652-2. PubMed PMID: 26002496.

Olson D. R., Konty, K. J., Paladini, M., Viboud, C., & Simonsen, L. Reassessing Google Flu Trends data for detection of seasonal and pandemic influenza: a comparative epidemiological study at three geographic scales. PLoS Computational Biology. 2013;9(10):e1003256. Epub 2013 Oct 17. doi: 10.1371/journal.pcbi.1003256. PubMed PMID: 24146603. PubMed Central PMCID: PMC3798275.

Renfrew MJ, McFadden A, Bastos MH, Campbell J, Channon AA, Cheung NF, et al. Midwifery and quality care: findings from a new evidence-informed framework for maternal and newborn care. The Lancet. 2014 Jun 22;384(9948):1129-45. doi: http://dx.doi.org/10.1016/S0140-6736(14)60789-3.

Ristevski B, Chen M. Big Data Analytics in Medicine and Healthcare. Journal of integrative bioinformatics. 2018 May 10.

Teng Y, Bi D, Xie G, Jin Y, Huang Y, Lin B, An X, Feng D, Tong Y. Dynamic forecasting of Zika epidemics using Google Trends. PloS one. 2017 Jan 6;12(1):e0165085.

ten Hoope-Bender P, de Bernis L, Campbell J, Downe S, Fauveau V, Fogstad H, et al. Improvement of maternal and newborn health through midwifery. The Lancet. 2014 Jun 22;384(9949):1226-35. doi: http://dx.doi.org/10.1016/S0140-6736(14)60930-2.

Van Lerberghe W, Matthews Z, Achadi E, Ancona C, Campbell J, Channon A, et al. Country experience with strengthening of health systems and deployment of midwives in countries with high maternal mortality. The Lancet. 2014 Jun 22;384(9949):1215-25. doi: http://dx.doi.org/10.1016/S0140-6736(14)60919-3.

International Federation of Gynecology and Obstetrics, International Confederation of Midwives, White Ribbon Alliance, International Pediatric Association, World Health Organization (2016). Corrigendum to "Mother-baby friendly birthing facilities"[Int J Gynecol Obstet 128 (2015) 95–9]. International Journal of Gynecology and Obstetrics. 2016;132:244. doi: http://dx.doi.org/10.1016/j.ijgo.2015.10.002.

World Health Organization [Internet]. The prevention and elimination of disrespect and abuse during facility-based childbirth: WHO statement [PDF]. 2014 Sept 3. Available from: http://www.who.int/reproductivehealth/topics/maternal_perinatal/statement-childbirth/en/.

World Health Organization [Internet]. World Health Statistics 2016: Monitoring Health for the SDGs Sustainable Development Goals [PDF]. 2016. Available from: http://www.who.int/gho/publications/world_health_statistics/2016/en/.

PART IV

Environments and architectures

CHAPTER 18

Designing space and place of birth

Neel Shah and *Nicoletta Setola*

Introduction

This chapter addresses the issue of architectural space in relation to healthcare in general, and place of birth in particular. It critiques the assumption that competent clinicians can provide excellent care no matter what the room or the building looks like, in the light of the fact that architecture could play an important part in the interaction between the form and function of the human body much as anatomy and physiology do. Life, activities, experiences and relationships occur in space for different users at the same time and this happens at different scales – the room, the service unit, the facility (see Figure 1). Although architectural space is not the only variable, the built environment can still impact behaviours, interactions, movements, and experiences (Lynch, 1960; Markus, 1993; Hamilton and Watkins, 2008; Hillier, 2007; Hillier et al, 1993). In healthcare buildings particularly, there is good evidence of this effect. Many studies have shown how the designed environment can alter stress levels, and, therefore, potentially affect human health, the experiences of users and the quality of care provided by the staff (Evans and Cohen, 1998; Del Nord, 2006; Edelstein, 2004; de Botton, 2006; Ulrich and Barach, 2006; Ulrich et al, 2008; Harte et al, 2016; Gesler et al, 2004).

Birthing facilities (birth centres, labour units, maternity wards) are usually considered to be healthcare buildings, part of hospital estates that deal with patients who are ill. However, it is necessary to reflect upon this classification, since we are referring in this case to 'health' spaces which have a specific function, which is not directly attuned to the usual assumptions about hospital settings. The users of these spaces are women, babies, partners, midwives and doctors, most of whom are not 'patients'. In fact, the main activity carried out in these places is in itself a natural event, birth, and thus not necessarily 'healthcare' in the strictest sense. The exact number of mothers who require clinical intervention to support healthy labour and birth is unknown, but it is widely believed that interventions in childbirth are frequently undertaken unnecessarily in some settings. As the recent *Lancet* commission on maternal health made clear, we sometimes provide too little care too late and other times provide too much care too soon (Miller et al, 2016). The challenge for clinicians is to find the right balance, in partnership with childbearing women. The challenge for designers is to create spaces that support this balance.

Figure 1:
The architecture approach through the design scales (Created by Setola N.)

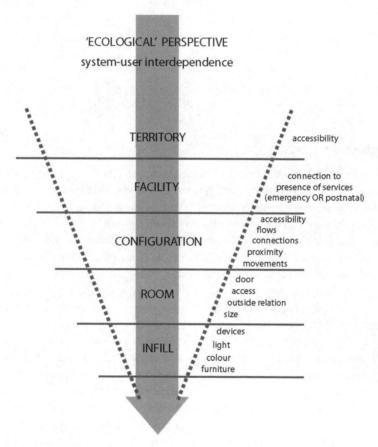

Birth space design

The design of formal institutional spaces for birth, from the second half of the 20th century, has been influenced by the fact that birth has been increasingly hospital based. Hospital birth spaces are sited in healthcare estates that are generally constructed to manage sickness and disease. Design, therefore, has followed efficiency-based models that are appropriate for all other functional areas of the hospital: general medicine, surgery, intensive care, diagnostics etc.

For the first time, in the 1990s, the architect Bianca Lepori began to introduce new reference categories for birth spaces (Lepori, 1994). Two decades later, there is still a lack of awareness of this work among architects today, for whom birth spaces are considered as medical speciality areas. Many buildings for birth are still being designed according to rules suitable for 'patients' and traditional wards. For example, rooms are designed around the bed as a central component.[*] They are generally rectangular and without curved lines. Spaces in which women are expected to labour physiologically are not differentiated from those designed for women with complications. Indeed, most EU countries do not have specific technical guidelines to differentiate different kinds of birth rooms, and therefore the default tends to be to design for high-risk scenarios. There are few official technical guidelines for birth centre building typologies, nor are there complete specific structural requirements or standards for these settings.[**]

All this suggests that a fundamental cultural change is needed in the field of architecture in order to understand what a normal physiological birth is, and which elements of architecture and space can support it and match the needs of the users. Although there is some recognition that soft furnishings and colourful walls or decorations recalling a family environment can help with this (Bowden, Sheehan and Foureur, 2016), a more fundamental rethink is required. This approach has specific reference to the creation of birth spaces both for healthy women and for those with complications, in which humanised, relationship-based approaches between women, their birth companions, and their caregivers can more easily be provided.

In this chapter we use our experience alongside studies carried out by interdisciplinary or other research groups (midwives, physicians, architects) to suggest the most important issues for architectural design in this field, and to suggest additional contributions that further research in the architectural field can provide.

The challenge of designing a space for birth

Designing the healthcare space is always a matter of compromise. In the same space, different users have different perceptions and experiences. The architect's work is to respond to all needs. For example, attention should be paid to the issue of privacy and at the same time to that of surveillance. In this case, the role of doors and partitions acquires significance. In terms of birth spaces, on the one hand the architect wants to create access to the outside for the woman and staff in order to allow direct natural light, and on the other hand, they need to design the space to separate the flows of visitors from that of staff. In this case, the design of the spatial layout is important. The architect also wants to respond to the need for humanisation for users, while not exceeding the standard number

---

[*]   The importance of the bed as a sign of acute care in maternity spaces has been referred to in many studies (Foureur et al, 2011; Bowden et al, 2016; Townsend et al, 2016)

[**] The more complete architectural guidelines tools in terms of planning dimensions, functional requirements and design environment for the birth centre model (MLU alongside and standalone) are the Australian Guidelines (AusHFG, 2017) and the UK Building Notes (Department of Health, 2013). The US Guidelines (FGI, 2018) and the Italian Ispsel Guidelines (Ispsel Guidelines, 2007) show a difference between physiological area/birth centre and the other traditional labour ward, mainly dealing with indications on the minimum birth room square metres.

of square metres required by standards and by the health authorities and other funding and governance agencies.

The architects continuously make choices, because they have to answer to different needs at the same time and when they build walls, doors, windows they have to consider how this either divides up spaces, and/or how it creates permeability between them. According to space syntax theory (Hillier, 2007), all these decisions have a consequence on the behaviour of people to a larger degree than might be assumed to be the case.

In this section, we address the following key concepts, which constitute a challenge for those who wish to design spaces for birth: *relationships, ecology, intimacy/presence, and nest/outside.*

Favouring relationships

In the birth space, it is particularly important to consider the set of human relationships that are created between users during the birthing event. This includes the direct relation/interactions between mothers and midwives, but also those between birth supporters (including doulas and partners) and midwives/obstetricians, and among obstetricians and midwives and other attending staff, such as paediatricians, and, in some settings, nurses. We are terming this a relationship-based approach, in which the focus is the relationships between users and the people and things that help them to flourish (Freeman et al, 2006; Iannuzzi, 2016; Setola, 2014; Longo and Setola, 2010). The set of these relationships between users is reflected in a certain way in the spatial relationships between spaces. The configuration of the layout plays a critical role since it influences the possibility of interaction and dialogue between people (Hillier and Hanson, 1984; Penn, 2008). In this context, Hillier (2007) defines the spatial configuration of a '*set of relationships which take into consideration other relationships*'.

Some studies in maternity care have examined the impact of different birth environments on the communication behaviour of users and in the provision of safe, high-quality care. For example, Foureur et al (2010a) highlight the way in which the design of the birth unit can influence the level of stress of both women and staff, which in turn can influence the quality of communication. Other studies have highlighted the importance of the presence of places that guarantee interactions and their accessible position within the unit. Williams (2003) identifies some spatial elements which favour communication; for example the central staff desk on a hospital ward. Berridge et al (2010) identify as important the spaciousness, the position and proximity between hub and desk as workplaces useful for communications. Hunt and Symonds (1995) identify the tea room, office and corridors as places essential to communication in maternity care settings.

The ecology of users and space

'Ecology' is the best word to indicate the symbiosis between users and space. In order to favour this symbiosis the space should be flexible, adaptable and adjustable to the needs of women, midwives, and other maternity carers, becoming a sort of 'ecological system' that changes according to preferences and situations. This kind of *flexibility* is crucial, and practical. For example, a long corridor may become a place for children to play, or a space where women can stroll during the first stage of labour as it is in the Margherita Birth Centre (IT) (see Figure 2). *Adaptability* is also essential for the birth space ecology. It happens when a space is modified through furnishings and infill elements in order to allow movements and position changes that are essential to women in labour (Frenk and Lepori, 2007). *Adjustability* can occur within the room space limits, by ensuring that lighting (both natural and artificial) is adjustable, and when the space provides a selection of auditory, visual and tactile sensory stimulation (Hodnett et al, 2009; Hauck et al, 2008).

Figure 2:
The multifunctional corridor: space for movements, seating, playing in the Margherita Birth Centre in Florence (IT) designed by the architect Bianca Lepori with the doctor Marco Santini (Created by Setola N.)

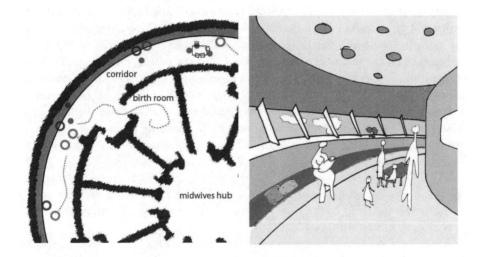

Enabling intimacy-presence

In the dichotomy of intimacy-presence, the proximity between spaces and the permeability level of partitions in the unit spatial layout play a significant role in favouring the perception of the 'presence' of the midwives and other carers for labouring women. Glass partitions, such as those used in intensive care units to allow surveillance of staff who are not in the direct company of patients, are not appropriate. In contrast, the birth space needs to be designed to facilitate the authentic 'presence' of the midwife or other maternity care provider. The creation of an undisturbed environment through a proper positioning of doors, lockable outer doors, the opportunity to see and experience warm water, comfortable furniture, quietness and adjustable lighting has important effects on the process of labour (Foureur, 2008). Additionally, women prefer, in the last stage of labour, a small, dim, quiet and 'protected area' (Lepori, 1994), and this is the finding of recent experiments carried out by Balabanoff (2016).

The nest and the outside

Linked to intimacy is the idea of building a nest, which is a space where the mother can feel at ease. This is particularly important for the moment of birth. Then, after the birth itself, the space needs to enable the woman to re-establish her relation with the outside, to celebrate the arrival of her baby with her birth partner and other chosen labour supporters, to see daylight, and a view of the world outside during the early postnatal period. Research on the impact of light in other health disciplines highlights how insufficient light is associated with an increase in the symptoms of depression (Evans, 2003). For patients recovering from illness, the amount of exposure to the light of day has an impact on physiological wellbeing, and reduces recovery times and physical and mental stress (Evans, 2003; Dalke, 2006; Edwards and Torcellini, 2002). People with Alzheimer's disease need an intense light to regulate their biological rhythm, and the elderly in general desire more light than they get. Light is therapy for bipolar patients, and it helps to avoid symptoms of delirium and, post-treatment depression in intensive care (Edwards and Torcellini, 2002). In terms of labour and the postpartum period, Jenkinson et al (2014) highlight how artificial lighting is associated with the release of adrenaline, inhibiting the normal physiological balance of the body. Lepori et al (2008) note that intense light stimulates and distracts the neocortex. Bright light encourages activity, whereas dimmer lights generate a relaxing atmosphere. All of these factors need to be considered, to ensure that the lighting in labour and postnatal spaces can be responsive to the changing needs of the woman as she labours, gives birth and then recovers from the birthing process, while building her relationship with her new baby.

All four of the concepts addressed above are related to each other. For them all, the role of the configuration of the unit is fundamental, including the relationship between spaces, their connecting systems (corridors), their proximity, and the possibility of movement they allow.

The contribution of architectural research

Many studies have been undertaken by researchers from a range of disciplines on the impact of maternity unit design on the level of satisfaction and expectation of women and on staff's perception of work performance (Newburn, 2003; Symon et al, 2008 a,b,c; Jenkinson et al, 2014). The next step in the architectural field is that of identifying more clearly which are the architectural elements and functions of space which facilitate an optimal experience of birth for everyone involved (see Figure 3). It is therefore important for architects to know the influence and implication of each environmental factor on people. Two important publications in this area were the guidelines developed by Forbes et al (2008) and a report on the birth environment, produced by the UK service user group, the National Childbirth Trust (NCT) (Newburn and Singh, 2003). However, many aspects remain which need further research. This includes the role of the midwives'/maternity care providers' desk/station, where to place it and why; the relationship between work activity and birth spaces; the role of opening doors in generating or interfering with an undisturbed environment; the accessibility of available spaces for all concerned and ideal dimensions of birth rooms. These are all issues regarding the configuration of space, confirmed also by the priorities of the women. For example, among the first seven elements identified in the UK NCT report, three related to a space configuration issue: *'ability to walk around'; 'not being in the sight of or overlooked by others', 'being able to control who comes into the room'* (Newburn and Singh, 2003).

Figure 3:
The spatial characteristics for an optimal birth space (Created by Setola N. and Naldi E.)

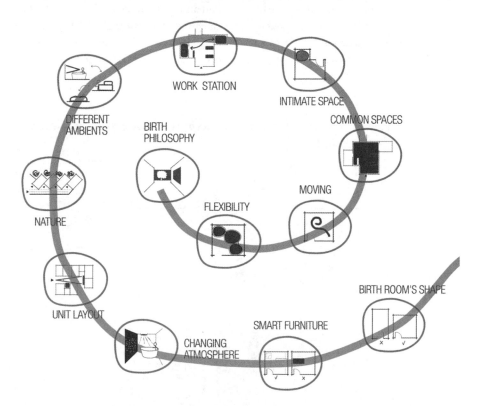

There is a need for tools which can guide design in this area. The only existing tool is the BUDSET* (Foureur et al, 2010b), which can be used as part of a Post Occupancy Evaluation POE process** or as a checklist for the planning and design of new birth spaces. However,

---

* The Birth Unit Design Spatial Evaluation Tool (BUDSET) is a tool to assess the optimality of birth units according to four domains with items describing the birth environment characteristics supporting optimal birth units. It was developed using a qualitative study including a literature review, interviews with key informants (architects, midwives and researchers) and consultation with an expert panel.

** POE aims to provide feedback on the quality of buildings in supporting their occupants' activities and perception by evaluating buildings 'in a systematic and rigorous manner after they have been built and occupied for some time' (Preiser, W.F., White, E., and Rabinowitz, H., 2015).

it still needs to be implemented and correlated to outcomes for women and staff (Foureur et al, 2011).

Another topic which currently needs to be addressed by architectural research is the issue of the impact that a space can have on intervention rates. There has been a steep rise in the rate of caesarean birth worldwide, making this the most common major surgery currently performed on humans. It would seem that the spatial characteristics of a birth setting can directly or indirectly influence birth outcomes (see Figure 4). This could be through suggestion that could influence the choices people make (for example, the presence of medical equipment in the birth room), or by indirect action on the cortisol levels of the woman (Jenkinson et al, 2014; Stenglin and Foureur, 2013; Foureur, 2010a; Priddis et al, 2012) and/or the midwives or other caregivers (Foureur et al, 2010a). There is some evidence that these kinds of factors could influence midwifery practice (Hammond et al, 2014). A recent literature review has just been published on this topic (Setola et al, 2019).

Figure 4:
The direct and indirect effect of spatial characteristics of a birth setting on birth outcomes
(Created by Setola N. and Cocina G.G.)

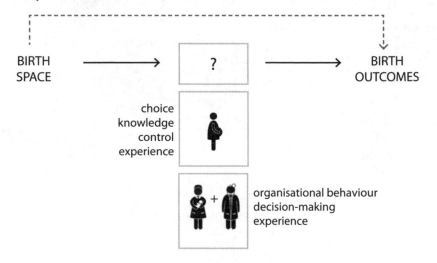

It is equally possible that design may impact care by either helping or hindering key processes, as suggested, for example, by the Pressure Tank Model (Plough et al, 2018a), which postulates that the design may influence outcomes by setting the physical capacity of a care unit, as well as by mediating the workflows of the care team. Some designs may enable flexibility or adaptability in responding to unexpected changes in the woman's needs, such as surges in the number of women in labour or acuity. Some designs may better facilitate knowledge-sharing or communication between key staff members by providing collaborative space or co-locating related service areas. Still others may create 'cognitive anchors' that reinforce certain patterns of work, for example, by prominently displaying centralised monitoring technology. There is evidence that in these dimensions, childbirth facilities vary widely. (Plough et al, 2018b).

Other methods in the architectural field for carrying out research on this phenomenon include 'space syntax', which includes a set of simulation tools for space configuration, people movement and behaviour analysis (Al-Sayed et al, 2014; Hillier and Raford, 2010) (see Figure 5). Its many applications for the healthcare environment are well known among architects (Khan, 2012, Setola, 2013; Peponis et al, 1996). Studies on workplace architecture could also be significant for a possible application to birthing facilities, for the purpose of identifying the effects of the spatial layout on organisational behaviour (Sailer, 2013; Sailer et al, 2009).

Figure 5:
The Space Syntax spatial analysis and the movements and activities observation in the hospital circulation spaces (Created by Setola N. and Borgianni S.)

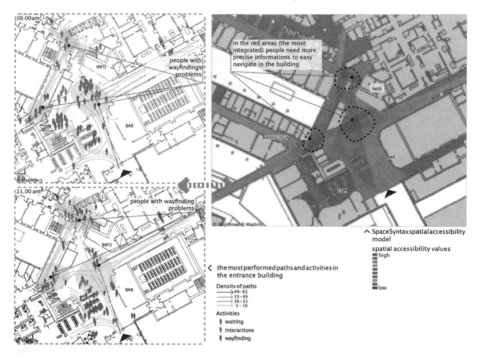

Conclusion

The importance of the configuration of space and its impact on the behaviour and practice of people in hospital design has been widely demonstrated (Haq and Luo, 2012; Setola and Borgianni, 2016; Sadek and Shepley, 2016), although specific studies on birth places are lacking. Understanding the importance of configuring birth spaces to permit effective relationships and activities is crucial. This includes the relationship between spatial layout and organisation, and which factors of space affect organisational behaviours in different ways, since organisational behaviours and culture are related to intervention rates (caesarean section, induction, episiotomy etc). This approach needs to be interdisciplinary in order to provide a real contribution, since there are many variables which influence the organisation. It needs to be developed at the scale of configuration in the unit, and it needs to integrate the perspectives of women using the service, their birth companions and maternity unit staff.

Architectural research in this field should also consider new findings on the ecology of birth settings at the level of materials, constructive elements and devices, to allow flexibility, adaptability and adjustability as well as the presence of an intimate space in the birth room.

Moreover, research should focus on identifying appropriate requirements and standard measures supporting the optimal birth room and unit layout as an addition to currently available design tools.

Key points for consideration

- Ensure clinicians, end-users (families) and architects collaborate when designing new facilities or renovating existing ones.
- Consider the impact of design on key care processes, including supporting communication and coordination among families and the care team.
- Consider ways the space can be used flexibly for labouring women with different or evolving needs, and in accordance with different or evolving volumes or acuities of service users.
- Consider how the labouring space facilitates necessary intimacy for the mother to feel at ease.

References

Aus HFG, 2017. Part B. Health Facility Briefing and Planning HPU 510 Maternity Unit; [Internet]. Available from: https://www.healthfacilityguidelines.com.au/health-planning-units [cited 2018, Oct 10].

Al-Sayed, K., Turner, A., Hillier, B., Iida, S. and Penn, A. (2014) Space Syntax Methodology. 4th edition. London: Bartlett School of Architecture, UCL.

Balabanoff Doreen. 2016. Light in the Reimagined Birth Environment PROCESS WORK. A document accompanying the doctoral dissertation submitted September 2, 2016 to University College Dublin. Available at: https://indd. adobe.com/view/3a35bb36-7f43-4e94-b79f-7ce4b989f452

Berridge Emma-Jane, Nicola J.Mackintosh, Della S.Freeth, 2010. Supporting patient safety: Examining communication with in delivery suite teams through contrasting approaches to research observation. Midwifery 26(2010)512–519

Bowden Calida, Athena Sheehan, Maralyn Foureur. 2016. Birth room images: What they tell us about childbirth. A discourse analysis of birth rooms in developed countries. Midwifery 35(2016)71–77

Dalke Hilary, Jenny Little, Elga Niemann, Nilgun Camgoz, Guillaume Steadman, Sarah Hill, Laura Stott. 2006. Colour and lighting in hospital design. Volume 38, Issues 4–6, June–September 2006, Pages 343–365

Del Nord R. (2006). Environmental stress prevention in children's hospital design. Technical guidelines and architectural suggestions. Milano: Motta Architettura

De Botton A., 2006, The Architecture of Happiness: the Secret Art of Furnishing Your Life, Penguin, New York

Department of Health, 2013. Health Building Note 09-02: Maternity care facilities; [Internet]. Available from: https://www.gov.uk/government/publications/ [cited 2018, Oct 10].

Edelstein E., 2004, Neuroscience and Architecture: Health Care Facilities, Erik Jonsson Center of the National Academy of Sciences, National Academy of Sciences, Woods Hole, Academy of Neuroscience for Architecture

Edwards L. and P.Torcellini. 2002. A Literature Review of the Effects of Natural Light on Building Occupants. Technical Report of National Renewable Energy Laboratory. Available at http://www.nrel.gov/docs/fy02osti/30769.pdf

Evans GW. 2003. The built environment and mental health. J Urban Health. 2003 Dec;80(4):536-55.

Evans GM., McCoy JM, 1998, When buildings don't work: the role of architecture in human health, Journal of Environmental Psycology 18, 85-94

FGI, 2018. Guidelines for Design and Construction of Hospitals; [Internet]. Available from: http://www.madcad. com/store/subscription/FGI-Guidelines-Hospital-2018/ [cited 2018, Oct 10].

Forbes, I, Homer, CSE, Foureur, M, Leap, N. Birthing Unit Design: Researching New Principles. Design & Health Scientific Review 1, 47–53. World Health Design, London; 2008

Foureur, M. 2008. Creating birth space to enable undisturbed birth. In: Birth Territory and Midwifery Guardianship: Theory for Practice, Education and Research, 1e 1st Edition by Kathleen Fahy, Maralyn Foureur, Carolyn Hastie. Elsevier Books for Midwifes. pp.57-77

Foureur Maralyn, Deborah Davis, Jennifer Fenwick, Nicky Leap, Rick Iedema,BA, Ian Forbes, Caroline S.E. Homer. 2010a. The relationship between birth unit design and safe, satisfying birth: Developing a hypothetical model. *Midwifery* 26(2010)520–525

Foureur MJ, Leap N, Davis D, Forbes I, Homer CSE. (2010b) Developing the Birth Unit Design Spatial Evaluation Tool (BUDSET): A qualitative study. *Health Environments Research and Design Journal*. 3(4): 43-57.

Foureur MJ, Leap N, Davis D, Forbes I, Homer CSE. (2011) Testing the Birth Unit Design Spatial Evaluation Tool (BUDSET) in Australia: A Pilot Study. HERD Volume 4, Number 2, pp 36-60

Freeman Lesa M., Vivienne Adair, Helen Timperley, Sandra H. West. 2006. The influence of the birthplace and models of care on midwifery practice for the management of women in labour. Women and Birth (2006) 19, 97

Franck, R. and Lepori Bianca. 2007. Architecture from the Inside Out: From the Body, the Senses, the Site and the Community, 2nd Edition. Wiley

Gesler W, Bell M, Curtis S, Hubbard P, Francis S. Therapy by design: evaluating the UK hospital building program. Health Place 2004;10 :117– 28.

Hamilton, D. K., Walkins, D.H., Evidence-Based Design for Multiple Building Types: Applied Research-Based Knowledge for Multiple Building Types, Ed. John Wiley & Sons, New York ,2008,

Hammond A. D., Homer C. S. E. & Foureur M. (2014). Messages from space: An exploration of the relationship between hospital birth environments and midwifery practice. Health Environments Research & Design Journal, 7(4), 81–95

Haq, S. and LUO, Y. (2012) Space Syntax in health-care facilities research: a review. Health Environments Research & Design. 5(4), pp. 98–117.

Harte, J. D., Sheehan, A., Stewart, S. C., & Foureur, M. (2016). Childbirth supporters' experiences in a built hospital birth environment: Exploring inhibiting and facilitating factors in negotiating the supporter role. Health Environments Research & Design Journal, 9(3), 135–161

Hauck Y., Rivers C, Doherty K. 2008, Women's experiences of using a Snoezelen room during labour in Western Australia, Midwifery 24, 460-470

Hillier, B., Penn, A., Hanson, J. and XU, J. (1993) Natural movement: or, configuration and attraction in urban pedestrian movement. Environment and Planning B: Planning and Design. 20, pp. 29–66.

Hillier, B. (2007) Space Is the Machine. [Online] London: Space Syntax. Available from: http://discovery.ucl. ac.uk/3881/1/SITM.pdf [accessed 14 December 2015].

Hillier, B. and Hanson, J. (1984) The Social Logic of Space. Cambridge: Cambridge University Press.

Hillier, B. and Raford, N. (2010) Description and discovery in socio-spatial analysis: the case of Space Syntax. In Walford, G. (eds) The Sage Handbook of Measurement. London: SAGE, pp. 265–281.

Hodnett ED, Stremler R, Weston JA, McKeever P., 2009, Re-conceptualizing the hospital labor room: the PLACE (Pregnant and Laboring in an Ambient Clinical Environment) pilot trial. Birth 36(2), 159-166

Hunt, S., & Symonds, A. (1995). The Social Meaning of Midwifery. New York: Palgrave MacMillan.

Khan, N. (2012) Analyzing patient flow: reviewing literature to understand the contribution of space syntax to improve operational efficiency in healthcare settings. In Greene, M., Reyes, J. and Castro, A. (eds) Proceedings: Eighth International Space Syntax Symposium. 8183, pp. 1–11. Santiago de Chile: PUC.

Iannuzzi, Laura (2016). An exploration of midwives' approaches to slow progress of labour in birth centres, using case study methodology. PhD thesis, University of Nottingham. Available on line at http://eprints. nottingham.ac.uk/37758/1/Iannuzzi%20PhD%20Thesis%20DEFINITIVE.pdf

Ispsel Guidelines, 2007. Linee guida per gli interventi di prevenzione relativi alla sicurezza e all'igiene del lavoro nel blocco parto. Istituto superiore per la prevenzione e la sicurezza del lavoro; [Internet]. Available from: https://appsricercascientifica.inail.it/ [cited 2018, Oct 10].

Jenkinson, B., Josey, N., & Kruske, S. (2014). BirthSpace: An evidence-based guide to birth environment design. Queensland Centre for Mothers & Babies, The University of Queensland.

Lepori B. 1994. Freedom of Movement in birth Places. Children's Environments 11(2): 1-12

Lepori B., Fourer M., Hastie C. 2008. Mindbodyspirit architecture: Creating Birth Space. In: Birth Territory and Midwifery Guardianship: Theory for Practice, Education and Research, 1e 1st Edition by Kathleen Fahy, Maralyn Foureur, Carolyn Hastie. Elsevier Books for Midwifes.pp.95-112

Lynch, K. (1960) Image of a City. Cambridge, MA: MIT Press.

Longo E., Setola N., "Towards a spatial dimension of social rights. New prospectives in architecture and law studies",

Interdisciplinary Themes Journal, Vol.1/2009. pp. 100-111.

Markus, T.A. (1993) Buildings and Power. Freedom and Control in the Origin of Modern Building Types. New York: Routledge.

Miller S, Abalos E, Chamillard Met al. 2016 Beyond too little, too late and too much, too soon: a pathway towards evidence-based, respectful maternity care worldwide. *Lancet* 388(10056):2176-2192.

Newburn M., Culture, control and the birth environment. *The Practising Midwife* [2003, 6(8):20-25]

Newburn M. and Debbie Singh, 2003, "Creating a Better Birth Environment. Women's views about the design and facilities in maternity units: a national survey". The National Childbirth Trust. London, UK

Penn, A. (2008) Architectural research. In Knight, A. and Ruddock, L. (eds) Advanced Research Methods in the Built Environment. Oxford: Wiley-Blackwell, pp. 14–27.

Peponis, J., Zimring, C. and Scanlon, M.M. (1996) New design technologies: using computer technology to improve design quality. Part I: Designing friendly hospital layouts – the contribution of Space Syntax. Journal of Healthcare Design. VIII, pp. 109–115.

Plough A, Polzin-Rosenberg D, Galvin G, Shao A, Sullivan B, Henrich N, T Shah N.2018a An Exploratory Study of the Relationship between Facility Design and the Provision of Childbirth Care. J Midwifery Womens Health. 2018 Nov 8. doi: 10.1111/jmwh.12920. [Epub ahead of print]

Plough A, Polzin-Rosenberg D, Galvin G, Shao A, Sullivan B, Henrich N, Shah NT. 2018b Assessing the Feasibility of Measuring Variation in Facility Design Among American Childbirth Facilities. HERD. 2018 Oct 3:1937586718796641. doi: 10.1177/1937586718796641. [Epub ahead of print]

Preiser, W. F., White, E., & Rabinowitz, H. (2015). Post-Occupancy Evaluation (Routledge Revivals). Routledge.

Priddis H., Hannah Dahlen, and Virginia Schmied. Juggling Instinct and Fear. INTERNATIONAL JOURNAL OF CHILDBIRTH Volume 1, Issue 4, 2011

Priddis Holly, Hannah Dahlen, Virginia Schmied, What are the facilitators, inhibitors, and implications of birth positioning? A review of the literature. Women and Birth (2012) 25, 100—106

Sadek AH, Shepley MM.2016. Space Syntax Analysis: Tools for Augmenting the Precision of Healthcare Facility Spatial Analysis. HERD. 2016 Oct;10(1):114-29.

Sailer, K. (2013). Organizational Learning and Physical Space: How Office Configurations Inform Organizational Behaviors. In A. Berthoin Antal, T. Meusburger, L. Suarsana (Eds.), Learning Organizations. Extending the Field (pp. 103-127). Dordrecht, The Netherlands: Springer Netherlands.

Sailer, K., Budgen, A., Lonsdale, N., Turner, A., & Penn, A. (2009). Comparative studies of offices pre and post – how changing spatial configurations affect organisational behaviours. Proceedings of the 7th International Space Syntax Symposium, 96. Stockholm, Sweden: Royal Institute of Technology (KTH).

Setola and Borgianni, 2016. Designing Public Spaces in Hospitals. Routledge, NY

Setola N., 2014, Quality of space and right to health. An interdisicplinary research in hospital facilities, *Techne* n.7/2014. pp. 157-164.

Setola, N. (2013) Percorsi, flussi e persone nella progettazione ospedaliera. L'analisi configurazionale, teoria e applicazione. Firenze: Firenze University Press.

Setola N., Naldi E., Cocina G.G., Bodil Eide L., Iannuzzi L., Daly D. (2019) The Impact of the Physical Environment on Intrapartum Maternity Care. Identification of Eight Crucial Building Spaces. HERD - Health Environments Research & Design Journal

Stenglin M, Foureur M. 2013. Designing out the Fear Cascade to increase the likelihood of normal birth. Midwifery. 2013 Aug;29(8):819-25.

Symon, Andrew; Paul, Jeanette; Butchart, Maggie; Carr, Val; Dugard, Pat. 2008a. Maternity Unit Design study part 2: perceptions of space and layout. In: British Journal of Midwifery, Vol. 16, No. 2, 2008, p. 110-114.

Symon, Andrew; Paul, Jeanette; Butchart, Maggie; Carr, Val; Dugard, Pat. 2008b. Maternity Unit Design part 3 : environmental comfort and control. In: British Journal of Midwifery, Vol. 16, No. 3, 2008, p. 167-171.

Symon, Andrew; Paul, Jeanette; Butchart, Maggie; Carr, Val; Dugard, Pat. 2008c. Maternity Unit Design part 4 : midwives' perceptions of staff facilities. In: British Journal of Midwifery, Vol. 16, No. 4, 2008, p. 228-231.

Townsend B., J. Fenwick , V. Thomson , M. Foureur. 2016. The birth bed: A qualitative study on the views of midwives regarding the use of the bed in the birth space. Women and Birth 29 (2016) 80–84

Ulrich, R.S. et al. (2008) A review of the research literature on evidence-based healthcare design. HERD. 1(3), pp. 61–125

Ulrich R., Barach P., 2006, Designing Safe Healthcare Facilities What are the Data and Where do we Go from Here? Healthcare Environments Research Summit, Robert Wood Johnson Foundation, Atlanta, GA

Williams, H. (2003). Storied births: narrative and organisational culture in a midwifery-led birth Centre. London: Kings College.

CHAPTER 19

Natural connections: biophilic birthplace design

Martin Brown and Tracey Cooper

Introduction

'We will have the ability in a very short time to create buildings that are literally as complex as a plant or a flower, that are biophilic in the true sense of the word.' (Paul Hawken[*])

Human beings have an innate relationship with nature. Yet, in a relatively short timeframe in terms of human evolution, humans have moved from the savannah to the jungle and from a natural to a built environment. Most people around the world now live, work and play in spaces comprised of concrete and glass, with little or no room for any living materials or connectivity with nature (Gelsthorp, 2017).

The lack of any meaningful connectivity with nature has been partly attributed to deteriorating physical, mental and social wellbeing (Gelsthorp, 2017). Anecdotally many people are aware, often unconsciously, of the power of nature and of 'being outside'. More pragmatically, there is some evidence that prescriptions for outdoor exercise can improve mood and wellbeing (Gladwell et al 2013).

Concepts of biophilia, biophilic design and biomimicry have become a dominant discourse for built environment sustainable design (Salingaros, 2015). There is an increased use of salutogenesis concepts within health building design (Peters, 2017 and see Chapter 17). This is not surprising, given the current shift in focus from notions of sustainability that have been too focused on energy and resources, to a concept of regenerative sustainability that now promotes health and wellbeing. This has resulted in a shift in thinking, from the need to reduce so-called 'sick building syndrome', to the promotion of buildings designed to improve health and healing (Brown, 2016).

In many counties, people spend 90% of their time within buildings (Klepeis, 2001). It is therefore not surprising that health has risen to the top of the corporate agenda,

---

[*] Hawken, P., Trim Tab Blog at International Living Future Institute trimtab.living-future.org

and given that staff account for 90% of an organisation's costs, this also makes very good financial sense. (WorldGBC, 2014). Major developers are currently preparing commercial and residential properties based on new building standards such as the Living Building Challenge* and the Well Build Standard**, recognising that 'well' designed facilities will be a future key prerequisite for buildings.

There is growing evidence that buildings designed on the basis of biophilic principles can improve health and reduce health costs (Ulrich et al, 2004; Browning et al, 2015). Buildings are being designed, built, and refurbished that not only reduce impact on occupant fatigue, and improve recovery times for sick people and foster a greater wellbeing, but also improve users' hope, health, happiness and wellbeing. (Peters, 2017).

Definitions and Insights

Biophilia literally means the love of nature. It suggests a deep, innate affinity between humans and nature. It is considered key to mental and health wellbeing (Williams, 2017). E.O. Wilson (1984) is recognised for popularising the concept of biophilia within his book of the same name. However, it is an area of study that has been around since the 16th century, when Swiss-German philosopher, physician and botanist Paracelsus suggested that sickness and health in the body relied on the harmony of humans (microcosm) and nature (macrocosm).***

Biophilic design is the application of biophilic principles that brings buildings 'alive' through recognising and improving bonds between the built environment and natural conditions. It is seen as a response to the human desire to regularly reaffirm contact with nature (Kellert, Calabrese, 2015).

Stephen Kellert, recognised as the 'Godfather of biophilia' has had a significant influence on the way spaces are created in the built environment. In his seminal book *Biophilic Design: The Theory, Science and Practice of Bringing Buildings to Life*, he defines biophilic design as *'building and landscape design that enhances human physical and mental wellbeing by fostering positive connections between people and nature'*.

Biophilic design remains an optional approach in today's building sustainability standards, with the exception of the Living Building Challenge (Sturgeon, 2017). As the most robust building standard globally, the Living Building Challenge calls for mandatory biophilic design considerations in its aim to create healthy buildings that are ecologically sound, socially just and culturally rich.

Florence Williams in *Nature Fix* (Williams, 2017) catalogues many co-benefits (health benefits that emerge as a consequence of design interventions) that are possible, or have been demonstrated through a designed connectivity with nature. Such design, referred to as Regenerative Design, takes a worldview approach, with humans as part of nature, rather than apart from nature. This is the core topic of EU Cost Action RESTORE (Brown et al, 2018).

Biomimicry is the principle that through understanding nature, people can mimic the way nature solves problems and apply natural solutions to everyday problems, in this case to buildings and spaces for work, life, play and, in terms of this book, to give birth in. Once

---

*   Living Building Challenge living-future.org/lbc

**   Well Build Standard www.wellcertified.com

***   www.revolvy.com/page/Paracelsus

seen as a revolutionary idea, biomimicry has recently gained traction and is now transforming many building designs and materials. Michael Palwyn (Palwyn, 2016) describes biomimicry as '*developing sustainable solutions that mimic the functional basis of nature*'. Janice Benyus (Benyus, 2009) introduced nine principles that significantly raised biomimicry's popularity through TED talks and social media presence. The nine principles describe how nature works and how nature can contribute to the way we approach design, based on asking the question 'How would nature solve this issue …?'

Regenerative sustainability: if sustainability is that 'do less harm' tipping point where humans give back as much as they take from nature, then regenerative sustainability is the 'healing' state where more is given back than is taken. From a health perspective, regenerative buildings, through biophilic patterns, circadian light and air quality can energise building users, enabling a 'healthier' feeling when leaving than when they arrived (Brown, 2016).

Biophilic components and benefits

One of the go-to guides for biophilic design is Terrapin Bright Green *Fourteen Patterns of Biophilic Design* (Browning et al, 2014), a guide that considers three aspects of nature – the presence of nature in the space, the presence of natural patterns or stimuli and the nature of the space.

Table 1:
14 Patterns of Biophilic Design

Nature in the Space
Nature in Space Patterns – Sensing nature
Visual Connection – the view to nature, from working and living places
Non Visual Connections – the sounds of nature
Non Rhythmic Sensory Stimuli – the brief, occasional, natural distraction, visual, sound, scent
Thermal and Airflow Variability – feeling the sense of natural environment, air, heat, humidity
Presence of Water – visual, sounds, suggestion of,
Dynamic and Diffuse Light – circadian, seasonal and diurnal change in light
Connection with Natural Systems – awareness of natural, seasonal or temporal changes
Natural Analogues
Biomorphic Forms and Patterns – textured internal finishes
Material Connection with Nature – natural objects
Complexity and Order – spatial layout, natural hierarchy to furnishings
Nature of the Space
Prospect – actual or sense of long-distance views
Refuge – a place of retreat from nature
Mystery – promise of more nature, encouraging exploration
Risk and Peril – a sense of natural threat and safety

Researcher Roger Ulrich (Ulrich et al, 2004) found that patients whose hospital window overlooked nature recorded shorter post-operative stays, required less pain medication and, interestingly, evaluated nursing staff more positively after gall bladder surgery than patients whose ward looked onto a brick wall. Other reported benefits from biophilia include: *,**

Table 2:
Benefits of Biophilic Design

Health	Productivity
• Reduced stress, blood pressure, heart rate	• Increased output and creativity
• Improved healing times following surgery	• Reduced boredom
• Improved mood and self-esteem	• Enhanced mental stamina and creative task performance
• Improved immune functions	**Good business**
• Improved attitude and happiness	
• Improved 'co-benefits'	• Increased productivity and profitability
Social	• Improved loyalty
	• Reduced staff costs through lower absenteeism, presentism and staff churn
• Fosters social cohesion	• Improved reputation as a responsible organisation
• Lower levels of crime and violence,	
• Enhanced safety performance	**Environment**
• Identification and attachment with place	
Learning	• Improved ecological literacy
	• Higher levels of sustainable behaviour and stewardship
• Improved attention and faster learning rates	
• Reduced symptoms of ADHD in children	
• Reduced school absenteeism	

---

*   *Light is Medicine* – Dyson Neonatal Intensive Care Unit, Bath RUH

**   *Biophilic Benefits*, collated (Brown, 2018) for keynotes from numerous sources (including those cited in references here)

Healthy materials, healthier birth spaces

'The materials we build with can affect our wellbeing as much as the food we eat, the water we drink and the air we breathe.' (Health Building Network [*])

While there is now recognition of the potential benefits of biophilic design for work, living, health and education spaces, it is not a sticking plaster to cover poor and unhealthy building design. If toxic materials are incorporated into the building (e.g. formaldehydes, PVCs or VOCs), or more often into the fittings and furnishings (formaldehyde glues, phthalates as fire retardants) then no measure of biophilic design can truly compensate.

For birth centre design, it is crucial to adopt the *precautionary principle*. Key to promoting healthier materials and eliminating toxic materials from buildings, the precautionary principle states that if a product has a suspected risk of causing harm, then the burden of proof that it is not harmful falls on those undertaking the design, specifying or procuring the products.

Biophilic design and birth space

Birth is a normal physiological process. Being surrounded by the sensation of a natural environment, even if it is technologically produced, may benefit the psychological state of all women in labour and birth, regardless of whether they have complications or not (Design Council 2013), and as indicated in Table 2, it may also be of benefit to birth partners and care providers (Kelly 2011). As described in Chapter 6, salutogenic theory provides a new framework for understanding women's positive health experiences of labour (Downe and McCourt, 2019). Chapter 5 describes how psychological wellbeing can affect physical bodily responses. Designing biophilic effects into buildings where birth takes place may salutogenically influence how the body works during labour if the mind and body are working together as one.

Using biophilia in practice

Fear and anxiety in labour can result in muscular tension and ischaemia, which intensifies the pain felt in childbirth, increasing pharmacological intervention. Women who experience these sensations often use epidural analgesia, even if this was not their original intention (Greer et al, 2014). Epidural analgesia is a very good form of pain relief, but it has also been associated with increased labour complications and interventions (Anim et al, 2018; Leap and Anderson, 2008, and see Chapter 16). These interventions include caesarean section, thus fear and anxiety could be contributing to increased rates globally. *The Lancet* optimising caesarean section series (Boerma et al, 2018) reported that globally caesarean section rates equated to 15% of births in 106 (63%) of 169 countries, whereas 47 (28%) countries had caesarean section rates of less than 10%. Interestingly they also found rates of caesarean section were almost five times more frequent in births in the richest versus the poorest quintiles in low-income

---

[*]   Healthy Building Network: Transforming the market for building materials to advance the best environmental, health and social outcomes. healthybuilding.net

and middle-income countries; markedly high caesarean use was observed among low obstetric risk births (Boerma et al, 2018).

Oxytocin and endorphins released by the body during labour and birth ensure progress of labour and reduce analgesic requirements (see Chapter 2). When these hormones are inhibited by the release of adrenaline and noradrenaline (stress hormones), pain experienced increases and progress may be delayed. They can pass across the placenta to the baby, and foetal compromise in some circumstances may be attributed to maternal fear or stress (British Neuroscience Association, 2013; Gilau et al, 1998).

In addition to the physical effects of fear and stress, 25–34% of women report that their births were traumatic, with studies demonstrating rates of PTSD that vary from 1.5–9% after childbirth (Beck and Indman, 2005; Cigoli et al, 2006; Czarnocka and Slade, 2000; Declercq et al, 2008; Gross et al, 2005; Soet et al, 2003; Szalay, 2011). See also Chapter 4. If diagnosed, women often need to access mental health services and other therapies, which can be distressing for them and their families. This also increases costs to health services.

Childbirth involves a dynamic physiological and psychosocial interplay between mother and foetus, but the exact nature of this complex process is not, as yet, well understood. It is recognised, however, that psychological and emotional factors influence the flow of hormones that affect the duration and experience of labour and birth. Reports of fear of birth are rising in pregnant women (Sheen et al, 2017; Roosevelt, 2016; Adams et al, 2012; Haines et al, 2012), and this is known to influence anxiety, pain and, consequently, labour progression.

Based on the studies discussed in the earlier sections of this chapter, biophilic design offers the potential to reduce stress and anxiety for labouring women, and to provide a positive working environment for staff working in labour and birth settings. However, there are few examples of the use of biophilia in birth environments. Moving Essence Nature Art Therapy (MENAT) has been used in other healthcare settings, for example critical care units and cancer care facilities, with good effects (Naylor et al, 2012; Kelly, 2011; Ulrich et al, 2004). Evidence from the settings where MENAT has been used suggested significant increases in pain threshold and reduced requirement of pain medication. Over three-quarters of patients who used MENAT reported reduction in anxiety, with feedback describing calming and relaxing benefits. Physical changes were noted, including reductions in pulse and blood pressure, and reports of reduced feelings of fear and stress (Design Council, 2013).

The evidence from other healthcare settings has demonstrated benefits including:

- 33%–52% increase in pain threshold without side effects (Tse et al, 2002)
- Fewer strong doses of pain medication needed with nature connection (Ulrich et al, 2004)
- 12% shorter hospital stays for patients with nature connection (Ulrich et al, 2004)
- 77% reported a reduction in anxiety (Kelly, 2011)
- 60% reported help with sleeping (Kelly, 2011)

- 24% longer for wound healing if patients are stressed (Design Council, 2013)
- 110% increase in care cost if cancer patients suffer from anxiety (Naylor et al, 2012)

This therapy was used in an Accident and Emergency setting, where a reduction of anger and fear, and an increase in pleasant feelings were reported, reducing stress within 3 to 5 minutes. Fewer negative reactions to treatment were recorded by staff. Blood pressure and pulse were lower on days when the therapy was available, compared to days with continuous daytime television programmes (Design Council, 2013).

Case study of using biophilic principles in labour and birth settings

Lancashire Teaching Hospitals Trust in the UK is a medium-sized facility, hosting 4,500 births a year. The Trust has one central hospital birth unit and two birth centres (one alongside the main unit and one sited 23 kilometres away). 1,100 births take place in the birth centres.

In 2016, funding was secured to introduce elements of biophilic design into the birth centres. This was extended into the hospital facility later in 2016. The intention was to create a calm and relaxing atmosphere in the birth room to improve the emotional, psychological and physiological state of the woman in labour and during birth, and reduce transfers between settings and improve clinical outcomes. Dynamic nature art therapy was used. This includes moving visual images projected onto the birthing room wall, and natural sounds and music controlled by the labouring woman. She can turn the system off if she doesn't want it on, or turn down the sound and use her own music on Bluetooth speakers in the rooms. When we first implemented this we could not find any evidence of it being used globally in a birth centre before.

To assess the acceptability of the use of MENAT in childbirth in the local setting, 15 labouring women and their birth companions were given the chance to use it before it was used more generally. The results are not comparative, so it isn't clear how far they reflect the use of the system over the use of the birth centre, or other unmeasured aspects of their care. With this caveat, all the women and their birth companions felt that the biophilic elements helped to reduce stress and anxiety and induce relaxation. All the women reported that labour and birth were easier than they had expected. Eight of them were having their first baby. Rebecca said:

'...the wall projections of nature next to the pool took me to that place. I really felt that I was by the sea listening and concentrating on the waves. It really helped me to concentrate on listening to my body and focusing on getting through labour. My baby was born to a stream running through a mountain, I can't think of a more beautiful way to be born in water next to a mountain stream. Jack was so calm and chilled when he was born he didn't cry just opened his eyes slowly as we introduced him to the world.'

In addition, five midwives who were with some of the women in the birthing room were asked for their opinions about the technology. All reported that they felt it had a positive effect on women during labour and birth, reducing stress and anxiety. They also felt that being in a calm, relaxed environment contributed to their job satisfaction.

Sadie (midwife) said:

> *'bringing nature scenes and sounds into the birthing nest really relaxes and calms both the woman and her birth partner down within the space of 20 minutes. It's as if they both just go 'ahh' and their shoulders relax, it's beautiful to see. It also makes a beautiful environment to practice in as a midwife, I feel like I am working in a spa!!'*

These results suggested that this innovation may reduce stress and anxiety during labour and birth. This is reinforced by data from other settings, as discussed above. However, the use of biophilia is in its infancy in maternity care, and further use of, and research into, this approach is required.

Conclusion

Biophilia and biophilic design offers immense opportunities to improve birth spaces for women, babies, partners, family and those that work within the spaces. However, while limited benefit can be attained through low-cost interventions (the plant in the corner, the forest wallpaper or video), real benefit can only be achieved through a holistic regenerative design approach that commences with a salutogenic mindset, to design and construct spaces that will maintain and improve health. We can and are increasingly designing for health, with biophilic-designed health facilities such as the Maternity Unit at Essen Hospital in Germany, the Maternity Waiting Village in Malawi, and the Dyson Neonatal Intensive Care Unit at Bath RUH pointing to a future of healthy buildings and spaces that are seen as medical instruments.

The potential for using biophilia to make a difference to women's experiences and those of their birth companions and all staff in the room are evident in this small sample. Further research is important as a small investment into the environment could have an effect not only on experiences, but also on birth outcomes, but this is yet to be proven. Due to the current resource challenges within the NHS it is difficult to obtain funding for what many view as 'a nice to do extra' and not as an essential part of care delivery. Simple additions like this can make a fundamental difference to the 'whole' person: mind, body and soul, of everyone experiencing it, not just the woman. *Better Births: A five Year Forward View* (National Maternity Review Team, 2016) focuses on personalisation and continuity, viewing the woman as a whole, and this concept fits perfectly into these elements. Maternity care needs to be delivered differently and this could be part of that fundamental change in how we view the childbirth experience.

Key points for consideration

- Think about the environment in any birth space. How can you make a biophilic connection with nature? There are a range of biophilic options open to you depending on your budget. The 'Creating Positive Spaces' white paper from Interface outlines options from No Budget to High Budget (Heath, 2018).
- The best inspiration for creating biophilic spaces is to go for a walk outside, in the forest, with your design team if designing spaces, with family and friends if considering birth space options.

- Connecting with nature through biophilia doesn't have to mean 'green' or 'living plants'. Be imaginative and inspirational, think about the space layout (prospect and refuge), shapes, sounds, lighting, presence of water, or even the sensing of natural thermal or air differences.

- Think 'people first': always think about the woman as a whole: mentally, physically and emotionally, and consider partners, family, visitors and importantly those who spend their working time in the environment.

- Work with Estates Departments to look at simple changes that could improve lighting, for example natural light, circadian light tubes, dimmer switches and biophilic wall murals if moving wall art is not possible.

- Apply to charity funds if capital investment sources will not fund your biophilic intentions. Use this chapter and references to support your application. Never give up. Use Voices Forum Partnerships to influence and help to develop environments. The '15 steps to better maternity experiences' toolkit (NHS England, 2018) could be used to help influence priorities within local maternity services systems.

References

Adams S, Eberhard-Gran M, Eskild A (2012) Fear of childbirth and duration of labour: a study of 2206 women with intended vaginal delivery. BJOG, 2012 Sep;119(10):1238-46. doi: 10.1111/j.1471-0528.2012.03433. Epub 2012 Jun 27.

Alder J, Stadlmayr W, Tschudin S, Bitzer J (2006) Post-Traumatic Symptoms after Childbirth: What Should we Offer? J Psychosom Obstet Gynaecol. Jun; 27(2):107-12.

Anim-Somuah M, Smyth RMD, Cyna AM, Cuthbert A (2018) Epidural versus non-epidural or no analgesia for pain management in labour (Review). Cochrane Database of Systematic Reviews. Link accessed 6/1/19: https://www.cochranelibrary.com/cdsr/doi/10.1002/14651858.CD000331.pub4/epdf/abstract

Beck CT, Indman P (2005) The many faces of postpartum depression. J Obstet Gynecol Neonatal Nurs 34(5):569-76

Beynus, J. (2009) Biomimcry: Innovation Inspired by Nature, Harper Collins

Boerma T, Ronsmans C, Melesse D, Barros A, Barros F, Juan L (2018) Global epidemiology of use of and disparities in caesarean sections. Optimising Caesarean Section Use Vol 392, Issue 10155,p 1341-1348. DOI:https://doi.org/10.1016/S0140-6736(18)31928-

British Neuroscience Association (2013). "Fetal exposure to excessive stress hormones in the womb linked to adult mood disorders." ScienceDaily. ScienceDaily, 7 April 2013. <www.sciencedaily.com/releases/2013/04/130407090835.htm>.

Brown, M.(2016) FutuREstorative: Working Towards a New Sustainability; 1st ed.; RIBA Publishing,

Brown, M.; Haselsteiner, E.; Apró, D.; Kopeva, D.; Egla, L.; Pulkkinen, K.-L.; Vula Rizvanolli, B., Eds (2018) Sustainability, Restorative to Regenerative; RESTORE.; Wien,

Browning, W.D., Ryan, C.O., Clancy, J.O., (2014) 14 Patterns of Biophilic Design. New York: Terrapin Bright Green, LLC

Browning, W.D, Garvin C, Ryan,C., Kallianpurkar, N., Labruto, L., Watson, S., Knop, T., (2015) Economics of Biophilia, Terrapin Bright Green, LLC

Cigoli V, Gilli G, Saita E (2006) Relational factors in psychopathological responses to childbirth. J Psychosom Obstet Gynaecol 27(2):91-7.

Czarnocka J, Slade P (2000) Br J Clin Psychol 39 (Pt 1):35-51. Prevalence and predictors of post-traumatic stress symptoms following childbirth.

Declercq E, Sakala C, Corry M, Applebaum S (2008) New Mothers Speak Out: National Survey Results Highlight Women's Postoartum Experiences. Childbirth Connection: New York

Gelsthorpe, J, 2017, Disconnect from nature and its effect on health and well-being A public engagement literature review. Natural History Museum. http://www.nhm.ac.uk/content/dam/nhmwww/about-us/visitor-research/Disconnect%20with%20nature%20Lit%20review.pdf

Gilau R, Comeron A, Fisk NM (1998) Fetal exposure to maternal cortisol. Lancet 1998;352(9129):707-8.

Gladwell VF, Brown DK, Wood C, Sandercock GR, Barton JL. The great outdoors: how a green exercise environment can benefit all. *Extrem Physiol Med*. 2013;2(1):3. Published 2013 Jan 3. doi:10.1186/2046-7648-2-3

Greer J, Lazenbatt A, Dunne L. (2014) 'Fear of childbirth' and ways of coping for pregnant women and their partners during the birthing process: a salutogenic analysis. *Evidence Based Midwifery* **12(3)**: 95-100

Gross MM, Hecker H, Keirse MJ (2005) An evaluation of pain and "fitness" during labor and its acceptability to women. Birth 32(2):122-8.

Haines H, Rubertsson C, Pallant J, Hildingsson I (2012) The influence of women's fear, attitudes and beliefs of childbirth on mode and experience of birth. BMC Pregnancy and Childbirth 201212:55 https://doi.org/10.1186/1471-2393-12-55

Heath O, Jackson V, Goode E, 2018 Creating Positive Spaces, Interface Design Lab Whitepaper

Hollowell J, Puddicombe D, Rowe R (2011). The Birthplace National Prospective Cohort Study: Perinatal and Maternal Outcomes by Planned Place of Birth. Birthplace in England Research Programme. Final Report Part 4. NIHR Service Delivery and Organisation prog http://www.sdo.nihr.ac.uk/projdetails.php?ref=08-1604-140

Kellert, Stephen R & Calabrese Elizabeth F., (2015). The Practice of Biophilic Design

Klepeis NE, Nelson WC, Ott WR, et al. The National Human Activity Pattern Survey (NHAPS): a resource for assessing exposure to environmental pollutants. Journal of exposure analysis and environmental epidemiology. 2001;11(3):231-252. https://www.nature.com/articles/7500165

Keswick, M, Maggies Architecture and Landscape Brief, https://www.maggiescentres.org/media/uploads/publications/other-publications/Maggies_architecturalbrief_2015.pdf

Leap N, Anderson T (2008) The Role of Pain in Normal Birth and the Empowerment of Women. In: S. Downe Normal Childbirth Evidence and Debate .Churchill Livingstone. London.

Maggioni C, Margola D, Filippi F (2006). PTSD, risk factors, and expectations among women having a baby: A two-wave longitudinal study. Journal of Psychosomatic Obstetrics & Gynecology. 27(2):81-90.

National Maternity Review Team (2016) Better Births: Improving outcomes of maternity services in England, A Five Year Forward View for Maternity Care. Available online at: https://www.england.nhs.uk/wp-content/uploads/2016/02/national-maternity-review-report.pdf

NHS England. 2018 https://www.england.nhs.uk/publication/the-fifteen-steps-for-maternity-quality-from-the-perspective-of-people-who-use-maternity-services/

Pawlyn, M., (2016) Biomimicry in Architecture (second edition), London, RIBA Publications

Peters, T., (2017) Design For Health: Sustainable Approaches for Therapeutic Architecture. Wiley

Roosevelt L, Kane Low L (2016) Exploring Fear of Childbirth in the United States Through a Qualitative Assessment of the Wijma Delivery Expectancy Questionnaire. Journal of Obstetric, Gynaecologic and Neonatal Nursing Volume 45, Issue 1, Pages 28–38. DOI: https://doi.org/10.1016/j.jogn.2015.10.005

Salingaros, Nikos A. (2015) "Biophilia and Healing Environments: Healthy Principles For Designing the Built World". New York: Terrapin Bright Green, LLC.

Sheen K, Slade P (2017) Examining the content and moderators of women's fears for giving birth: A meta-synthesis Journal of Clinical Nursing Volume 27, Issue 13-14 Pages: 2517-2916, e1686-e1688. https://doi.org/10.1111/jocn.14219

Soet JE, Brack GA, Dilorio C (2003) Prevalence and predictors of women's experience of psychological trauma during childbirth. Birth 30(1):36-46.

Sturgeon, A. (2017) Creating Biophilic Buildings, EcoTone Publishing.

Szalay S (2011) Post-Traumatic Stress Disorder after Childbirth in an Out-of-Hospital Birth Population. Presentation at Annual Conference of Midwives Association of Washington State, Seattle, Washington (unpublished).

Ulrich, R, Xiaobo Quan, Center for Health Systems and Design, Craig Zimring, Anjali Joseph, Ruchi Choudhary,(20014) The Role of the Physical Environment in the Hospital of the 21st Century: A Once-in-a-Lifetime Opportunity https://www.healthdesign.org/system/files/Ulrich_Role%20of%20Physical_2004.pdf

Walsh D (2009) Pain and Epidural Use in Normal Childbirth. Evidence Based Midwifery: Sept 2009. Royal College of Midwives. London.

Williams, F. (2017) The Nature Fix: Why Nature Makes Us Happier, Healthier, and More Creative. Norton Publishing

Wilson, E.O. (1984) *Biophilia*, Cambridge MA, Harvard University Press.

World Green Building Counsel Report (2014) Health, Wellbeing & Productivity in Offices, http://www.worldgbc.org/sites/default/files/compressed_WorldGBC_Health_Wellbeing__Productivity_Full_Report_Dbl_Med_Res_Feb_2015.pdf

Acknowledgements

Thank you to Mark Minnard for helping provide information for this chapter: MENNAT www.movingessence.org

Thank you to Cathy Atherton, Head of Midwifery at Lancashire Teaching Hospitals Trust for giving permission to share information from the Trust.

CHAPTER 20

Healthy settings and birth

Mark Dooris and *Lucia Rocca-Ihenacho*

Introduction

The 'healthy settings' approach supports a shift in focus from a pathogenic and often reductionist model of disease to a salutogenic 'whole system' model concerned to harness and release health potential within the contexts of everyday life. It is focused on what makes people thrive and flourish in the physical and environmental settings in which humans live their lives. The approach has been applied within hospitals and health services and holds strong potential for maternity care, in relation to the experiences of both service users and staff. Childbirth is still the single most common reason for hospital admission, even though there is strong evidence suggesting that centralised facility-based care is inappropriate for healthy women and babies in well-resourced healthcare contexts.[1]

This chapter introduces the healthy settings approach, and outlines its application within health service environments in general, before considering the elements that make a birth place a healthy setting. It concludes by exploring the synergistic interaction between physical and organisational cultural environments; the application of learning within wider hospital-based maternity care; and promising directions for future research.

Healthy settings: background and overview

The healthy settings approach has become a key element of the current public health discourse, with programmes spanning contexts as diverse as cities, universities, schools, hospitals and prisons. Its roots lie in the 1986 Ottawa Charter for Health Promotion, which contended that:

'health is created and lived by people within the settings of their everyday life; where they learn, work, play and love'.[2]

The approach has a number of key characteristics:[3]

- It goes beyond prevention to embrace 'salutogenesis',[4] which is concerned with what creates and sustains wellbeing, and what makes people thrive and flourish in the places they live their lives.

- It adopts an ecological model, appreciating that health is determined by a complex interaction of factors operating at different levels, highlighting the interrelationships between people and place, and addressing human health in relation to ecosystem health.

- It views settings as systems, acknowledging interconnectedness, interdependency and synergy between different components, and recognising that settings are 'nested'[5] and connected to one another by a flow of people and by their remit and operations.

- It adopts a holistic change focus, moving beyond disconnected ad hoc approaches and using multiple interconnected interventions to embed health in the ethos and culture of organisations and other settings.

- It appreciates that most settings do not have health as their main *raîson d'être* and that it is therefore essential to advocate for health in terms of impact on, or outflow from, 'core business'.

This means harnessing the multi-dimensional nature of settings, and within this the relationship between place and people, and between the structural dimension provided by their contexts, facilities, services and programmes, and the human agency within them. By so doing, those working in this field are better placed to take a comprehensive approach to human flourishing.[6] This includes the creation of healthy, supportive and sustainable environments; integrating health into routine life (whether this is quality of patient care in hospitals, education in schools or rehabilitation in prisons); and contributing to the wellbeing of the wider community (Figure 1).

Kickbusch has commented: *'the "settings approach" became the starting point for WHO's lead health promotion programmes...shifting the focus from the deficit model of disease to the health potentials inherent in the social and institutional settings of everyday life'.*[8,5] The popularity of healthy settings is not difficult to understand. Physical, social, economic, political, organisational and cultural contexts influence health,[6] and people don't compartmentalise their lives into specific risk factors or behaviours. The settings approach is thus widely seen to have a range of benefits compared to narrowly-focused topic-based and disease-specific interventions. It contributes a richness and coherence that is perceived to make health promotion more relevant, appropriate and efficacious.[9] However, it remains true that it: *'has been legitimated more through an act of faith than through rigorous research and evaluation studies...much more attention needs to be given to building the evidence.'*[10]

There are three inter-related challenges in building the evidence base.[11] First, the diversity of concepts and practice brought together under the label of healthy settings makes it difficult to generate heterogenous research that allows for comparability and transferability. Second, the established public health evidence system retains a primary focus on specific diseases, problems and single risk factor interventions rather than multiple interventions and settings. Third, evaluation of the settings approach is complex, characterised as it is by a whole system ecological perspective. This complexity has reinforced a tendency to evaluate only discrete projects. It has mitigated against the generation of credible evidence of effectiveness for the settings approach as a whole. However, there are some important relevant studies within healthcare, and these are summarised in the next section.

Figure 1:
The Whole System Healthy Settings Approach (Adapted from: Dooris et al, 2010)[7]

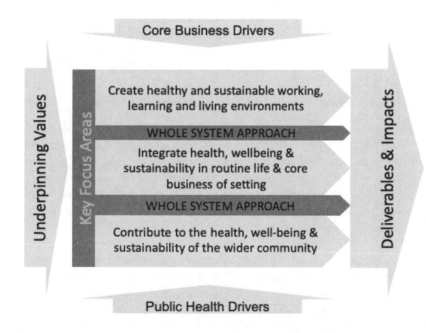

Application of the healthy settings approach to healthcare services

Health services were quick to adopt the settings approach. WHO initially focused on hospitals, in part because of their size, reach and potential to re-orient from sickness to health and promote patient, staff and community wellbeing. Additionally, there was recognition of their influence on professional education and potential as large-scale organisations to develop socially and environmentally responsible procurement and institutional management practices.[11]

The WHO European Network of Health Promoting Hospitals was launched in 1990, four years after the Ottawa charter. The network embraced principles of holism, equity, participation and partnership, and emphasised integration of these principles into core management processes. It also promoted coordination with parallel agendas such as quality, corporate social responsibility and sustainability.[12] Responding to worldwide interest and appreciating the potential to apply the settings approach across the whole healthcare system, the European Network evolved into the International Network of Health Promoting Hospitals and Health Services. With membership comprising 24 national/regional networks and a total of 600 hospital and health service members, it currently works in partnership with WHO through two collaborating centres, with the aim of improving health gain for patients, staff, and communities.[13] A European review carried out in 2000 concluded that a health promoting hospital initiative may strengthen the ethos of health promotion and facilitate the introduction of specific interventions.[14] Later research found '*stronger evidence for many health promotion interventions directed at patients, staff and the community*', but noted that '*the process of extending and incorporating these activities at a broader level has been slow*'.[15]

In considering what characterises a Health Promoting Health Service (as distinct from delivering health promotion activities within healthcare organisations), two particular aspects are relevant – the built environment and the organisational culture.

The influence of the built environment and organisational culture

The word 'hospital' comes from the Latin 'hospes', meaning a host who welcomes a guest. However, with their soulless maze of corridors, harsh lighting, bland decor and systems that tend to anonymise by making patients feel little more than a number to be processed, hospitals are frequently anything but hospitable. Historically, healthcare has prioritised functionality over quality and aesthetics, with an overriding focus on clinical processes rather than the creation of 'place' supportive to wellbeing.[16] More recently, there has been growing appreciation that the design, construction and operation of buildings profoundly impacts wellbeing of people and planet,[17] and an associated engagement with salutogenic and regenerative frameworks such as the Well Building Standard[18] and Living Building Challenge[19] (see the other chapters in this section for more details). It is increasingly recognised that good design is fundamental to the future of health services, enhancing not only delivery of medical and surgical procedures, but also (in the context of whole-life costing) overall productivity, efficiency and value for money. Good-quality well-designed buildings enable more rapid recovery from illness and surgery, promote positive health and wellbeing, improve staff wellbeing and performance, increase connectedness to the local community and contribute to sustainable development.[16, 20-22]

The integration of 'health' into the culture and fabric of the healthcare system is pivotal to success. Reflecting on the evaluation of Scotland's Health Promoting Health Services framework, Johnson and Paton[23] stress the importance of the organisational culture. They highlight managerial commitment, transformational leadership, co-ordination and training, and comment that meaningful progress is dependent not just on the delivery of health promotion interventions, but also on developing infrastructures to support programme delivery and facilitate appropriate organisational change.

What makes a birth place a healthy setting?

Birth places are not only environments where women give birth. They are also working environments for the staff assisting and supporting those women. Growing evidence suggests that the environment plays not only a crucial role in determining women's experiences of birth and the physiological process of labour, but that it also affects staff wellbeing.[24-31]

Since the 1970s birth in most high-income countries has been centralised in large obstetric units which have been designed with a view to the functionality of the space, using industrial production line principles.[32]

For women, birth settings which facilitate nesting and a sense of privacy and safety are associated with positive birth experiences and wellbeing. Hammond, Homer and Foureur[31] suggest that friendliness, functionality and freedom are three core characteristics of healthy maternity care settings in hospital. Friendliness of an environment can be associated with a space which makes service users and staff feel welcome and reduces a sense of fear. Functional rooms have the ability to support the activities which are happening within that space and to enable choice. Freedom refers to a space which allows its user the liberty of movement and fits with the needs of the users rather than imposing restrictions. These elements have been associated with positive experiences and wellbeing by staff and service users both in hospital[31] and birth centre settings.[30,33,34] They seem to offer a sound basis on which to further develop knowledge and understanding of healthy settings and their influence on birth place.

Birth centres as healthy settings

The healthy settings approach resonates with the concept of the birth centre (also known as midwifery units in countries where they are run by midwives). These are small maternity units that are either based in the community ('freestanding units'), at a distance from the nearest central maternity unit or in hospital grounds or buildings near to a secondary or tertiary maternity unit ('alongside units').[34] They are usually staffed by midwives, though in some countries, such as Canada, they can be led by general practitioners. They are designed for healthy women experiencing uncomplicated pregnancies. The organisational culture of such units tends to have a family and community focus, and to be orientated towards maximising the potential for physiological birth.[32,35] The positive effects of giving birth in such units may be partly generated by the physiological effects of feeling safe and relaxed. In this state, stress hormones such as catecholamines are down-regulated and oxytocin and endorphins are up-regulated. Environments that allow a 'working with pain' approach are more likely to minimise the production of catecholamines and adrenaline in labour, and, therefore, to support optimal labour processes.[36-37]

Birth centres focus on the healthy transition to parenthood, informed by a salutogenic perspective that stresses the importance of the creation of health as well as the minimising of pathology.[4] This reflects Kickbusch[7] in highlighting the shift away from a deficit disease model and a concern to harness the health potentials offered by the re-orientation of physical, organisational and cultural environments within settings. The philosophy of care that characterises birth centres is based on the concept of optimum birth: supporting women to achieve a positive birth experience, maximising the potential for physiological birth and intervening only when justified.[30] This philosophy is grounded in the knowledge of the processes of what facilitates or inhibits physiological labour and birth. It acknowledges that in the absence of pre-existing pathology, normal labour can present wide variations. Downe and McCourt ([38]: see also Chapter 6) refer to this as 'unique normality'. It also embraces the idea of creating a space and place in which the woman can labour undisturbed.[36]

One model of a healthy birth setting has been developed, based on the needs expressed by women using freestanding midwifery units (Figure 2). The model could be applied to any setting, but is particularly likely to describe what actually happens in birth centres in the community. Core features include building rapport and trusting the midwife or other primary caregiver.

Figure 2.
Healthy birth: the woman's dimension

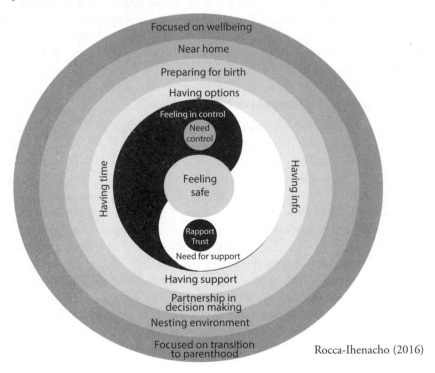

Focused on wellbeing

Near home

Preparing for birth

Having options

Feeling in control

Need control

Having time

Feeling safe

Having info

Rapport Trust

Need for support

Having support

Partnership in decision making

Nesting environment

Focused on transition to parenthood

Rocca-Ihenacho (2016)

The research underpinning this model suggests that, when women identify an environment as 'friendly', they are referring to both physical and emotional/psychological elements. Echoing the wider literature on healthy settings and health-promoting health services,[16,21] and the observations made earlier in this chapter, the physical element refers to the design of the unit, while the emotional/psychological aspects refer to the 'ambience' created by the organisational culture. In birth centres, this is specifically typified by the relationships established by staff and birth supporters who are working with the labouring woman.[30,33] Both Walsh[33] and Rocca-Ihenacho[30] refer to staff in freestanding units doing 'vicarious nesting' for the women – for example by getting the room ready before her arrival, ensuring the lights are dimmed, getting the birth pool ready, using aromatherapy and collecting together pillows and other birth equipment that the woman might use to help her to feel comfortable. Limited evidence exists about the interaction between the physical and the organisational environment, but they seem to synergise and enhance each other.[30] It is possible that a sensitively-designed homely environment with a negative organisational culture and unfriendly staff would not function well; and that, likewise, a positive organisational culture and friendly staff within a poorly-designed unfriendly environment would be limited in its influence. This hypothesis remains to be tested in future studies.

Impact of birth centre settings on staff

As well as considering the direct impact of the birth setting on labouring women, the physical and organisational aspects of the environment also impact on staff.[28] This, in turn, has an impact on the way staff respond to the women they are working with.[28] Understanding what contributes to a healthy work environment is a growing field of enquiry.[39] This work could counter burnout and sickness among healthcare staff in general, and maternity services staff in particular.[40] The challenge is to ensure that any impact is, as far as possible, salutogenic. Evidence indicates that staff working in birth centres feel healthier than those working in obstetric settings, and that they are better able to provide the emotional and psychosocial support women need in labour.[28-30] This may be a function of workload, of the capacity to form positive relationships in salutogenic settings, or some other set of circumstances.

Conclusion

Appreciating that health is created in the contexts of everyday life, the healthy settings approach has become integral to public health theory and practice. The approach articulates an ecological and salutogenic 'whole system' perspective, which is concerned with ensuring supportive and health-enhancing physical and organisational environments, and with increasing understanding of the relationships between people, place and planet.

Healthcare provision, through the Health Promoting Hospitals and Health Services movement, represents one major focus and application of the healthy settings approach. While they have largely emerged independently of this movement, birth centres, and especially freestanding birth centres, reflect and illustrate the healthy settings approach, concerned as they are to provide a social model of maternity care focused on creating homely, family-focused environments that are truly salutogenic.

Birth centres offer the potential to impact positively on both service users and staff. Looking ahead, this potential is most likely to be realised with increased understanding of how physical environment and organisational culture interact to create positive or negative synergies. There are also wider lessons to be learned about the relationship between environment, culture and power relations with childbearing women, which could be brought back to and applied to obstetric services, in order to maximise the potential for optimum birth for childbearing women experiencing complex pregnancies, and for healthy women who would prefer hospital settings for their labour. These are important areas for future research.

The lessons learned about healthy maternity care settings can and must be spread to all maternity settings and not only birth centres. It is crucial that the benefits and advantages of salutogenic birth environments are implemented and offered to women who have complex pregnancies in order to maximise their opportunities for optimal birth, including maximising physiological functions and positive birth experiences.

The concepts of friendliness, functionality and freedom can be incorporated in the design or improvement of all maternity units. As previously discussed, these concepts do not only refer to the design of the space, but also to a philosophy of care which reflects knowledge and understanding of the physiology of labour and birth, women's need for control over the environment and decision-making and the need for both staff and service users to be able to establish meaningful relationships.

Key points for consideration

- Design birth settings which facilitate nesting and a sense of privacy and safety.
- Ensure that birth settings balance and facilitate friendliness, functionality and freedom.
- Consider how physical and organisational aspects of birth settings impact staff wellbeing and performance.
- Combine design considerations that reduce negative impacts while also maximising positive and salutogenic potentials.
- Ensure that the bio-psycho-social model of care is reflected in both the design and the organisational/team culture.

References

1   Birthplace in England Collaborative Group, Brocklehurst, P., Hardy, P., Hollowell, J., Linsell, L., Macfarlane, A., McCourt, C., Marlow, N., Miller, A., Newburn, M., Petrou, S., Puddicombe, D., Redshaw, M., Rowe, R., Sandall, J., Silverton, L., Stewart, M. (2011) 'Perinatal and maternal outcomes by planned place of birth for healthy women with low risk pregnancies: The Birthplace in England national prospective cohort study', British Medical Journal, 2011; 343.

2   World Health Organization (WHO). Ottawa charter for health promotion. Geneva: World Health Organization; 1986.

3   Dooris M. Bridging the silos: towards healthy and sustainable settings for the 21st Century. Health & Place. 2013;20:39-50.

4   Antonovsky A. Unraveling the mystery of health. San Francisco: Jossey-Boss; 1987

5   Bronfenbrenner U. Ecological models of human development. In: Husen T, Postlethwaite T, editors.

International Encyclopedia of Education. 2nd ed. 1994;3:1643-1647. Oxford: Elsevier

6   Dooris, M. (2009) Holistic & sustainable health improvement: the contribution of the settings-based approach to health promotion. Perspectives in Public Health. 2009;129:29-36

7   Dooris, M., Cawood, J., Doherty, S. & Powell, S. Healthy Universities: Concept, Model and Framework for Applying the Healthy Settings Approach within Higher Education in England. Final Project Report, 2010, Preston: UCLan / London: RSPH. https://healthyuniversities.ac.uk/healthy-universities/model-and-framework-for-action/ Dooris, M., Poland, B., Kolbe, L., de Leeuw, E.,McCall,D.,Wharf-Higgins,J. Healthy settings: building evidence for the effectiveness of whole system health promotion—challenges and future directions. In: McQueen, D., Jones, C. (Eds.), Global Perspectives on Health Promotion Effectiveness, 2007, Springer Science and Business Media, New York.

8   Kickbusch I. Tribute to Aaron Antonovsky – 'what creates health'? Health Promot Int. 1996;11:5-6.

9   Dooris M. Healthy settings: challenges to generating evidence of effectiveness. Health Promot Int. 2006;21:55-65.

10   St Leger L. Health promoting settings: from Ottawa to Jakarta. Health Promot Int. 1997;12:99-101.

11   Dooris M. Settings for promoting health. In: Jones L, Douglas J. *Public health: building innovative practice*. London: Sage/Milton Keynes: Open University Press; 2012, p.346-376.

12   Pelikan J. Health Promoting Hospitals – Assessing developments in the network. Italian Journal of Public Health. 2007;4:261-270.

13   hphnet.org [Internet]. The International Network of Health Promoting Hospitals and Health Services. Copenhagen: Clinical Health Promotion Centre, University of Copenhagen [cited 2017 Mar 14]. Available from http://hphnet.org/.

14   McKee M. Settings 3 – Health promotion in the health care sector. In: International Union for Health Promotion and Education. The evidence of health promotion effectiveness. shaping public health in a new Europe. Part Two: Evidence book. Brussels – Luxembourg: ECSC-EC-EAEC; 2000, p.123-133.

15   Groene O, Garcia-Barbero M, editors. Health promotion in hospitals: evidence and quality management. Copenhagen: WHO Regional Office for Europe; 2005, p. 11, 17.

16   Prasad S. Changing hospital architecture. London: RIBA Publishing; 2008.

17   Fedrizzi R. Foreword in: Guenther R, Vittori G. Sustainable Healthcare Architecture. 2nd ed. Chichester: Wiley; 2008, pxiii.

18   wellcertified.com [Internet]. Well Building Standard. Washington DC: International Well Building Institute. Available from https://www.wellcertified.com/our-standard.

19   living-future.org/lbc/ [Internet] Living Building Challenge. Seattle: International Living Future Institute. Available from https://living-future.org/lbc/.

20   Ulrich R. View through a window may influence recovery from surgery. Science. 1984;224:420-421.

21   Commission for Architecture and the Built Environment (CABE) Designed with care: design and neighbourhood healthcare buildings. London: CABE; 2006.

22   Hancock T. Greening healthcare: looking back, looking forward. Healthcare Quarterly. 2005;8:40-41.

23   Johnson A, Paton K. Health promotion and health services: management for change. Oxford: Oxford University Press; 2007

24   Foureur, M., Davis, D., Fenwick, J., Leap, N., Iedema, R., Forbes, I. & Homer, C. (2010) 'The relationship between birth unit design and safe, satisfying birth: Developing a hypothetical model', *Midwifery*, vol. 26, no. 5, pp. 520-5.

25   Hammond, A., Foureur, M., Homer, C. & Davis, D. (2013) 'Space, place and the midwife: Exploring the relationship between the birth environment, neurobiology and midwifery practice', *Women and Birth*, vol. 26, pp. 277-81.

26   Jenkinson, B., Josey, N. and Kruske, S. (2013) BirthSpace: An evidence-based guide to birth environment design. Queensland: Centre for Mothers & Babies, The University of Queensland.

27   Hammond, A., Foureur, M. and Homer, C.S. (2014) The hardware and software implications of hospital birth room design: a midwifery perspective. *Midwifery*, *30*(7), pp.825-830.

28   Hammond, A.D., Homer, C.S. and Foureur, M., 2014. Messages from space: an exploration of the relationship between hospital birth environments and midwifery practice. *HERD: Health Environments Research & Design Journal*, *7*(4), pp.81-95.

29   McCourt, C., Rayment, J., Rance, S. and Sandall, J. (2016) Place of birth and concepts of wellbeing: an analysis from two ethnographic studies of midwifery units in England. Anthropology in Action, 23(3), pp.17-29.

30   Rocca-Ihenacho, L (2017) *An ethnographic study of the philosophy, culture and practice in an urban freestanding midwifery unit.* PhD Thesis. City University of London

31   Hammond, A., Homer, C. and Foureur, M. (2017) Friendliness, functionality and freedom: design characteristics that support midwifery practice in the hospital setting. Midwifery, 50, pp.133-138.

32   Walsh, D. (2006a) 'Subverting assembly-line birth: Childbirth in a free-standing birth center', *Social Science & Medicine*,62, 1330-1340. doi:10.1016/j.socscimed.2005.08.013

33   Walsh, D. (2005) 'Nesting' and 'Matrescence' as distinctive features of a free-standing Birth   Centre   in   the

U.K.', *Midwifery,* 22, 228-239. Elseiver. doi:10.1016/j.midw.2005.09.005.25.

34   Rowe, R. and Birthplace in England Collaborative Group (2011) *Birthplace terms and definitions: consensus process. Birthplace in England research programme.* Final report part 2: NIHR Service Delivery and Organisation programme. Available at: https://www.npeu.ox.ac.uk/birthplace (Accessed: 28 October 2014).

35   Walsh, D., (2006b) 'Birth centres, community and social capital', *MIDIRS Midwifery Digest,* 16:1, pp.7-15.

36   Leap, N. and Hunter, B. (2016) *Supporting Women for Labour and Birth: A Thoughtful Guide.* Oxon: Routledge.

37   Leap,N ., Anderson, T. (2008) The role of pain in normal birth and the empowerment of women', in Downe, S. ed. (2008) *Normal Childbirth: evidence and debate* (second edition). London: Churchill Livingstone

38   Downe, S., McCourt, C. (2004). From Being to Becoming: Reconstructing Childbirth Knowledges In: Downe, S. (2004) *Normal Childbirth Evidence and Debate.* London: Churchill Livingstone.

39   Parkinson MD 2018 The Healthy Health Care Workplace: A Competitive Advantage.Curr Cardiol Rep. 31;20(10):98. doi: 10.1007/s11886-018-1042-3.

40   Hunter, B., Fenwick, J., Sidebotham, M., Pallant, J. (2018) *Work, Health and Emotional Lives of   Midwives in the United Kingdom: The UK WHELM study.* Cardiff: Cardiff University.

PART V

Making change happen

CHAPTER 21

Implementation science in maternity care

James Harris, Michelle Newton, Kate Dawson and *Jane Sandall*

Introduction

Since its inception, 'evidence-based healthcare' has attempted to provide a scientific justification for the treatments and care provided within healthcare systems (Haynes, 2006). This approach has been guided by a traditional view of the hierarchy of evidence, culminating with meta-analyses and randomised controlled trials (Evans, 2003). However, despite the near-complete respect for evidence-based healthcare that is routinely expressed by healthcare agencies and practitioners, many practices and procedures followed in healthcare services lack, or are actively contrary to, the actual evidence base (Lau, Stevenson, Ong et al, 2014). At times this is because the evidence does not yet exist and researchers are yet to ask and/or answer questions about certain practices. However, even where the evidence does exist, practice often directly contravenes the relevant research findings.

Implementation science aims to address this evidence to practice gap through '*the scientific study of methods to promote the uptake of research findings into routine healthcare in clinical, organisational or policy contexts*' (Eccles, Foy, Sales, Wensing and Mittman, 2012). Implementation science studies differ from clinical research in many ways (Figure 1). It can take as long as 17 years for a piece of research evidence to directly impact patient care (Morris, Wooding and Grant, 2011). The evidence-translation gap is influenced by a multitude of interrelated factors, which can arise from individuals, organizations, and/or society. Implementation scientists aim to develop innovative approaches to identifying, understanding and overcoming barriers to the adoption, adaption, integration, scale-up and sustainability of evidence-based interventions, tools, policies and guidelines (Brownson, Colditz and Proctor, 2012). This chapter will provide a practical guide to some of these approaches, using the example of midwifery-led continuity of care (MLCC) as an illustration.

Figure 1.
Outlining the difference between empirical and implementation research

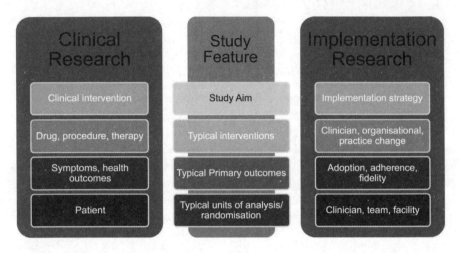

Evidence and change in maternity care

Innovations are common within maternity care, which has seen many technological, practice, and policy changes. However, the degree to which appropriate implementation – or 'de-implementation' (when evidence suggests stopping a certain practice) occurs has varied. At times, adoption of evidence-based guidelines has supported practitioners who view pregnancy and birth as a 'normal' event. For example, the routine practice of episiotomies was readily de-implemented within the UK following publication of supportive evidence (Thacker and Banta, 1983). However, other practices appear deeply entrenched despite a wealth of evidence against them. A prime example is admission cardiotocographic monitoring of the foetus where there is no medical or obstetric indication (Blix, 2013).

At times, support for effective practices has been withdrawn prematurely, such as the very large reduction in rates of vitamin K administration to neonates following the publication of evidence linking it to childhood cancers (Jean Golding, Greenwood, Birmingham and Mott, 1992; Jean Golding, Paterson and Kinlen, 1990). This occurred even though the initial findings were promptly refuted by other studies (Klebanoff, Read, Mills and Shiono, 1993; McKinney, Juszczak, Findlay and Smith, 1998). In other situations, changes have been adopted readily, apparently driven by a respect for technological advancements and client desire (e.g. ultrasound scans, Down's syndrome screening). It seems to be more difficult for maternity care organisations and providers around the world to implement changes that support a low-technology, normality agenda. For example, despite the convincing evidence published in studies demonstrating the safety of non-obstetric unit births (De Jonge, Van Der Goes, Ravelli et al, 2009; Birthplace in England Collaborative et al, 2011; Tracy, Hartz, Tracy et al, 2013), home birth and out-of-hospital midwife unit rates remain lower than alternatives (McLaren, 2013). In terms of clinical practice, for example, while both scientific evidence and public policy now support optimal cord clamping, its uptake around the world remains unclear (McAdams, 2014).

Implementation science as a solution

Implementation science aims to explore these issues, and to achieve sustainable change in practice. This can work on a micro level – changing the behaviours of individual women or healthcare professionals; a meso level – addressing localised structural and organisational barriers to facilitate and encourage organisational change; or a macro level – addressing the governmental, policy and financial concerns that may act as barriers to the effective implementation of innovations. Implementation science also brings a multidisciplinary approach, with healthcare professionals, service users, social scientists, managers, policy-makers and bench scientists working in partnership to bring about change. Implementation scientists uses theories, frameworks and models to gauge how best to bring about the desired change, and to attempt to explain consequent successes (and failures).

Implementation theories, models and frameworks – the tools of the trade

Implementation science is relatively new and many differing theories, frameworks and models have been proposed, each purporting to be the next 'best' way to encourage or measure change for a particular setting. Indeed, over 60 implementation frameworks have been identified (Birken et al, 2017). Within the scope of this chapter we will consider three of the main frameworks with a strong citation history that support their use. Table 1 identifies specific practical examples used within maternity, and directs readers on where to find further help.

Changing the individual – micro level behavioural change

Changing the behaviour of consumers or clinicians is often the desire of implementation scientists. For these micro level changes, the health psychology theory of COM-B (Michie, van Stralen and West, 2011), provides a useful starting point. COM-B (capability, opportunity, motivation and behaviour) is an overarching theory that incorporates a series of popular tools and frameworks for behaviour change work. The theory recognises that a combination of motivation (the brain processes that energise and direct behaviour), capability (an individual's capacity to engage in the activity concerned) and opportunity (the factors outside the individual that make a behaviour possible) encourage a behaviour. The theory suggests that both opportunity and capability can influence motivation, that the three components generate behaviour, while behaviours themselves can influence the three factors (Figure 2).

Figure 2.
The COM-B system for understanding behaviour

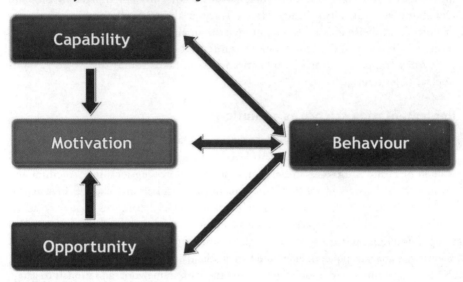

To encourage a certain behaviour intervention designers need to consider firstly what the behavioural target would be, and then what components of the behavioural system would need to be changed to achieve that. Once identified, the 'behaviour change wheel' (Figure 3) can be used to identify which intervention functions and policy categories are pertinent to change the behaviour.

Figure 3.
The Behaviour Change Wheel

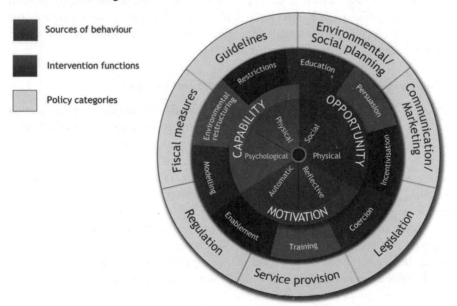

An additional tool, the Theoretical Domains Framework (Cane, O'Connor and Michie, 2012), highlights 14 clearly defined domains, each with constructs that outline the various barriers and facilitators to changing behaviours. An individual can discover the pertinent TDF domains for their behavioural target (e.g. increasing physical activity, delaying clamping of the umbilical cord) through qualitative or quantitative methods. The TDF domains are mapped onto the behaviour change wheel, which in turn identifies which intervention and policy functions can influence those constructs. The proposed intervention can then be piloted and assessed for efficacy. The URL links for this framework, and for others discussed in this chapter, are given in Table 1.

Changing the system – meso level organisational change

While COM-B can explain the actions of individuals, this is often not sufficient when dealing with the complexities of whole systems, such as maternity care. Outside of individual behaviour, social interactions and organisational dynamics may also impact on implementation and acceptance (Reeves, Albert, Kuper and Hodges, 2008) and may assist in anticipating the mechanisms that will influence the process of change in specific circumstances (Craig et al, 2008). Care models or techniques that appear valuable in principle or in carefully controlled randomised trials often don't work as well when they are rolled out to other settings. Effective implementation relies on the social organisation of any interventions, of embedding these interventions into routine elements of everyday life in specific situations, and sustaining the intervention within social contexts (May and Finch, 2009). Normalisation Process Theory (NPT) aims to consider these points (May et al, 2009). It was developed from a desire not just to evaluate the success or failure of why interventions work, but rather what the mechanisms of an effect are. It aims to identify how interventions become normalised within healthcare settings, and why some are more effective than others. It considers the joint concerns of the process issues of implementation, with the structural issues of integrating that new way of working into existing settings. It recognises the need to effectively plan and evaluate the implementation of policy and innovations into practice (Figure 4).

The NPT outlines four core constructs – coherence (making sense of the intervention), cognitive participation (building a community of practice), collective action (operational issues) and reflexive monitoring (appraising the work). NPT is designed to be used in many ways, including the design of an initial intervention, planning and reflecting during an implementation cycle, and in terms of both academic and clinical practice perspectives. The team behind the NPT have developed a toolkit to support its use. This toolkit asks 16 questions that facilitate thinking through the implementation problem. Following completion teams can view a report that includes graphical representation on the strengths of the proposed plan in relation to the core constructs of the theory.

Table 1.
Summary of theories, their uses and practical examples

Theory (and source reference)	Explanation	Maternity examples	Further advice
COM-B (Michie et al., 2011)	Individual behaviour is influenced – and influences – that individuals' capacity, opportunity and motivation to perform that behaviour	• Used to develop a smartphone app for pregnant smokers (Tombor et al., 2016). • Used to consider how midwives can promote healthy behaviours to women during pregnancy (Olander, Darwin, Atkinson, Smith, & Gardner, 2016)	http://www.behaviourchangewheel.com
Normalisation process theory (May et al., 2009)	Successful implementation relies on social organisation, of them becoming embedded into routine, and part of the social context.	• Exploration of healthcare professionals' attitudes to providing a HPV vaccine to postnatal women (Gross et al., 2016). • Development of screening tool for intimate partner violence (Taft et al., 2015; Taft et al., 2012).	http://www.normalizationprocess.org
Consolidated framework for Implementation Research (Damschroder et al., 2009)	Implementation is reliant on a combination of factors related to the intervention itself, the inner and outer settings of the intervention, the individuals that require change, and the process of implementation.	• Used to design and evaluate a five-step intervention to prevent mother-to-child HIV transmission across Africa (Sherr et al., 2014). • Used to strengthen the Midwifery professional role in Morocco (Abou-Malham, Hatem, & Leduc, 2015).	http://cfirguide.org

Figure 4.
The Normalisation Process theory

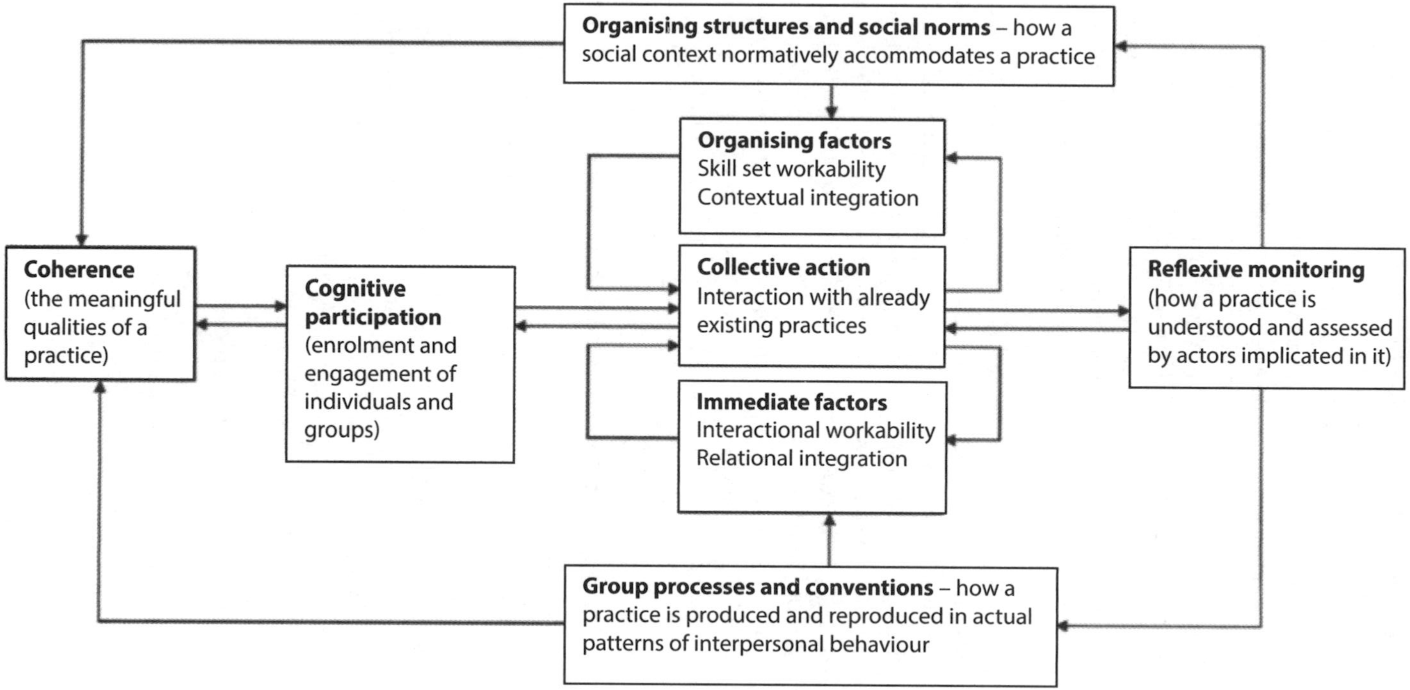

Changing policy – macro level policy change

Above we have outlined two approaches, one from psychology (COM-B) and one from sociology (NPT). While both the behaviour of an individual maternity care provider, and the social organisation of the workplace are important, so are the larger external factors such as governmental and economic will (Ashton, 2015). An integrative approach, which also accounts for policy-level changes is sometimes required when considering large, complex, multifaceted interventions. One such framework is the consolidated framework for implementation research (CFIR) (Damschroder et al, 2009). The CFIR consists of five domains – the intervention (the characteristics of the change being implemented), the inner setting (the local setting of the change), the outer setting (the economic, political and social contexts), the individuals involved (including their professional mindsets, norms and affiliations) and the implementation process (the various steps taken to encourage uptake of the intervention). The authors recognise the interaction between the different domains.

The framework encourages those wanting to implement change to consider issues such as the adaptability of the intervention, external policies and incentives, internal cultures, and individual knowledge and beliefs about the intervention, and argues that each factor is important to bring about sustainable and scalable implementation. An extensive toolkit is available to help researchers use the CFIR, for those either designing new interventions or evaluating those already in place. A strength of this framework is the recognition of both qualitative and quantitative methods, with the CFIR team providing advice for either approach on their website.

Implementation science in maternity care: the example of midwife-led continuity of care (MLCC)

The evidence base supporting the need for implementation – the case for continuity

Women's access to MLCC in developed countries is varied, despite high-level evidence that continuity of care by a primary midwife is associated with reduced childbirth intervention, improved neonatal outcomes, reduced costs to organisations and the healthcare system (McLachlan et al, 2012; Sandall, Soltani, Gates, Shennan and Devane, 2016; Tracy et al, 2013), increased maternal satisfaction (Forster et al, 2016; Sandall et al, 2016) and evidence of positive outcomes for midwives working in these models (Collins, Fereday, Pincombe, Oster and Turnbull, 2010; Jepsen, Juul, Foureur, Sørensen and Nøhr, 2017; Newton, McLachlan, Willis and Forster, 2014). Implementation of this model of care varies widely: some countries have limited uptake and acceptance, while in other countries MLCC is well established and long standing. In the presence of compelling evidence of the benefits of midwife-led continuity, why is there such diversity of availability of this model in high-income countries? Does implementation science have potential in exploring this question? Reflecting on the micro, meso and macro levels, the remainder of this chapter will illustrate the potential of using implementation science to explain how and why quality evidence is, or is not, successfully transferred into practice using the example of implementation of MLCC.

Caseload and midwives – the micro level in MLCC

Successful implementation of midwife-led continuity models (MLCC) requires midwives being willing to work in them (ten Hoope-Bender, 2013). Since working in MLCCs requires a move from shift work to more flexible rostering, midwives may require support structures and strategies to avoid burnout by helping them to achieve a work-life balance (Newton, McLachlan, Forster and Willis, 2016; Newton et al, 2014). Numerous studies have explored the experiences of midwives working in MLCC models (Damschroder et al, 2009; Dawson, McLachlan, Newton and Forster, 2016; Newton et al, 2016; Sandall, Davies and Warwick, 2001) and others have reported the willingness of students to work in this way upon graduation (Dawson, Newton, Forster and McLachlan, 2015; Gray, Taylor and Newton, 2016; McLachlan, Newton, Nightingale, Morrow and Kruger, 2013). However, reluctance to assume MLCC work has also been reported (Collins et al, 2010; Fereday and Oster, 2008; Newton et al, 2014), as has difficulty in recruiting to the model (Dawson, Newton, Forster and McLachlan, 2013; C.S. Homer, 2016) and it has been suggested that a lack of understanding of how the model operates and the actual (rather than perceived) impact on midwives' personal and professional time could be influential in how midwives view MLCC work (Newton et al, 2016). Beyond the midwife response, there is very little work on how other key stakeholders, such as obstetricians and paediatricians, react to and influence the success or otherwise of midwife-led models of care.

There is therefore an opportunity to further advance understanding of the role of the individual in the successful uptake and upscale of MLCCs. Consideration of the behavioural changes required in this work for all stakeholders (as described in COM-B or similar theories) may provide valuable insight into factors such as the capability, opportunity and motivation of midwives choosing (or being allocated to) MLCC work, and of other maternity providers' response to this change. Applying such models may also catalyse behavioural changes as individuals adapt to a different way of working. This approach to research about MLCCs may help organisations to be better informed about the nature of MLCC work by clearly articulating the behavioural adaptations that are required, thus fostering a more sustainable workforce.

Organisational change – the meso level in MLCC

Within an organisation, the introduction of a new model of care is a complex intervention, (Forster, Newton, McLachlan and Willis, 2011; C. Homer, Brodie and Leap, 2008; Sandall, Hatem, Devane, Soltani and Gates, 2009; Tracy et al, 2013) and maternity care settings are themselves complex (Hawe, Shiell and Riley, 2009). Organisational readiness for change is contingent on local conditions

(Burau and Overgaard, 2015). The introduction of MLCC models may not only involve a change in the nature of the work of midwives (Newton et al, 2016), but also impacts on how midwives are managed, how the midwives working in this way interact with other health professionals, and how the workload is reorganised within the service. Organisations considering implementation of MLCC have identified issues such as the need for funding to establish the model, the interest and availability of staff to work in the model, organisational support and consumer demand (Dawson et al, 2016). Successful implementation and sustainability of MLCC requires both collaboration and consultation by midwives, managers and other key stakeholders within the organisation (Burau and Overgaard, 2015; C. Homer et al, 2008). Over 26 different organisational readiness tools have been identified (Khan et al, 2014). Their appropriateness is context specific, and a tool has been developed to help identify the most appropriate for each context (see Table 2 – additional resources for link).

Research into complex interventions should address how and why an intervention may function within a specific context and how to address structural and organisational barriers. Normalisation process theory (NPT), or other similar sociological implementation theories, can help to identify the organisational barriers to change. With detailed knowledge of the local context (which often requires multidisciplinary collaboration), the 16 questions within the NPT toolkit could identify what areas require addressing to facilitate successful implementation. Although NPT has been applied to studies to evaluate the outcome of implementation and acceptance of MLCC (Newton et al, 2016), assessing a particular organisation's readiness for change is key to achieving sustainable implementation. For further expansion and sustainability of MLCC models, using tools such as NPT in the planning and implementation stages of MLCC may assist in overcoming barriers that have been shown to impact on organisational outcomes.

Whole system change – the macro level in MLCC

How a country organises its maternity services is dependent on a number of factors, including division of labour, consumer group mobilisation and gendered dynamics alongside competing interests, professional boundary struggles, funding and insurance models and changing consumer interests (Benoit et al, 2005).

Internationally there are valuable examples of how macro-level change can be key to widespread implementation of MLCC. Access to midwife-led continuity models (i.e. caseload) may be reflected in public policy and legislation, as is the case of the Netherlands (Amelink-Verburg and Buitendijk, 2010) and New Zealand (NZ) (Benoit et al, 2005; Guilliland and Tracy, 2015). In these countries, MLCC is the predominant model (Benoit et al, 2005; Perdok et al, 2016; Wiegers, Warmelink, Spelten, Klomp and Hutton, 2014), available for all low-risk women in the Netherlands (de Jonge and Sandall, 2016), while more than 85% of women access MLCC in NZ (Ministry of

Table 2.
Additional resources

Name and reference	Location	Information
What are the effects of interventions to improve the uptake of evidence from health research into policy in low and middle-income countries? (Clar, Campbell, Lisa, & Wendy, 2011)	https://assets.publishing.service.gov.uk/media/57a08ab3ed915d3cfd0008c2/SR_EvidenceIntoPolicy_Graham_May2011_MinorEditsJuly2011.pdf	Systematic review exploring the uptake of interventions within low and middle income countries.
Developing and evaluating complex interventions: the new Medical Research Council guidance. (Craig et al., 2008)	http://www.mrc.ac.uk/documents/pdf/complex-interventions-guidance/	Detailed guidance from the MRC on the development-evaluation-implementation process when developing interventions with several interacting components
Evaluating improvement and Implementation for health (Ovretveit, 2014)	Book – Open University Press – ISBN 0335242774	Excellent text book on implementation evaluation approaches, challenging some of the assumptions of the evidence based healthcare movement
Implementation research in health: a practical guide (Peters, Tran, & Adam, 2013)	http://who.int/alliance-hpsr/alliance hpsr_irpguide.pdf	Freely available step-by-step guide to implementation work authored by the World Health Organization
Writing implementation research grant proposals: ten key ingredients (Proctor, Powell, Baumann, Hamilton, & Santens, 2012)	http://implementationscience.biomedcentral.com/articles/10.1186/1748-5908-7-96	Guide for applying for funding for implementation work
Complex interventions in Health: An overview of research methods	Book – Routledge – ISBN 0415703166	Textbook that focuses on the development, implementation and evaluation of complex interventions
Rameses jiscmail list	https://www.jiscmail.ac.uk/cgi-bin/webadmin?A0=RAMESES	JISCMAIL list is for researchers interested in learning about realist and meta-narrative reviews
The EPOC Taxonomy (Effective Practice and Organisation of Care (EPOC, 2015)	http://epoc.cochrane.org/epoc-taxonomy	Repositories of evidence- based implementation strategies
Ready, set change! (Timmings et al., 2016)	http://readiness.knowledgetranslation.ca	Resource that helps researchers select from the many different types of organisational readiness for change tools available

Health, 2015). The New Zealand example illustrates the complexity of macro-level changes that have resulted in the widespread availability of this model, which included amendment to the Nurses Act, a strong consumer movement, a sympathetic Prime Minister, a campaigning professional midwifery organisation and funding reform that culminated in legislative changes (Guilliland and Tracy, 2015) to allow women to select their own lead maternity carer (LMC).

However, in closely related countries with similar economic profiles, there is fragmented implementation of MLCC. In Denmark 61% of public maternity units have implemented caseloading practice for the minority of childbearing women, with reports of up to 24% of childbearing women accessing caseload midwifery in north and central Denmark (Jepsen et al, 2017). In Australia 31% of public maternity care services offer midwifery-led continuity models with an estimated 8% of women able to access the model (Dawson et al, 2016).

Explaining this difference is challenging. The context of funding for maternity care, community demand for specific models, policy and legislation are all significant in the realisation of innovation. Policy alone does not result in change. In Australia there have been decades of governmental documents supporting increased access to MLCC for women, yet the numbers, although increasing, remain low (Dawson et al, 2016). Similarly, in the UK the National Maternity Review (NHS England, 2016) has recommended that every woman should have a midwife, who can provide continuity throughout the pregnancy, birth and postnatally. However, in the USA and Canada only a small percentage of births are attended by midwives (Kozhimannil, Attanasio, Yang, Avery and Declercq, 2015) and only a minority of women receive continuity of care from a midwife throughout the maternity episode in the UK.

An appraisal of the broader issues that can influence the introduction of an effective innovation in a specific setting may be best undertaken by using an approach such as the Consolidated Framework for Implementation Research (CFIR) (Dramschroder, Aron, Keith et al, 2009). Instead of focusing on these factors as an 'outcome' of the research, a first step in implementation trials can be to fully explore and describe the policy, economic, consumer, professional and healthcare context in which the maternity services are positioned.

Conclusions

It can be argued that when considering change in practice that no one level alone (micro, meso or macro) can explain why innovations have or have not been successfully introduced and sustained. Each are inter-related, and successful implementation of an innovation is unlikely without consideration of how each of these impacts on the proposed change. Implementation science could be the next 'wave' of research that is needed, not only in the case of MLCC, but also anywhere the gap between the evidence and its translation into practice is evident.

While the 2016 Cochrane systematic review of midwife-led continuity models recommends further research into how the model influences specific neonatal morbidity and mortality outcomes, the overwhelming evidence of benefit for MLCC is strong (Sandall et al, 2016; WHO, 2016). What is lacking is a clear understanding of why there is a disparate uptake and scale-up of these models. Well-designed implementation studies that consider each of these factors in describing the implementation and then reporting on the success (or not) of implementation strategies, instead of just the impact of the intervention on the target population (Pinnock et al, 2017) could be the much-needed next body of work in maternity care research to support growth in MLCC.

Key points for consideration

- Despite the evidence-based practice agenda, effective maternity care practices are still not implemented, and non-effective practices are commonplace.
- Implementation science aims to address this evidence to practice gap.
- This requires action at the micro (practitioner, individual) meso (organisational) and macro (policy) level.
- There are a range of models that can help with this process.
- Midwife-led continuity of care offers an example both of lack of implementation in some situations, and of effective change in others.
- Those planning to implement effective practice/models of care, or to deimplement those that are ineffective, need to consider all three levels of the organisation/communities they want to influence, and the inter-relationships between them.

References

Abou-Malham, S., Hatem, M., & Leduc, N. (2015). Analyzing barriers and facilitators to the implementation of an action plan to strengthen the midwifery professional role: a Moroccan case study. *BMC health services research, 15*(1), 382.

Amelink-Verburg, M. P., & Buitendijk, S. E. (2010). Pregnancy and Labour in the Dutch Maternity Care System: What Is Normal? The Role Division Between Midwives and Obstetricians. *The Journal of Midwifery & Women's Health, 55*(3), 216-225. doi:10.1016/j.jmwh.2010.01.001

Ashton, T. (2015). Implementing integrated models of care: the importance of the macro-level context. *Int J Integr Care, 15*, e019.

Benoit, C., Wrede, S., Bourgeault, I., Sandall, J., Vries, R. D., & Teijlingen, E. R. v. (2005). Understanding the social organisation of maternity care systems: midwifery as a touchstone. *Sociology of Health & Illness, 27*(6), 722-737. doi:10.1111/j.1467-9566.2005.00471.x

Birken, S. A., Powell, B. J., Presseau, J., Kirk, M. A., Lorencatto, F., Gould, N. J., . . . Yu, Y. (2017). Combined use of the Consolidated Framework for Implementation Research (CFIR) and the Theoretical Domains Framework (TDF): a systematic review. *Implementation Science, 12*(1), 2.

Birthplace in England Collaborative, G., Brocklehurst, P., Hardy, P., Hollowell, J., Linsell, L., Macfarlane, A., . . . Stewart, M. (2011). Perinatal and maternal outcomes by planned place of birth for healthy women with low risk pregnancies: the Birthplace in England national prospective cohort study. *BMJ, 343*, d7400. doi:10.1136/bmj.d7400

Blix, E. (2013). The admission CTG: is there any evidence for still using the test? *Acta obstetricia et gynecologica Scandinavica, 92*(6), 613-619.

Brownson, R. C., Colditz, G. A., & Proctor, E. K. (2012). *Dissemination and implementation research in health: translating science to practice*: Oxford University Press.

Burau, V., & Overgaard, C. (2015). Caseload midwifery as organisational change: the interplay between professional and organisational projects in Denmark. *BMC Pregnancy & Childbirth, 15*(1), 1.

Cane, J., O'Connor, D., & Michie, S. (2012). Validation of the theoretical domains framework for use in behaviour change and implementation research. *Implement Sci, 7*, 37. doi:10.1186/1748-5908-7-37

Clar, C., Campbell, S., Lisa, D., & Wendy, G. (2011). What are the effects of interventions to improve the uptake of evidence from health research into policy in low and middle-income countries. *Systematic review)(pp. 107pp)*: University of Aberdeen (UoA).

Collins, C. T., Fereday, J., Pincombe, J., Oster, C., & Turnbull, D. (2010). An evaluation of the satisfaction of midwives' working in midwifery group practice. *Midwifery, 26*(4), 435-441. doi:10.1016/j.midw.2008.09.004

Craig, P., Dieppe, P., Macintyre, S., Michie, S., Nazareth, I., & Petticrew, M. (2008). Developing and evaluating complex interventions: the new Medical Research Council guidance. *BMJ, 337*, a1655.

Damschroder, L. J., Aron, D. C., Keith, R. E., Kirsh, S. R., Alexander, J. A., & Lowery, J. C. (2009). Fostering implementation of health services research findings into practice: a consolidated framework for advancing implementation science. *Implement Sci, 4*, 50. Damschroder, L.J., Aron, D.C., Keith, R.E., Kirsh, S.R., Alexander, J.A. and Lowery, J.C., 2009. Fostering implementation of health services research findings into practice: a consolidated framework for advancing implementation science. *Implementation science, 4*(1), p.50.

Dawson, K., McLachlan, H., Newton, M., & Forster, D. (2016). Implementing caseload midwifery: Exploring the views of maternity managers in Australia – A national cross-sectional survey. *Women and Birth, 29*(3), 214-222. doi:http://dx.doi.org/10.1016/j.wombi.2015.10.010

Dawson, K., Newton, M., Forster, D., & McLachlan, H. (2013). Exploring the introduction, expansion and sustainability of caseload midwifery in Australia. *Women and Birth 26(Supplement 1):S4.*

Dawson, K., Newton, M., Forster, D., & McLachlan, H. (2015). Exploring midwifery students' views and experiences of caseload midwifery: A cross-sectional survey conducted in Victoria, Australia. *Midwifery, 31*(2), e7-e15.

De Jonge A, van der Goes BY, Ravelli AC, Amelink-Verburg MP, Mol BW, Nijhuis JG, et al. Perinatal mortality and morbidity in a nationwide cohort of 529,688 low-risk planned home and hospital births. BJOG2009;116:1177-84

de Jonge, A., & Sandall, J. (2016). Improving Research into Models of Maternity Care to Inform Decision Making. *PLoS Med, 13*(9), e1002135.

Eccles, M. P., Foy, R., Sales, A., Wensing, M., & Mittman, B. (2012). Implementation Science six years on--our evolving scope and common reasons for rejection without review. *Implement Sci, 7*, 71. doi:10.1186/1748-5908-7-71

Effective Practice and Organisation of Care (EPOC). (2015). EPOC Taxonomy. Retrieved from Available at: https://epoc.cochrane.org/epoc-taxonomy

Evans, D. (2003). Hierarchy of evidence: a framework for ranking evidence evaluating healthcare interventions. *J Clin Nurs, 12*(1), 77-84.

Fereday, J., & Oster, C. (2008). Managing a work-life balance: the experiences of midwives working in a group practice setting. *Midwifery, 26*(3), 311 - 318.

Forster, D., McLachlan, H., Davey, M.-A., Biro, M. A., Farrell, T., Gold, L., . . . Waldenström, U. (2016). Continuity of care by a primary midwife (caseload midwifery) increases women's satisfaction with antenatal, intrapartum and postpartum care: results from the COSMOS randomised controlled trial. *BMC pregnancy and childbirth, 16*(1), 1.

Forster, D., Newton, M., McLachlan, H., & Willis, K. (2011). Exploring implementation and sustainability of models of care: Can theory help? *Women & Birth, 24*, S14-S14. doi:10.1016/j.wombi.2011.07.059

Golding, J., Greenwood, R., Birmingham, K., & Mott, M. (1992). Childhood cancer, intramuscular vitamin K, and pethidine given during labour. *BMJ, 305*(6849), 341-346.

Golding, J., Paterson, M., & Kinlen, L. (1990). Factors associated with childhood cancer in a national cohort study. *British Journal of Cancer, 62*(2), 304.

Gray, J., Taylor, J., & Newton, M. (2016). Embedding continuity of care experiences: An innovation in midwifery education. *Midwifery, 33*, 40-42.

Gross, T. T., Rahman, M., A, M. W., J, M. H., Sarpong, K. O., Rupp, R. E., . . . Berenson, A. B. (2016). Implementation of a Postpartum HPV Vaccination Program in a Southeast Texas Hospital: A Qualitative Study Evaluating Health Care Provider Acceptance. *Matern Child Health J, 20*(Suppl 1), 154-163. doi:10.1007/s10995-016-2030-0

Guilliland, K., & Tracy, S. (2015). Australian and New Zealand midwifery and maternity services. In S. Pairman, J. Pincombe, C. Thorogood, & S. Tracy (Eds.), *Midwifery Preparation for Practice* (Third ed.). Sydney: Elsevier.

Hawe, P., Shiell, A., & Riley, T. (2009). Theorising interventions as events in systems. *American journal of community psychology, 43*(3-4), 267-276.

Haynes, R. B. (2006). Of studies, syntheses, synopses, summaries, and systems: the "5S" evolution of information services for evidence-based healthcare decisions. *Evid Based Med, 11*(6), 162-164. doi:10.1136/ebm.11.6.162-a

Homer, C., Brodie, P., & Leap, N. (2008). *Midwifery Continuity of Care: A practical guide.* Sydney: Elsevier Australia.

Homer, C. S. (2016). Models of maternity care: evidence for midwifery continuity of care. *The Medical journal of Australia, 205*(8), 370.

Jepsen, I., Juul, S., Foureur, M., Sørensen, E. E., & Nøhr, E. A. (2017). Is caseload midwifery a healthy work-form? – A survey of burnout among midwives in Denmark. *Sexual & Reproductive Healthcare, 11*, 102-106. doi:http://dx.doi.org/10.1016/j.srhc.2016.12.001

Khan, S., Timmings, C., Moore, J. E., Marquez, C., Pyka, K., Gheihman, G., & Straus, S. E. (2014). The development of an online decision support tool for organizational readiness for change. *Implementation Science, 9*(1), 56.

Klebanoff, M. A., Read, J. S., Mills, J. L., & Shiono, P. H. (1993). The risk of childhood cancer after neonatal exposure to vitamin K. *N Engl J Med, 329*(13), 905-908. doi:10.1056/NEJM199309233291301

Kozhimannil, K. B., Attanasio, L. B., Yang, Y. T., Avery, M. D., & Declercq, E. (2015). Midwifery Care and Patient–Provider Communication in Maternity Decisions in the United States. *Maternal and Child Health Journal, 19*(7), 1608-1615. doi:10.1007/s10995-015-1671-8

Lau, R., Stevenson, F., Ong, B.N., Dziedzic, K., Eldridge, S., Everitt, H., Kennedy, A., Kontopantelis, E., Little, P., Qureshi,

N. and Rogers, A., 2014. Addressing the evidence to practice gap for complex interventions in primary care: a systematic review of reviews protocol. *BMJ open, 4*(6), p.e005548.May, C., & Finch, T. (2009). Implementing, embedding, and integrating practices: an outline of normalization process theory. *Sociology, 43*(3), 535-554.

May, C., Mair, F., Finch, T., MacFarlane, A., Dowrick, C., Treweek, S., . . . Rogers, A. (2009). Development of a theory of implementation and integration: Normalization Process Theory. *Implementation Science, 4*(1), 29.

McAdams, R. M. (2014). Time to implement delayed cord clamping. *Obstet Gynecol, 123*(3), 549-552. doi:10.1097/AOG.0000000000000122

McKinney, P. A., Juszczak, E., Findlay, E., & Smith, K. (1998). Case-control study of childhood leukaemia and cancer in Scotland: findings for neonatal intramuscular vitamin K. *BMJ, 316*(7126), 173-177.

McLachlan, H., Forster, D., Davey, M. A., Farrell, T., Gold, L., Biro, M. A., . . . Waldenstrom, U. (2012). Effects of continuity of care by a primary midwife (caseload midwifery) on caesarean section rates in women of low obstetric risk: the COSMOS randomised controlled trial. *BJOG: An International Journal of Obstetrics & Gynaecology, 119*(12), 1483-1492.

McLachlan, H., Newton, M., Nightingale, H., Morrow, J., & Kruger, G. (2013). Exploring the 'follow-through experience': A statewide survey of midwifery students and academics conducted in Victoria, Australia. *Midwifery, 29*, 1064-1072.

McLaren, E. (2013). Births in England and Wales by Characteristics of Birth 2, 2011.

Michie S, Atkins L, West R. (2014) The Behaviour Change Wheel: A Guide to Designing Interventions. London: Silverback Publishing. www.behaviourchangewheel.com

Michie, S., van Stralen, M. M., & West, R. (2011). The behaviour change wheel: a new method for characterising and designing behaviour change interventions. *Implement Sci, 6*, 42. doi:10.1186/1748-5908-6-42

Minstry of Health. (2015). *Report on Maternity 2014*. Wellington, New Zealand.

Morris, Z. S., Wooding, S., & Grant, J. (2011). The answer is 17 years, what is the question: understanding time lags in translational research. *Journal of the Royal Society of Medicine, 104*(12), 510-520.

Newton, M., McLachlan, H., Forster, D., & Willis, K. (2016). Understanding the 'work' of caseload midwives: A mixed-methods exploration of two caseload midwifery models in Victoria, Australia. *Women and Birth, 29*(3), 223-233. doi:http://dx.doi.org/10.1016/j.wombi.2015.10.011

Newton, M., McLachlan, H., Willis, K., & Forster, D. (2014). Comparing satisfaction and burnout between caseload and standard care midwives: findings from two cross-sectional surveys conducted in Victoria, Australia. *BMC Pregnancy and Childbirth, 14*(426).

NHS England. (2016). National Maternity Review. Better Births; Improving Outcomes of Maternity Services in England. *NHS England, London*.

Olander, E. K., Darwin, Z. J., Atkinson, L., Smith, D. M., & Gardner, B. (2016). Beyond the 'teachable moment'–A conceptual analysis of women's perinatal behaviour change. *Women and Birth, 29*(3), e67-e71.

Ovretveit, J. (2014). *Evaluating improvement and implementation for health*: McGraw-Hill Education (UK).

Perdok, H., Jans, S., Verhoeven, C., Henneman, L., Wiegers, T., Mol, B. W., . . . de Jonge, A. (2016). Opinions of maternity care professionals and other stakeholders about integration of maternity care: a qualitative study in the Netherlands. *BMC Pregnancy and Childbirth, 16*(1), 188. doi:10.1186/s12884-016-0975-z

Peters, D. H., Tran, N. T., & Adam, T. (2013). *Implementation research in health: a practical guide*: World Health Organization.

Pinnock, H., Barwick, M., Carpenter, C. R., Eldridge, S., Grandes, G., Griffiths, C. J., . . . Patel, A. (2017). Standards for Reporting Implementation Studies (StaRI) Statement. *BMJ, 356*, i6795.

Proctor, E. K., Powell, B. J., Baumann, A. A., Hamilton, A. M., & Santens, R. L. (2012). Writing implementation research grant proposals: ten key ingredients. *Implementation Science, 7*(1), 96.

Reeves, S., Albert, M., Kuper, A., & Hodges, B. D. (2008). Why use theories in qualitative research. *BMJ, 337*(7670), 631-634.

Sandall, J., Davies, J., & Warwick, C. (2001). *Evaluation of the Albany Midwifery Practice*. Retrieved from London:

Sandall, J., Hatem, M., Devane, D., Soltani, H., & Gates, S. (2009). Discussions of findings from a Cochrane review of midwife-led versus other models of care for childbearing women: continuity, normality and safety. *Midwifery, 25*, 8-13.

Sandall, J., Soltani, H., Gates, S., Shennan, A., & Devane, D. (2016). Midwife-led continuity models versus other models of care for childbearing women. *Cochrane Database of Systematic Reviews*(4). doi:10.1002/14651858.CD004667.pub5

Sherr, K., Gimbel, S., Rustagi, A., Nduati, R., Cuembelo, F., Farquhar, C., . . . Gloyd, S. (2014). Systems analysis and improvement to optimize pMTCT (SAIA): a cluster randomized trial. *Implementation Science, 9*(1), 55.

Taft, A. J., Hooker, L., Humphreys, C., Hegarty, K., Walter, R., Adams, C., . . . Small, R. (2015). Maternal and child health nurse screening and care for mothers experiencing domestic violence (MOVE): a cluster randomised trial. *BMC medicine, 13*(1), 150.

Taft, A. J., Small, R., Humphreys, C., Hegarty, K., Walter, R., Adams, C., & Agius, P. (2012). Enhanced maternal and child health nurse care for women experiencing intimate partner/family violence: protocol for MOVE, a cluster randomised trial of screening and referral in primary health care. *BMC public health, 12*(1), 811.

ten Hoope-Bender, P. (2013). Continuity of maternity carer for all women. *The Lancet, 382*(Nov), 1685-1687.

Tracy S, Hartz D, Tracy M, Allen J, Forti A, Hall B, et al. Caseload midwifery care versus standard maternity care for women of any risk: M@NGO, a randomised controlled trial. Lancet 2013;382(November):1723–32.

Thacker, S. B., & Banta, H. D. (1983). Benefits and risks of episiotomy: an interpretative review of the English language literature, 1860-1980. *Obstetrical & gynecological survey, 38*(6), 322-338.

Timmings, C., Khan, S., Moore, J. E., Marquez, C., Pyka, K., & Straus, S. E. (2016). Ready, Set, Change! Development and usability testing of an online readiness for change decision support tool for healthcare organizations. *BMC medical informatics and decision making, 16*(1), 24.

Tombor, I., Shahab, L., Brown, J., Crane, D., Michie, S., & West, R. (2016). Development of SmokeFree Baby: a smoking cessation smartphone app for pregnant smokers. *Translational Behavioral Medicine, 6*(4), 533-545.

Tracy, S., Hartz, D., Tracy, M., Allen, J., Forti, A., Hall, B., . . . Kildea, S. (2013). Caseload midwifery care versus standard maternity care for women of any risk: M@NGO, a randomised controlled trial. *The Lancet, 382*(November 23), 1723-1732.

Wiegers, T. A., Warmelink, J. C., Spelten, E. R., Klomp, T., & Hutton, E. K. (2014). Work and workload of Dutch primary care midwives in 2010. *Midwifery, 30*(9), 991-997.

WHO Reproductive Health Library. WHO recommendation on midwife-led continuity of care during pregnancy. (November 2016). The WHO Reproductive Health Library; Geneva: World Health Organization.

Illustrations

Figure 2: Reproduced from Michie S, Atkins L, West R. (2014) The Behaviour Change Wheel: A Guide to Designing Interventions. London: Silverback Publishing. www.behaviourchangewheel.com with permission

Figure 3: Reproduced from Michie, S., Atkins, L., West, R. (2014) *The Behaviour Change Wheel: A Guide to Designing Interventions*. London: Silverback Publishing. www.behaviourchangewheel.com with permission

CHAPTER 22

Optimising physiological birth for women and babies with complex needs

Shawn Walker

Introduction

Childbirth is not always straightforward, but it is always an event of great significance in the lives of a woman and her family, and it influences the future for all of them. When there are medical and/or obstetric considerations, it is important to maintain awareness of the birthing woman as an individual undergoing a transformative experience. Retaining as much normality as possible can help prevent the challenges becoming the overwhelming focal point for either the woman or her caregivers. This chapter explores *complex normality*: ways of optimising physiological birth processes for women with complex needs, so that childbirth remains as normal as possible, as the birthing woman defines it. It begins with my personal experience of advocating for women seeking support for a vaginal breech birth. Following this, I will discuss some guiding principles and further examples of how others are providing women-centred care despite the challenges of greater complexity. This chapter shows how obstetric care, in particular, can be flexible and empowering, rather than rigid and reducing.

My background

My interest in complex normality originated in my work with women experiencing a breech pregnancy. Beginning in 2010, while working as an independent midwife, I became aware that a significant number of women were feeling their care in the UK National Health Service did not meet their needs, particularly when they were seeking a vaginal breech birth. As a consequence, I and my managers pioneered an integrated care pathway and a new role, the Breech Specialist Midwife (Plested and Walker, 2014). This project was complex and demanding. At the time, the available training was largely based on experience rather than evidence. Locally, all professional and managerial groups agreed that developing experience to support vaginal breech birth was a good idea, but there was no blueprint for how to do this safely. Recognition of this need and a deep desire to balance safety with true choice and autonomy for women led me to my research path (Walker et al, 2018a, 2018b).

Nine years and a PhD later, the result has been an evidence-based training programme (Walker et al, 2017b) and a community interest company that delivers training internationally. Centres across Europe and further afield have developed successful breech clinics and care pathways. Frankfurt is well known for the work of Drs Frank Louwen and Anke Reitter (Louwen et al, 2017; Reitter et al, 2014). But the model has been implemented effectively in many other places: by Dr Kamilla Gerhard Nielsen in Aabenraa, Denmark; Dr Caroline Daelemans in Brussels, Belgium; Dr Leonie van Rheenan-Flach in Amsterdam, Netherlands to name a few. The cornerstone of a good breech service is a healthy obstetric-midwifery partnership, and I am honoured to have provided training to these centres to help them build their services. I feel deeply grateful to consider these women-centred teams my colleagues and for the opportunity to continue learning from them. The work continues to make breech birth safer due to the many obstetricians, midwives and women who share with me their breech triumphs and tribulations.

Physiological breech birth: developing specialist expertise

All obstetricians are expected to lead care for women with a wide variety of medical and obstetric needs. Although breech guidelines (Impey et al, 2017; Kotaska et al, 2009) recognise that skill and experience are safety factors for vaginal breech birth, evidence indicates that a significant proportion of consultant obstetricians do not feel experienced or confident enough to facilitate this approach (Carcopino et al, 2007; Chinnock and Robson, 2007; Devarajan et al, 2011; Dhingra and Raffi, 2010; Walker et al, 2017b). As a result, limited system and clinical support result in 'stress, anger, fear and injustice' among women who wish to birth their breech babies physiologically (Petrovska et al, 2017), and introduce significant risks to future pregnancies (Sandall et al, 2018; Vlemmix et al, 2013). External cephalic version can significantly reduce caesarean section for breech presentation (Hofmeyr et al, 2015), but the procedure is not always successful. And because outcomes for babies turned this way are similar to those who are born in the breech position (Hofmeyr et al, 2015; Melo et al, 2018; Vlemmix et al, 2014), not all women choose external cephalic version (Guittier et al, 2011; Watts et al, 2016). In the context of modern maternity care, offering women a choice of mode of childbirth, and maximising the potential to safely achieve a planned vaginal breech birth, requires innovative and flexible approaches (Catling et al, 2015).

Qualitative research with experienced breech providers suggests a multi-disciplinary team approach as a way to balance the need for maternal choice with the need for safety, with the emphasis on continuity with women and the team (Walker et al, 2018a, 2018b). In line with evidence about the effects of compassionate leadership on innovation (West et al, 2017), evidence-based support of physiological breech births is pushing providers to reconsider the organisational structures of care provision. In addition to greater continuity from the obstetric team, teams which have successfully reintroduced a reliable vaginal breech birth service are also taking account of the positive effect of trusting midwifery relationships in the physiological birth process (Allen et al, 2017; Tracy et al, 2013). In areas across the UK, such as Belfast (Hickland et al, 2018), Oxford, London and Sheffield (Dresner-Barnes and Bodle, 2014), breech care is led by experienced midwives with support from designated obstetricians in a dedicated clinic. An organised care pathway ensures an offer of external cephalic version at term from an experienced provider, which also increases the likelihood of effectiveness of this procedure (Andrews et al, 2017; Bogner et al, 2012; Walker et al, 2015). When unsuccessful, women can rely on a genuine choice of how they birth their breech babies.

In areas where vaginal breech birth skills are being revived, breech birth is being retaught as a complex physiological birth skill (Walker et al, 2016a, 2016b). Women are supported to birth in the position they choose, often in an upright, forward-leaning kneeling posture, without an epidural. Evidence indicates that for breech babies, maternal upright positioning results in shorter second stages, fewer maternal and neonatal injuries, fewer manoeuvres performed and lower rates of intrapartum caesarean section (Bogner et al, 2015; Louwen et al, 2017). Local breech leaders, such as midwife Emma Spillane at St George's Hospital in London, are developing the confidence to introduce these new skills by frequently teaching them with experienced providers in a thoroughly evaluated training programme (Walker et al, 2017b, 2017a). The frequent repetition in simulation, alongside pattern recognition through birth video study, supports enhanced consolidation of skills that would otherwise take years to acquire (Walker et al, 2018a). Physiological skills are spreading through the use of modern educational technology and generous gifts of videos from women who have birthed their breech babies vaginally and feel passionately that the skills should be shared. Currently, in the Netherlands and Canada midwives are taught upright physiological breech skills as standard (Association of Ontario Midwives and contributors, 2019; Aten et al, 2017).

Flexible obstetrics follows the woman: birth after caesarean section and instrumental births

Following the results of the Birthplace study (Birthplace in England Collaborative Group, 2011) and subsequent changes in national guidance (NICE, 2014), most women in the UK assessed at 'low risk' of complications are given a choice of where to give birth: home, freestanding midwifery-led birth centre, alongside midwifery-led unit or consultant-led unit. Many women who require additional medical or obstetric input during pregnancy also like to decide on their birth setting according to their own needs and values, and it is their right to do so (GMC, 2008). In the UK East Lancashire Hospitals Trust, honouring this right of women to make their own decisions in birth means facilitating choice of birth place in complex situations as well as where labour and birth are straightforward.

Care for women planning a birth after caesarean section is one example. Once controversial and innovative (Garrard, 2011), clinics offering women consistent, balanced information about benefits and risks have now become mainstream in the UK and are most often run by senior midwives (David et al, 2010; White et al, 2016), alongside obstetric clinics for those who require additional input. In East Lancashire, many women choosing to birth their babies vaginally after a previous caesarean section are also drawn to the option of a midwifery-led birth centre because they feel their bodies will work best in this setting and model of care. Additionally, the most recent evidence indicates that women who have previously birthed both vaginally and by caesarean are at no greater risk when birthing in a community setting (Bovbjerg et al, 2017).

Obstetricians like Rineke Schram strive to work in collaboration with women's instincts and choices by mitigating potential risks with low intervention strategies appropriate for birth centre settings. Instead of insisting on intravenous cannulation and continuous monitoring throughout labour, based on a predictive risk profile, this relational model of care requires learning new ways to identify potential scar rupture, alongside intermittent foetal heart rate monitoring. These include observation of the woman's respiratory rate, behaviour and description of abdominal pain. Obstetric input focuses on supporting midwives to recognise abnormality in this type of complex physiological birth, enabling rapid response with careful transfer plans, and increasing confidence throughout the team to provide care centred on the woman, rather than her potential risk.

Some women need help to birth vaginally. Schram and her team also work with physiological principles to ensure operative births remain as dignified and satisfying as possible. They regularly assist births with ventouse or forceps in non-lithotomy positions, such as left lateral and even standing. Following individualised assessment, the woman maintains the position in which she feels strong, centred and safe. The goal is to bring the baby's head to crown on the perineum and then to remove the instrument, avoiding an episiotomy wherever possible. The woman then finishes by herself, pushing her baby out under her own steam. The birth remains an achievement by her, for her, and it is kept as *normal* as possible. She then picks her baby up when she is ready, or with assistance as she requests. This strategy may be particularly helpful to women who have experienced prior sexual traumas or women who have felt disempowered and abused in previous experiences, and may have a great fear of lithotomy positioning and/or loss of control (Montgomery, 2013; Montgomery et al, 2015). Similar physiology-informed techniques are also used in the Anterior Non-Episiotomy Forceps technique pioneered by Stelios Myriknas at Chelsea and Westminster Hospital in London (Myriknas and Papadakis, 2018). Working with supine maternal positioning, Myriknas has reduced rates of both episiotomies and severe tears, while enabling women to experience the powerful moment of 'finishing' the birth themselves.

Crucial to the success of flexible pathways and innovative obstetric practices is the presence of a consultant who is comfortable and confident with high-risk obstetric care (Lundgren et al, 2015). Evidence from twin and birth after caesarean studies indicates that continuity of care in specialist clinics, and intrapartum care by specialised obstetricians, increases the likelihood of a planned vaginal birth and improves outcomes

(Gardner et al, 2014; Henry et al, 2015). The presence of consultants focused on woman-centred obstetric care enables obstetric specialist trainees to develop the confidence and flexibility to use their skills in new ways, following the lead and needs of the women they care for (Reitter et al, 2018).

Physiology-informed caesarean section

Not every physiological labour ends with a vaginal birth, and some women require or choose a planned caesarean section (Schiller, 2018). Consultant obstetrician Liz Martindale works with Rineke Schram in East Lancashire. Undoubtedly, having supportive colleagues and a compassionate leadership culture (West et al, 2017) increases individual clinicians' ability to be flexible to address women's unique needs, practising in a way that is informed by guidelines rather than dictated by them. As David Haslam, chair of NICE says, they are 'guidelines, not tramlines'. In response to women's requests for more physiological aspects of care during planned (or even emergency) caesarean sections, Martindale and her colleagues began to enhance the support of physiological processes alongside the surgical procedure (Korteweg et al, 2017). Evidence-based non-surgical practices are implemented alongside the routine of evidence-based surgical practices which guide the performance of caesarean surgery (Dahlke et al, 2013). These include optimal cord clamping (McDonald et al, 2013), immediate skin-to-skin contact with the mother (Moore et al, 2016), and assistance to initiate early breastfeeding. Skin-to-skin contact and breastfeeding have often been delayed following caesarean birth, with implications for the future success of the breastfeeding relationship (Hakala et al, 2017). Although sometimes called 'gentle' caesarean section, these procedures should be standard at all caesareans without the moniker of being 'gentle' – they are just 'better', and certainly don't make the surgery any less invasive for the mother.

Nevertheless, facilitating these changes has involved a number of practical adjustments requiring the support of obstetric, anaesthetic, theatre team and midwifery colleagues – a challenge because it required educating a wide range of health professionals about the benefits (Zwedberg et al, 2015). Prior to starting the operation, maternal heart monitoring leads are placed on the birthing woman's back rather than her chest, one arm is removed from the gown, and the cannula and blood pressure cuffs are positioned in a way that will not interfere with immediate skin-to-skin contact. The screen is left down during the birth, enabling the mother to be involved in her own birth experience rather than just having an operation done to her behind a screen. Cord clamping is not performed immediately, waiting until pulsation stops, to optimise neonatal blood volume (Rana et al, 2019). After the birth, the screen is replaced, partly to maintain the sterile field, but also because it affords the family some privacy in their first moments together. Dimmer lighting behind the screen also makes it easier on the baby's eyes than bright theatre lights, as the baby gazes at his or her mother for the first time. Weighing is postponed until after this initial period of skin-to-skin bonding has taken place, as it would be following a physiological birth. For Martindale, enhancing physiological processes alongside surgical deliveries replaces some aspects of the early relationship with her baby which are lost when a woman does not labour.

Continuity is an instrument of care

The examples illustrated in this chapter resonate with a shift in maternity care away from systems of care characterised by prediction and control, back towards models of care based on relationship and response (Walker et al, 2016b). The 'critical importance of continuity of carer and high quality relationships', highlighted in research about midwives' and obstetricians' experiences of supporting women planning a vaginal birth after caesarean section (Foureur et al, 2017), is a recurrent theme in the support of complex physiological birth. Ample high-quality evidence exists to support midwifery-led continuity of care for women at all risk levels (Sandall et al, 2018; see also Chapter 11). Results include reductions in preterm birth, stillbirth, epidural use and interventions during birth (Sandall et al, 2016). Less work has been done to explore issues of continuity in obstetric care. Even describing what continuity in obstetric care means is challenging. Midwifery-led continuity entails a consistent relationship between the woman and her midwife or small team of midwives. Continuity of obstetric care at a basic level is similar, entailing a relationship between the woman and her named obstetrician. But coordinating complex care necessarily involves multiple health professionals. Obstetricians often create plans for care which will be provided by or with others, for example midwives, obstetric nurses in some settings, anaesthetists and theatre practitioners, other specialists or other obstetricians depending on rotas. Their ability to deliver individualised care inevitably depends on trust and respect in their leadership, the quality and consistency of their relationships with professional colleagues and the clarity of forward-looking plans that cover all eventualities.

Continuity also enables the development of significant levels of skill in a particular aspect of care, leading to levels of expertise which would be considered specialist. Specialist clinics are associated with improved health outcomes, more efficient and guideline-centred care, and less use of inpatient services (Gruen et al, 2003). Mounting evidence supports their use in obstetrics (Angood et al, 2010). The development of specialist clinics is also mirrored in the development of specialist midwife roles, such as work with twins (Henry et al, 2015), diabetes (NHS Diabetes, 2010), mental health (Royal College of Midwives, 2015) and perineal care (Priddis et al, 2014; Shore, 2015).

Conclusion

Further research in the area of complex normality should explore women's experiences of physiological processes in complex care, including caesarean deliveries, and the outcomes associated with innovative models of care provision. The role of continuity and of specialists, both midwifery and obstetric, should also be evaluated in the context of complex normality. Finally, relationships and continuity within small specialist teams should be considered a relevant factor in the provision of high-quality care. Its effect on maternal/neonatal outcomes, professional resilience and the ability to innovate should be studied further.

Key points for consideration

- Get to know the pregnant woman, her character and family, her values and preferences, fears and fantasies, and coping strategies. If competent, she is a respect-worthy adult with a backstory. This is her life, her baby, her future and her responsibility.

- Don't assume anything – always lay out all courses of action, starting with 'doing nothing' (natural history) and awaiting events.

- Risks are not amorphous, only existing on one side of a decision calculus, and are not 'trump cards' for a certain course of action – they have prevalence rates, predictors, symptoms and signs, and if they eventuate, they can be ameliorated by advance planning.

- Be clear about your professionalism. You are not the pregnant woman's friend. You are obliged to spell out unwelcome relevant information, but you must remain compassionate, polite and completely unthreatening. You must not abandon her.

- In cases where a way forward is not clear, allow time, repeat conversations, and use second opinions to guide a plan.

- Document your advice: make forward-looking plans with their 'safety' parameters, and who should do what, when, and why.

References

Allen, J., Kildea, S., Hartz, D.L., Tracy, M., Tracy, S., 2017. The motivation and capacity to go 'above and beyond': Qualitative analysis of free-text survey responses in the M@NGO randomised controlled trial of caseload midwifery. Midwifery 50, 148–156. https://doi.org/10.1016/j.midw.2017.03.012

Andrews, S., Leeman, L., Yonke, N., 2017. Finding the breech: Influence of breech presentation on mode of delivery based on timing of diagnosis, attempt at external cephalic version, and provider success with version. Birth 44, 222–229. https://doi.org/10.1111/birt.12290

Angood, P.B., Armstrong, E.M., Ashton, D., Burstin, H., Corry, M.P., Delbanco, S.F., Fildes, B., Fox, D.M., Gluck, P.A., Gullo, S.L., Howes, J., Jolivet, R.R., Laube, D.W., Lynne, D., Main, E., Markus, A.R., Mayberry, L., Mitchell, L. V, Ness, D.L., Nuzum, R., Quinlan, J.D., Sakala, C., Salganicoff, A., 2010. Blueprint for action: steps toward a high-quality, high-value maternity care system. Womens. Health Issues 20, S18-49. https://doi.org/10.1016/j.whi.2009.11.007

Association of Ontario Midwives & Contributors, 2019. Emergency Skills Workshop Manual, 6th ed. AOM.

Aten, L., Beers, L., Bijsterveld-Smid, B., Goodarzi, B., Hageraats, E., Theeuwen, K., 2017. LVOV richtlijn Baring in stuit.

Birthplace in England Collaborative Group, 2011. Perinatal and maternal outcomes by planned place of birth for healthy women with low risk pregnancies: the Birthplace in England national prospective cohort study. BMJ 343, d7400–d7400. https://doi.org/10.1136/bmj.d7400

Bogner, G., Strobl, M., Schausberger, C., Fischer, T., Reisenberger, K., Jacobs, V.R., 2015. Breech delivery in the all fours position: a prospective observational comparative study with classic assistance. J. Perinat. Med. 43, 707–13. https://doi.org/10.1515/jpm-2014-0048

Bogner, G., Xu, F., Simbrunner, C., Bacherer, A., Reisenberger, K., 2012. Single-institute experience, management, success rate, and outcome after external cephalic version at term. Int. J. Gynecol. Obstet. 116, 134–137. https://doi.org/10.1016/j.ijgo.2011.09.027

Bovbjerg, M.L., Cheyney, M., Brown, J., Cox, K.J., Leeman, L., 2017. Perspectives on risk: Assessment of risk profiles and outcomes among women planning community birth in the United States. Birth. https://doi.org/10.1111/birt.12288

Carcopino, X., Shojai, R., D'Ercole, C., Boubli, L., 2007. French trainees in obstetrics and gynaecology theoretical training and practice of vaginal breech delivery: a national survey. Eur J Obs. Gynecol Reprod Biol 135, 17–20.

https://doi.org/10.1016/j.ejogrb.2006.10.023

Catling, C., Petrovska, K., Watts, N., Bisits, A., Homer, C.S.E., 2015. Barriers and facilitators for vaginal breech births in Australia: Clinician's experiences. Women Birth 29, 138–143. https://doi.org/10.1016/j.wombi.2015.09.004

Chinnock, M., Robson, S., 2007. Obstetric trainees' experience in vaginal breech delivery: implications for future practice. Obstet. Gynecol. 110, 900–3. https://doi.org/10.1097/01.AOG.0000267199.32847.c4

Dahlke, J.D., Mendez-Figueroa, H., Rouse, D.J., Berghella, V., Baxter, J.K., Chauhan, S.P., 2013. Evidence-based surgery for cesarean delivery: an updated systematic review. Am. J. Obstet. Gynecol. 209, 294–306. https://doi.org/10.1016/j.ajog.2013.02.043

David, S., Fenwick, J., Bayes, S., Martin, T., 2010. A qualitative analysis of the content of telephone calls made by women to a dedicated 'Next Birth After Caesarean' antenatal clinic. Women and Birth 23, 166–171. https://doi.org/10.1016/j.wombi.2010.07.002

Devarajan, K., Seaward, P.G., Farine, D., 2011. Attitudes among Toronto obstetricians towards vaginal breech delivery. J. Obstet. Gynaecol. Can. 33, 437–42.

Dhingra, S., Raffi, F., 2010. Obstetric trainees' experience in VBD and ECV in the UK. J. Obstet. Gynaecol. (Lahore). 30, 10–12. https://doi.org/10.3109/01443610903315629

Dresner-Barnes, H., Bodle, J., 2014. Vaginal breech birth – the phoenix arising from the ashes. Pract. Midwife 17, 30–33.

Foureur, M., Turkmani, S., Clack, D.C., Davis, D.L., Mollart, L., Leiser, B., Homer, C.S.E., 2017. Caring for women wanting a vaginal birth after previous caesarean section: A qualitative study of the experiences of midwives and obstetricians. Women and Birth 30, 3–8. https://doi.org/10.1016/j.wombi.2016.05.011

Gardner, K., Henry, A., Thou, S., Davis, G., Miller, T., 2014. Improving VBAC rates: The combined impact of two management strategies. Aust. New Zeal. J. Obstet. Gynaecol. 54, 327–332. https://doi.org/10.1111/ajo.12229

Garrard, N. and, 2011. Rethinking provision of care: a radical restructuring of antenatal care services for women with complex pregnancies. MIDIRS Midwifery Dig. 21, 279–285.

GMC, 2008. Consent: patients and doctors making decisions together. General Medical Council, London.

Gruen, R.L., Weeramanthri, T.S., Knight, S.S.E., Bailie, R.S., 2003. Specialist outreach clinics in primary care and rural hospital settings. Cochrane Database Syst. Rev. Art. No.: CD003798. https://doi.org/10.1002/14651858.CD003798.pub2

Guittier, M.-J., Bonnet, J., Jarabo, G., Boulvain, M., Irion, O., Hudelson, P., 2011. Breech presentation and choice of mode of childbirth: a qualitative study of women's experiences. Midwifery 27, e208-13. https://doi.org/10.1016/j.midw.2010.08.008

Hakala, M., Kaakinen, P., Kääriäinen, M., Bloigu, R., Hannula, L., Elo, S., 2017. The realization of BFHI Step 4 in Finland – Initial breastfeeding and skin-to-skin contact according to mothers and midwives. Midwifery 50, 27-35. https://doi.org/10.1016/j.midw.2017.03.010

Henry, A., Lees, N., Bein, K.J., Hall, B., Lim, V., Chen, K.Q., Welsh, A.W., Hui, L., Shand, A.W., 2015. Pregnancy outcomes before and after institution of a specialised twins clinic: A retrospective cohort study. BMC Pregnancy Childbirth 15, 217. https://doi.org/10.1186/s12884-015-0654-5

Hickland, P., Gargan, P., Simpson, J., McCabe, N., Costa, J., 2018. A novel and dedicated multidisciplinary service to manage breech presentation at term; 3 years of experience in a tertiary care maternity unit. J. Matern. Neonatal Med. 31, 3002–3008. https://doi.org/10.1080/14767058.2017.1362382

Hofmeyr, G.J., Kulier, R., West, H.M., 2015. External cephalic version for breech presentation at term. Cochrane database Syst. Rev. CD000083. https://doi.org/10.1002/14651858.CD000083.pub3

Impey, L., Murphy, D., Griffiths, M., Penna, L., on behalf of the Royal College of Obstetricians and Gynaecologists, 2017. Management of Breech Presentation. BJOG. https://doi.org/10.1111/1471-0528.14465

Korteweg, F.J., de Boer, H.D., van der Ploeg, J.M., Buiter, H.D., van der Ham, D.P., 2017. [Skin-to-skin caesarean section: a hype or better patient care?]. Ned. Tijdschr. Geneeskd. 161, D582.

Kotaska, A., Menticoglou, S., Gagnon, R., Maternal Fetal Med, C., 2009. Vaginal delivery of breech presentation No. 226, June 2009. Int. J. Gynecol. Obstet. 107, 169–176. https://doi.org/10.1016/j.ijgo.2009.07.002

Louwen, F., Daviss, B., Johnson, K.C., Reitter, A., 2017. Does breech delivery in an upright position instead of on the back improve outcomes and avoid cesareans? Int. J. Gynecol. Obstet. 136, 151–161. https://doi.org/10.1002/ijgo.12033

Lundgren, I., van Limbeek, E., Vehvilainen-Julkunen, K., Nilsson, C., 2015. Clinicians' views of factors of importance for improving the rate of VBAC (vaginal birth after caesarean section): a qualitative study from countries with high VBAC rates. BMC Pregnancy Childbirth 15, 196. https://doi.org/10.1186/s12884-015-0629-6

McDonald, S.J., Middleton, P., Dowswell, T., Morris, P.S., 2013. Effect of timing of umbilical cord clamping of term infants on maternal and neonatal outcomes, in: McDonald, S.J. (Ed.), Cochrane Database of Systematic Reviews. John Wiley & Sons, Ltd, Chichester, UK. https://doi.org/10.1002/14651858.CD004074.pub3

Melo, P., Georgiou, E., Hedditch, A., Ellaway, P., Impey, L., 2018. External cephalic version at term: a cohort study of 18 years' experience. BJOG An Int. J. Obstet. Gynaecol. 1–7. https://doi.org/10.1111/1471-0528.15475

Montgomery, E., 2013. Feeling Safe: A Metasynthesis of the Maternity Care Needs of Women Who Were Sexually Abused in Childhood. Birth 40, 88–95. https://doi.org/10.1111/birt.12043

Montgomery, E., Pope, C., Rogers, J., 2015. The re-enactment of childhood sexual abuse in maternity care: a qualitative study. BMC Pregnancy Childbirth 15, 194. https://doi.org/10.1186/s12884-015-0626-9

Moore, E.R., Bergman, N., Anderson, G.C., Medley, N., 2016. Early skin-to-skin contact for mothers and their healthy newborn infants, in: Moore, E.R. (Ed.), Cochrane Database of Systematic Reviews. John Wiley & Sons, Ltd, Chichester, UK. https://doi.org/10.1002/14651858.CD003519.pub4

Moss, E.L., Redman, C.W.E., Arbyn, M., Dollery, E., Petry, K.U., Nieminen, P., Myerson, N., Leeson, S.C., 2015. Colposcopy training and assessment across the member countries of the European Federation for Colposcopy. Eur. J. Obstet. Gynecol. Reprod. Biol. 188, 124–128. https://doi.org/10.1016/j.ejogrb.2015.03.012

Myriknas, S., Papadakis, K., 2018. Anterior non-episiotomy or natural forceps delivery: refining the technique and improving communication as a way of reducing obstetric anal sphincter injuries in instrumental deliveries. J. Pelvic, Obstet. Gynaecol. Physiother. 122, 50–55.

NHS Diabetes, 2010. Lead Midwife in Diabetes: Standards, Role and Competencies. NHS Diabetes, London.

NICE, 2014. Intrapartum Care: care of healthy women and their babies during childbirth. NICE Guideline, CG190.

Petrovska, K., Watts, N.P., Catling, C., Bisits, A., Homer, C.S., 2017. 'Stress, anger, fear and injustice': An international qualitative survey of women's experiences planning a vaginal breech birth. Midwifery 44, 41–47. https://doi.org/10.1016/j.midw.2016.11.005

Plested, M., Walker, S., 2014. Building confident ways of working together around higher-risk birth choices. Essentially MIDIRS 5, 13–16.

Priddis, H.S., Schmied, V., Kettle, C., Sneddon, A., Dahlen, H.G., 2014. "A patchwork of services" – caring for women who sustain severe perineal trauma in New South Wales – from the perspective of women and midwives. BMC Pregnancy Childbirth 14, 236. https://doi.org/10.1186/1471-2393-14-236

Rana, N., KC, A., Målqvist, M., Subedi, K., Andersson, O., 2019. Effect of Delayed Cord Clamping of Term Babies on Neurodevelopment at 12 Months: A Randomized Controlled Trial. Neonatology 115, 36-42. https://doi.org/10.1159/000491994

Reitter, A., Daviss, B.-A., Bisits, A., Schollenberger, A., Vogl, T., Herrmann, E., Louwen, F., Zangos, S., 2014. Does pregnancy and/or shifting positions create more room in a woman's pelvis? Am. J. Obstet. Gynecol. 211, 662. e1-662.e9. https://doi.org/10.1016/j.ajog.2014.06.029

Reitter, A., Döhring, N., Maden, Z., Hessler, P., Misselwitz, B., 2018. Is it reasonable to establish an independent obstetric leadership in a small hospital and does it result in measurable changes in quality of maternity care? Z. Geburtshilfe Neonatol.

Royal College of Midwives, 2015. Caring for Women with Mental Health Problems: Standards and Competency Framework for Specialist Maternal Mental Health Midwives [WWW Document]. URL https://www.rcm.org.uk/sites/default/files/Caring for Women with Mental Health Difficulties 32pp A4_h.pdf (accessed 5.17.17).

Sandall, J., Coxon, K., Mackintosh, N., Rayment-Jones, H., Locock, L., Page, L., 2016. Relationships: the pathway to safe, high-quality maternity care. Report from the Sheila Kitzinger symposium at Green Templeton College October 2015. Green Templeton College, Oxford.

Sandall, J., Soltani, H., Gates, S., Shennan, A., Devane, D., 2016. Midwife-led continuity models versus other models of care for childbearing women. Cochrane Database Syst. Rev. Art. No.: CD004667. https://doi.org/10.1002/14651858.CD004667.pub5

Sandall, J., Tribe, R.M., Avery, L., Mola, G., Visser, G., Homer, C., Gibbons, D., Kelly, N., Kennedy, H.P., Kidanto, H., Taylor, P., Temmerman, M., 2018. Short-term and long-term effects of caesarean section on the health of women and children. Lancet. https://doi.org/10.1016/S0140-6736(18)31930-5

Schiller, R., 2018. Maternal Request Caesarean.

Shore, C., 2015. A day in the life of a specialist perineal care clinic. Pract. Midwife 18, 21–3.

Tracy, S.K., Hartz, D.L., Tracy, M.B., Allen, J., Forti, A., Hall, B., White, J., Lainchbury, A., Stapleton, H., Beckmann, M., Bisits, A., Homer, C., Foureur, M., Welsh, A., Kildea, S., 2013. Caseload midwifery care versus standard maternity care for women of any risk: M@NGO, a randomised controlled trial. Lancet 382. https://doi.org/10.1016/S0140-6736(13)61406-3

Vlemmix, F., Bergenhenegouwen, L., Schaaf, J.M., Ensing, S., Rosman, A.N., Ravelli, A.C.J., van der Post, J.A.M., Verhoeven, A., Visser, G.H., Mol, B.W.J., Kok, M., 2014. Term breech deliveries in the Netherlands: did the increased cesarean rate affect neonatal outcome? A population-based cohort study. Acta Obstet. Gynecol. Scand. 93, 888–896. https://doi.org/10.1111/aogs.12449

Vlemmix, F., Kazemier, B., Rosman, A., Schaaf, J., Ravelli, A., Duvekot, H., Kok, M., Mol, B., 2013. 764: Effect of increased caesarean section rate due to term breech presentation on maternal and fetal outcome in subsequent pregnancies. Am. J. Obstet. Gynecol. 208, S321. https://doi.org/http://dx.doi.org/10.1016/j.ajog.2012.10.102

Walker, S., Breslin, E., Scamell, M., Parker, P., 2017a. Effectiveness of vaginal breech birth training strategies: An integrative review of the literature. Birth 44, 101–109. https://doi.org/10.1111/birt.12280

Walker, S., Parker, P., Scamell, M., 2018a. Expertise in physiological breech birth: A mixed-methods study. Birth 45, 202–209. https://doi.org/10.1111/birt.12326

Walker, S., Perilakalathil, P., Moore, J., Gibbs, C.L., Reavell, K., Crozier, K., 2015. Standards for midwife practitioners of external cephalic version: A Delphi study. Midwifery 31, e79–e86. https://doi.org/10.1016/j.midw.2015.01.004

Walker, S., Reading, C., Siverwood-Cope, O., Cochrane, V., 2017b. Physiological breech birth: Evaluation of a training programme for birth professionals. Pract. Midwife 20, 25–28.

Walker, S., Scamell, M., Parker, P., 2018b. Deliberate acquisition of competence in physiological breech birth: A grounded theory study. Women and Birth 31, e170–e177. https://doi.org/10.1016/j.wombi.2017.09.008

Walker, S., Scamell, M., Parker, P., 2016a. Standards for maternity care professionals attending planned upright breech births: A Delphi study. Midwifery 34, 7–14. https://doi.org/10.1016/j.midw.2016.01.007

Walker, S., Scamell, M., Parker, P., 2016b. Principles of physiological breech birth practice: A Delphi study. Midwifery 43, 1–6. https://doi.org/10.1016/j.midw.2016.09.003

Watts, N.P., Petrovska, K., Bisits, A., Catling, C., 2016. This baby is not for turning: Women's experiences of attempted external cephalic version. BMC Pregnancy Childbirth 16, 248. https://doi.org/10.1186/s12884-016-1038-1

West, M., Eckert, R., Collins, B., Chowla, R., 2017. Caring to change: How compassionate leadership can stimulate innovation in health care.

White, H.K., le May, A., Cluett, E.R., 2016. Evaluating a Midwife-Led Model of Antenatal Care for Women with a Previous Cesarean Section: A Retrospective, Comparative Cohort Study. Birth 43, 200–208. https://doi.org/10.1111/birt.12229

Zwedberg, S., Blomquist, J., Sigerstad, E., 2015. Midwives' experiences with mother–infant skin-to-skin contact after a caesarean section: 'Fighting an uphill battle'. Midwifery 31, 215–220. https://doi.org/10.1016/j.midw.2014.08.014

Acknowledgements

Thank you to Dr Susan Bewley for reviewing and commenting on two drafts of this chapter.

Thank you to Drs Liz Martindale, Niamh McCabe, Rineke Schram and Leonie van Rhennan-Flach for contributing their thoughts and experiences to this chapter.

CHAPTER 23

Quality midwifery care for all women and all infants: learning from and using the *Lancet* Series on Midwifery

Mary Renfrew and *Petra ten Hoope-Bender*

Introduction

The Lancet Series on Midwifery is the most comprehensive and high-profile examination of midwifery to date. It has positively influenced the strengthening of midwifery across the world, in low, middle and high-income countries, and it is being used as a powerful tool by decision-makers and advocates. In this chapter we will describe why the series was needed, what it has to say about the type of care that women, infants and families want and require, and how it is being used to transform maternal and newborn care and services across the world.

What is *The Lancet* Series on Midwifery and why does it matter?

The Lancet Series on Midwifery is a series of five papers (Renfrew et al, 2014; Homer et al 2014; van Lerberghe et al, 2014; ten Hoope-Bender et al, 2014; Kennedy et al, 2016) together with an editorial and commentaries from a range of stakeholders (www. thelancet.com/series/midwifery). When planning for the Series began in 2011 it was clear that, despite progress over the previous decade, rates of maternal and newborn death and stillbirth remained unacceptably high in many areas. A range of other challenges was also identified, many of which remain to be addressed. Not only was there a lack of appropriate evidence-informed care for many women and newborn infants, but there was also a lack of compassion, with neglect and physical and emotional abuse occurring in many countries. The importance of pregnancy, labour and birth and the early weeks after birth to longer-term health and wellbeing and to establishing family relationships was often overlooked. Escalating over-medicalisation was resulting in interventions being seen increasingly as normal and routine, even when they were unnecessary. At the same time, midwifery was inconsistently implemented across the world, despite examples of its important role.

The international author team was tasked with answering the question: what can midwifery contribute to improving survival, health and wellbeing, and what are the conditions needed to implement it at scale? The 50 series co-authors, drawn from different disciplines and experience in low, middle and high-income countries in five continents, and including advocates and lay co-authors, brought a new and challenging perspective to the five papers in the Series.

A rigorous and innovative way to analyse, synthesise and use evidence from very diverse sources was developed to build connections between different bodies of knowledge, drawing on critical synthesis of systematic reviews, meta-syntheses, case studies and modelling, and including consensus-building among a group of interdisciplinary and international experts. Fundamentally important to this was the integration of evidence on women's views and experiences together with evidence on effectiveness. The needs of women, infants and families across the whole continuum of care was the focus of our work at all times.

The findings of this critical synthesis of hundreds of different sources of evidence were used to build a framework for the quality care that all women and all newborn infants need (the QMNC framework, Figure 1).

The framework summarises the evidence arising from the critical synthesis, and shows that women and newborn infants need specific practices, for care to be organised to meet their needs, and that this care should be founded on the values of respect and human rights, and a philosophy that optimises normal process and builds women's own capabilities. It also shows that care providers must work together to provide the skills and care to meet the needs of all. By distinguishing between *what* care is needed, *how* it should be provided, and *by whom*, the Series was able to use all the available evidence from low, middle, and high-income countries alike, on specific practices as well as on midwifery as a package of care, and on women's own views. This approach avoided the trap of being drawn into competing discourses around, for example, safety versus choice or home versus facility birth, demonstrating that all of these factors matter in different ways in different situations. Using a human rights approach with a focus on the care needed by *all* women, infants and families, the evidence showed that care should be tailored to the individual, and not pre-planned according to routine risk pathways. Preventive and supportive care was shown to be essential to avoid complications, as was early recognition and effective response to complications as they develop. By using all the available evidence – qualitative, quantitative, and case studies – the debate broadened from a traditional focus on essential interventions for emergencies and on workforce coverage to one where the overall quality of care was central.

The strong evidence base that emerged showed that a combination of key components of care – evidence-informed practices, providing continuity across the woman's journey

Figure 1:

The framework for quality maternal and newborn care: maternal and newborn health components of a health system needed by childbearing women and newborn infants (Renfrew et al, 2014)

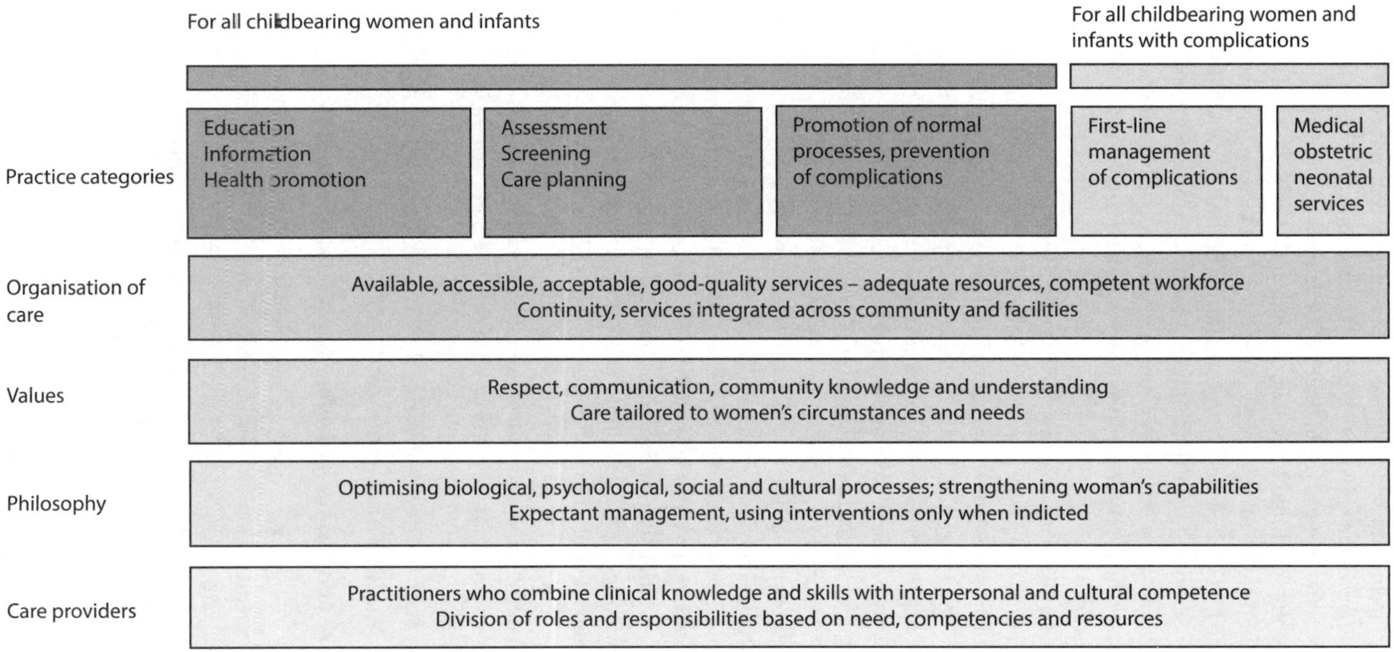

For all childbearing women and infants

For all childbearing women and infants with complications

| Practice categories | Education Information Health promotion | Assessment Screening Care planning | Promotion of normal processes, prevention of complications | First-line management of complications | Medical obstetric neonatal services |

Organisation of care: Available, accessible, acceptable, good-quality services – adequate resources, competent workforce. Continuity, services integrated across community and facilities

Values: Respect, communication, community knowledge and understanding. Care tailored to women's circumstances and needs

Philosophy: Optimising biological, psychological, social and cultural processes; strengthening woman's capabilities. Expectant management, using interventions only when indicted

Care providers: Practitioners who combine clinical knowledge and skills with interpersonal and cultural competence. Division of roles and responsibilities based on need, competencies and resources

281

to motherhood, respectful care, optimising normal processes of reproduction and early life, and effective interdisciplinary working – are critically important in saving lives and improving health and wellbeing, as well as preventing unnecessary interventions and strengthening women's own capabilities. The combined evidence from the Series papers showed the extensive reach and scale of the impact of midwifery – and specifically the work of professional midwives – on the survival, health and wellbeing of women and infants. The impact of full scope midwifery provided by professional midwives who are educated, regulated and integrated into the health system dwarfs the impact of other interventions. Its universal implementation could reduce stillbirths and deaths of women and newborn infants by more than 80%, as well as substantively improving the lives of those who survive. It truly is a vital solution needed by all women and all infants in all countries.

The evidence showed that over 70% of effective practices within the scope of midwifery promote normal processes. This brings balance to the system and challenges the current direction of maternity provision globally where the use of unnecessary interventions is escalating (Boerma et al, 2018). It demonstrates the limitations of the deployment of less-skilled health workers who do not provide the full scope of midwifery care. It shows the need for a paradigm shift in maternal and newborn care provision, from a focus on identifying and treating pathology to providing skilled and compassionate care for all. Midwifery is core to any quality strategy for maternal and newborn services. Through preventing maternal and newborn deaths and improving health and wellbeing its impact reaches through individuals and families to communities and beyond.

The evidence in the Series has demonstrated that midwifery is a fundamental way to fulfil the human rights of childbearing women and of infants. Without access to full-scope, high-quality midwifery, women and infants – and by extension, families and communities – are much more vulnerable. Integrating high-quality midwifery that works across communities and facilities into the health system is a cost-effective way to enable the rights of all women and children. It will result in lives saved, damage avoided, more effective and efficient use of health services, improved attachment within the family, and thus improved long-term outcomes for society.

How can this evidence be used to improve the lives of women, infants, families and communities?

Being clear about what midwifery is, and its contribution

Midwifery is inconsistently implemented internationally, with strong care models in some, predominantly high-income, countries, weak models in other settings, and a complete absence in many countries (UNFPA, 2014). In many settings, care for childbearing women and newborn infants is provided by other professional and non-professional staff, including doctors, nurses, community health workers, and traditional birth attendants. Even where midwives do exist, their work can be constrained in scope. They may not be fully integrated into the health system, and their core contribution to the interdisciplinary team is often not recognised. The work of midwives is often poorly understood, and midwives themselves report barriers to their work including lack of respect and remuneration, bullying, and unsafe working conditions (WHO, 2016). As a consequence, decision-makers often have a limited or inaccurate knowledge of midwifery and what it can contribute, and it can be difficult for advocates and colleagues to argue for the strengthening of midwifery or the importance of professional midwives. A key part of the Series that is being used widely across the world is the definition of midwifery as the universal care that *all* childbearing women, infants and families need:

'Skilled, knowledgeable and compassionate care for childbearing women, newborn infants and families across the continuum from pre-pregnancy, pregnancy, birth, postpartum and the early weeks of life. Core characteristics include optimising normal biological, psychological, social and cultural processes of reproduction and early life, timely prevention and management of complications, consultation with and referral to other services, respecting women's individual circumstances and views, and working in partnership with women to strengthen women's own capabilities to care for themselves and their families' (Renfrew et al, 2014)

This definition, and the framework for Quality Maternal and Newborn Care (Figure 1) map completely to the core competencies of the professional midwife as described by the International Confederation of Midwives (ICM, 2018), thus providing a compelling evidence base for the effectiveness and efficiency of midwives who are educated to that standard and fully supported by and integrated into the health system. The evidence presented in the Series shows that midwives can provide care in any setting, most effectively when they have access to a fully functioning health system that includes referral to other care providers when needed. With the capacity to support and strengthen the normal processes of pregnancy, birth, postpartum and the early weeks of life, midwifery puts the principles of people-centred care into practice, adapting care to the need of each woman and infant, respectfully and deliberately. Quality midwifery has a key role in helping to fulfil the human rights of women and infants for life, health, and dignity, and for freedom from fear and discrimination (UN 1948, 1979, 1989, 2000).

Informing policy development, building the case for investment

Building on the evidence from the Series, *The State of the World's Midwifery Report 2014* then showed that midwives can provide 87% of the essential care that women and newborns need (UNFPA, 2014), and it also showed that midwifery makes a contribution to health throughout the life-course of women and families. As a result, this report called for substantial investment in midwifery education, and for the deployment of midwives as a cost-effective development.

Informing education and system development

The Series has made an important contribution to midwifery education, demonstrating that midwives need to be skilled in what they do, including in practices, tasks, and interventions, and crucially, in how they do it; with respect, promoting normal processes, and strengthening women's own capabilities. This helps to clarify what is needed in midwifery education, and can be used to develop standards, guidance and curricula. It has also shown that the challenge of providing high-quality midwifery care is a challenge for the whole system. Midwives alone cannot organise and provide this care. The system needs to be organised to ensure professional regulation, high-quality education and full integration into the health economy to enable midwives to work closely with others as part of effective interdisciplinary teams to meet the needs of all women and newborn infants.

Informing the research agenda

In an important development, the Series moved beyond examining current evidence to considering the future research agenda (Kennedy at al, 2016). The QMNC framework was used to analyse the topics addressed by existing maternity care research. This analysis showed that the majority of research to date has focused on the treatment of complications, with much less research on the key topics of preventive and supportive care, or on ways of providing respectful care, or of promoting effective teamwork. This final paper in the Series reported the findings of a structured priority-setting exercise to establish priorities for new research programmes that, if funded, would redress the balance and inform the future implementation of quality maternal and newborn care. The three top priorities identified were i) to examine the effectiveness of the midwifery model of care (as defined by the Series), ii) to examine the processes of care that optimise or disturb biological processes, and iii) to determine which indicators, measures and benchmarks are most valuable in planning and evaluating care provision. Substantial investment in research in these priority areas would fill key gaps in the provision of cost-effective quality care for women, infants and families worldwide, and would help to expedite progress towards the SDGs. A call to action has been published (Kennedy et al, 2018), and work directly to inform funding agencies about the importance of these research topics is ongoing.

The global impact of the *Lancet* Series on Midwifery

New perspectives on maternal and infant health and care and on quality, equity, and dignity

Knowledge evolves and develops over time, and is used in different ways in different contexts. The perspectives developed in the *Lancet* Series on Midwifery are informing new work in many different disciplines and countries. The Series papers have already been cited many hundreds of times, in studies ranging widely on topics including early childhood development, health system planning, sustainability and interventions to improve outcomes for women and infants. It has informed other *Lancet* Series, on newborn care, stillbirth, and maternal health, for example, and is cited in a number of chapters in this volume.

The evidence presented in the Series has both initiated and helped to inform changes that are taking place at local, national, regional and global levels. It has helped to open minds to thinking differently about what women want, and has generated discussions on how services should be organised. It is supporting the recognition of the midwife as core to the interdisciplinary maternal and newborn health team, and to the provision of quality, equity, and dignity for all.

This evidence shows that midwives sit at the heart of primary healthcare, public health and clinical care, and that they are core to the successful implementation of universal health coverage (WHO, 2017). It demonstrates that midwifery is an essential foundation for the United Nations' (UN) mandate to transform individuals, communities and societies, and to successful implementation of the UN's Global Strategy for Women's Children's and Adolescents' Health (UN, 2015a). Midwifery is key to making progress on many of the UN's Sustainable Development Goals (SDGs: UN, 2015b) especially SDG 3, which aims '*to ensure healthy lives and promote well-being for all ages*'.

An evidence base for action

Advocacy and action across the world, at local, national, regional and global levels, is now being informed by the evidence and analyses presented in the Series. Effective action is usually the result of a combination of factors, and that is certainly the case in the way the Series is being used. Organisations and colleagues have reported that the Series is being used to inform work on quality maternal and newborn care, to shape the development of regulatory standards and of educational curricula for students and for educators, to argue for new priorities for research funding and to strengthen or introduce professional midwives. Some examples of many actions that we are aware of include:

- The World Health Organization has used the Series to inform discussions with governments, and to develop guidance and technical documents on quality care, and on midwifery education. One consequence of this the decision to present a key report on the importance of midwifery at the World Health Assembly in 2019.
- The QMNC framework has been integrated into WHO quality of care work and the new WHO antenatal, intra-partum and postnatal guidelines. It has helped to broaden the focus from specific interventions to include how care is provided and organised, and how it is experienced by women and families.
- The International Confederation of Midwives has used the Series to inform the development of the Midwifery Services Framework (Nove et al, 2018), now being used in many low and middle-income countries to measure, improve or establish midwifery services.
- In the USA, advocates and midwives are using the evidence to make the case for strengthening midwifery and the deployment of midwives both nationally and in local areas.
- In the UK, the evidence has been used to inform national reviews of maternity and neonatal services, and to shape new national regulatory standards for the education of midwives. It is being used for service planning and monitoring by specific health services.
- In Australia, the Series has been used in several universities to inform the development of new curricula for student midwives.

- In India, the Series has been used to inform discussions with the national government, which has resulted in support for the introduction of professional midwives and the development of national guidance.
- Across south-east Asia, the Series has been used to inform regional planning to strengthen midwifery.
- In Bangladesh, the Series is being used to inform a national education programme for midwife educators.
- In Malawi and other sub-Saharan countries, the Series is being used to inform plans to strengthen midwifery.

An international group, led by Yale University and supported by other academic and advocacy partners, has been established to take forward advocacy and action on the funding of new research priorities. This group has already participated in discussions with the WHO and other global funders, as well as a range of national research funders.

Conclusion

The evidence presented in the *Lancet* Series on Midwifery demonstrates that investment in quality midwifery care during pregnancy, childbirth and beyond will enable women's capacity to transform their family, their community and society at large. Midwifery can make a unique contribution to fulfilling the vision of the UN Global Strategy for Women's, Children's and Adolescents' Health. This is for a world in which every woman, adolescent and child everywhere realise their rights to physical and mental health and wellbeing, have social and economic opportunities, and are able to participate fully in shaping prosperous and sustainable societies. The aim is for them to survive (ending preventable deaths), thrive (have health and wellbeing) and then transform their communities and nations through expanded enabling environments.

This new perspective on the evidence demonstrates that a paradigm shift is needed in how maternity care is valued and provided. There would be a substantive return on investment from quality maternal and newborn care provided by the interdisciplinary team and with midwives at its heart. This would be manifest across the Sustainable Development Goals. This includes not just the obvious health and gender goals, but all of those where the lives and capabilities of women and children make a contribution, such as economic empowerment, universal health coverage, access to and use of education, financial participation and development, reducing the impact and increase of climate change, reducing poverty and hunger, the return of peaceful and inclusive societies and revitalising global partnerships. Quality midwifery for all would result in a radical transformation across the globe.

The *Lancet* Series on Midwifery situates midwifery as central to the quality care of all women and children, essential for the effective working of the interdisciplinary team. It demonstrates that midwives make a unique contribution to a range of important and often contentious discourses, including safety, choice, respect and the sustainability of health systems. The Series identifies and describes a philosophy of care that is respectful, promotes normal processes and builds women's own capabilities. It also offers a strongly evidenced and detailed description of a model of care, and provides a practical approach to care provision, system planning, monitoring, advocacy and education for all countries. It is an invaluable tool for decision-makers and advocates in their work to implement midwifery, both to introduce professional midwives into health systems and to strengthen their role where they already exist.

Key points for consideration

- Analysis of quantitative and qualitative evidence from low, middle, and high-income countries has demonstrated the essential contribution that midwifery can make to the survival, health and wellbeing of all women and infants, to their communities, and to the sustainability of health services.
- The evidence-informed definition of midwifery and the quality framework show the combination of factors needed to provide quality care for childbearing women and newborn infants across the whole continuum of care.
- The impact of high-quality midwifery is extensive, dwarfing the impact of other interventions. It can improve clinical and psycho-social outcomes for both the woman and the newborn infant, reduce the use of unnecessary interventions, and save resources. Midwives make a unique contribution to a range of challenging discourses, including safety, choice, respect, and the sustainability of health systems.
- This evidence demonstrates that work is urgently needed to tackle the barriers to midwifery care and to integrate high-quality midwifery provided by well-educated and supported midwives into the health system in all countries.
- There are examples from across the world of this evidence being used to strengthen midwifery through informing policy, practice, guidance and strategy development in low, middle, and high-income countries.
- Use current best evidence drawn from all relevant quantitative and qualitative sources to inform practice and policy.
- Always focus first on the needs of women and newborn infants, and work to plan and provide high-quality care and services that best meet their needs; always involving women, families and communities in the development and monitoring of midwifery services.
- High-quality care for all women and newborn infants needs a combination of the right practices with appropriate organisation of care to reach all women and infants and maximise continuity, respectful care tailored to individual needs, a shared philosophy that optimises normal processes and builds women's own capabilities, and interdisciplinary working with the appropriate skill mix.
- Midwifery is central to the quality care of all women and children, essential for the effective working of the interdisciplinary team, and to tackling the challenges of survival, health and wellbeing of women and infants and to the unsustainable over-medicalisation of services; care by well-educated and well-supported midwives brings balance to health systems, offering preventive and supportive care to avoid complications as well as the knowledge and skills to respond quickly and appropriately when complications occur.

- Work to implement high-quality midwifery care for all is urgently needed. This evidence provides a powerful tool for decision-makers and advocates to inform strategies to implement large-scale change.

References

Boerma T, Ronsmans C, Melesse D, Barros A, Barros F, Juan L et al. Global epidemiology of use of and disparities in caesarean sections. The Lancet. 2018;392(10155):1341-1348.

Homer C, Friberg I, Dias M, ten Hoope-Bender P, Sandall J, Speciale A et al. The projected effect of scaling up midwifery. The Lancet. 2014;384(9948):1146-1157.

International Confederation of Midwives. Essential competencies for midwifery practice. ICM 2018. www. internationalmidwives.org/assets/files/general-files/2018/10/icm-competencies---english-document_final_ oct-2018.pdf

Kennedy H, Yoshida S, Costello A, Declercq E, Dias M, Duff E et al. Asking different questions: research priorities to improve the quality of care for every woman, every child. The Lancet Global Health. 2016;4(11):e777-e779.

Kennedy H, Cheyney M, Dahlen H, Downe S, Foureur M, Homer C et al. Asking different questions: A call to action for research to improve the quality of care for every woman, every child. Birth. 2018;45(3):222-231.

Nove A, ten Hoope-Bender P, Moyo N, Bokosi M. The Midwifery services framework: What is it, and why is it needed? Midwifery. 2018;57:54-58.

Renfrew M, McFadden A, Bastos M, Campbell J, Channon A, Cheung N et al. Midwifery and quality care: findings from a new evidence-informed framework for maternal and newborn care. The Lancet. 2014;384(9948):1129-1145.

ten Hoope-Bender P, de Bernis L, Campbell J, Downe S, Fauveau V, Fogstad H et al. Improvement of maternal and newborn health through midwifery. The Lancet. 2014;384(9949):1226-1235.

UN General Assembly, Universal Declaration of Human Rights, 10 December 1948, 217 A (III), available at: https://www.refworld.org/docid/3ae6b3712c.html [accessed 8 January 2019]

UN General Assembly, Convention on the Elimination of All Forms of Discrimination Against Women, 18 December 1979, United Nations, Treaty Series, vol. 1249, p. 13, available at: www.refworld.org/docid/3ae6b3970.html [accessed 8 January 2019]

UN General Assembly, Convention on the Rights of the Child, 20 November 1989, United Nations, Treaty Series, vol. 1577, p. 3, available at: https://www.refworld.org/docid/3ae6b38f0.html [accessed 8 January 2019]

UN Committee on Economic, Social and Cultural Rights (CESCR), General Comment No. 14: The Right to the Highest Attainable Standard of Health (Art. 12 of the Covenant), 11 August 2000, E/C.12/2000/4, available at: www.refworld. org/docid/4538838d0.html [accessed 8 January 2019]

UN Global Strategy for Women's, Children's and Adolescent's Health 2016-2030. New York: United Nations, 2015. https://www.who.int/life-course/partners/global-strategy/en/

UN Sustainable Development Goals (SDGs). New York: United Nations, 2015. https://sustainabledevelopment. un.org

UNFPA. The State of the World's Midwifery 2014: a universal pathway, a woman's right to health. New York: UNFPA

Van Lerberghe W, Matthews Z, Achadi E, Ancona C, Campbell J, Channon A et al. Country experience with strengthening of health systems and deployment of midwives in countries with high maternal mortality. The Lancet. 2014;384(9949):1215-1225.

World Health Organization. Midwives' voices, midwives' realities: findings from a global consultation on providing quality midwifery care. 2016. Geneva, WHO

World Health Organization 2017. Together on the Road to Universal Health Coverage. WHO, Geneva. WHO/HIS/ HGF/17.1 https://www.who.int/universal_health_coverage/road-to-uhc/en/

From disrespect and abuse to respectful and compassionate care: a global perspective

Nicholas Rubashkin and *Elena Ateva*

Introduction

Wherever and whenever births have moved into hospitals, debates about gender, power, and the humanisation of care have flourished. In her 18th-century treatise on midwifery, English midwife Elizabeth Nihell penned a forceful critique of 'men-midwives', a document that may contain the earliest discussion of 'abuse' in childbirth in the English language literature.[1] More recently, over the last two decades many groups around the world have worked to improve the experience of childbirth for women, families and communities. In the 1980s in Latin America the Humanization of Childbirth movement emerged as a reaction against the overmedicalisation of childbirth.[2] In the1990s after the fall of Communism new civil society organisations in Eastern Europe, starting with the Dignity in Childbirth movement in Poland, similarly challenged the substandard treatment of pregnant women in birth facilities.[3,4] More recently, in 2007 and 2010 respectively, human rights organisations like the Center for Reproductive Rights and Amnesty International put the spotlight on violations of women's rights in childbirth in Kenya and the United States.[5,6] This human-rights focus gave birth to the movement for respectful maternity care.

What started as a community of concern focused on 'respectful maternity care' has now expanded to encompass a global, multi-sectoral network of more than 100 organisations, representing 300 members, including researchers, clinicians, advocates, professional associations, non-governmental organisations, UN agencies and donors. The Global Respectful Maternity Care Council coordinated by the White Ribbon Alliance serves as the hub for identifying, implementing and advocating for strategies to define disrespect and abuse,[7,8] influence stakeholders to take a position on the issue,[9-11] and propose viable solutions.[12,13] Human rights and gender equity have remained at the core of the RMC movement with the compilation of the Respectful Maternity Care charter, a list of human rights based on universally recognised international instruments to which most countries are signatories, thus providing potential avenues for accountability efforts and, ultimately, the empowerment of pregnant women the world over.

In summary, various forms of evidence about mistreatment in birth facilities, spanning the clinical research, legal, and advocacy worlds, have long existed and have already catalysed positive change. In this chapter, we discuss our observations regarding recent calls for more formal types of 'evidence' of the mistreatment of women in childbirth.[8] We believe that such evidence was critical during the early stages of the RMC movement in order to strengthen the research, advocacy and implementation agendas. However, we argue below that formal evidence, such as that accepted as authoritative in the clinical research world, has the potential to dominate other forms of evidence, including women's interpretations of their experiences. To support this point, we review examples of where 'reliable and valid' evidence from randomised controlled trials (and other large cohort studies) have become dominant in other areas of global public health. We finish by reviewing other forms of evidence that were used to create positive change. We conclude that rather than investing in the most resource-intensive forms of evidence of mistreatment, we should instead be strategic and thoughtful about when other forms of evidence might be applicable.

Hierarchies of evidence in global health policy

In 2010 Bowser and Hill published a framework detailing seven categories of disrespect and abuse (D&A) of pregnant women in childbirth: physical abuse, non-consented care, non-confidential care, non-dignified care, discrimination, abandonment of care and detention in facilities.[7] Bowser and Hill's typology has proven extremely influential; nearly every study since has been grounded in their seven categories. A follow-up systematic review by WHO refined the Bowser and Hill categories.[8] Efforts to standardise the definitions of disrespect and abuse are underway, as are interventions that target D&A for reduction.[14]

The calls for 'high-quality' trials to reduce disrespect and abuse of pregnant women in birth facilities may be following a familiar path of evidence production in global public health,[15] namely a faithful pursuit of 'hierarchies of evidence'. At the top of this hierarchy sits systematic reviews, or an analysis that summarises all existing intervention trials into a single estimate of effectiveness. Systematic reviews are followed by the single randomised controlled trial (RCT), largely accepted as the 'gold standard' for proving clinical effectiveness because researchers are able to control for unmeasured factors that can cause spurious associations. Under the RCT we find evidence that results from cohort studies, and below cross-sectional studies. The two study designs listed below RCTs are progressively more prone to errors that cannot be measured, and therefore are more likely to yield unreliable and invalid results for a given intervention. Reliable and valid measurements are then implemented into sufficiently powered trials to follow the effect of an intervention compared to a control group.[16] As the logic goes, researchers should progress up the ladder to discover the most 'reliable and valid' evidence to inform policy change.[17] This hierarchy is not inherently bad or morally wrong. As Petticrew and Roberts observe, the hierarchy debates narrowly focus our attention on the subject of study design. They instead propose a 'matrix of knowledge' to generate a range of questions and methodologies that can inform not only effectiveness trials, but implementation and acceptability.[18]

The rigid implementation of the hierarchy in global health has been much criticised for how it affects the kinds of questions that get asked and the types of knowledge produced. The three-step ladder of evidence with its origins in the clinical sciences now heavily informs global health policy, from deciding which studies to fund and which NGOs are successful.[19] For instance, at the behest of funders a safe motherhood program in rural Tibet had to abandon a plan to train health workers. Funders were more in favour of conducting an RCT that compared a traditional Tibetan postpartum haemorrhage medication to a Western medication regimen. The result of the RCT was 'negative' in that the Tibetan medication was not found to be superior. However, with the safe motherhood program delayed until it found alternative funding, the most tangible health 'benefit' was that Tibetan scientists became trained in Western ethical standards to conduct clinical research.[19]

A rigid application of the RCT gold standard is especially problematic when applied to complex social problems like the mistreatment of women. A full understanding of the mistreatment of women demands multiple forms of evidence that sit lower on the hierarchy: rigorous qualitative data, legal testimony, stories and direct action. A rigid application of the 'RCT gold standard' to the mistreatment of women could potentially direct attention away from women themselves, in favour of more complex statistical models.[19] The RCT gold standard raises some troubling ethical questions as well: would it be ethical to randomise women to no treatment? Would areas of high prevalence of abuse but low numbers of women be overlooked in order to obtain 'statistical power' to detect a difference? Would forms of abuse that only fit the established taxonomies be recognised as abuses and targeted for intervention?

In summary, we are concerned about the potential for a rigid application of the hierarchy of evidence to the mistreatment of women. If women's experiences don't fit the accepted categories, they may not speak out. If certain experiences of mistreatment are not amenable to context-independent measurement, researchers may overlook forms of mistreatment that are highly local and laden with meaning. Providers may feel disempowered to change their local conditions, lacking as they may the knowledge of how to conduct resource-intensive trials. Finally, the phenomenon of disrespect and abuse could 'disappear' according to outcome measures designed for controlled trials, but outside the context of a clinical trial women and providers may still not be equipped to prevent new forms of abuse as they emerge. In the next section we review how evidence like simple surveys, civil society actions and storytelling – all forms of evidence that would be considered 'weak' from a clinical effectiveness standpoint – helped to build the political will needed to address the mistreatment of women in birth facilities.[20]

Examples of diverse forms of evidence creating positive change

Evidence for advocacy takes many forms and depends on whom you are trying to convince and the type of evidence your targets consider to be convincing. Sometimes high-quality research evidence is needed to change the mind of a policy-maker. Often, however, evidence generated by ordinary people, focusing on their lived reality and experiences, can be a powerful tool when working together with elected officials. A single story of an abusive childbirth or even the quiet presence of pregnant women in the house of parliament can change the policy discourse. More importantly, these other forms of evidence may have a greater ability than formal evidence to amplify women's own voices and to ensure that any policy changes actually serve the needs of the people. Other forms of evidence also contribute to building a movement of people who are invested in the improvement of maternal and newborn health in their own countries, whereas an exclusive focus on more formal evidence runs the risk of relying on external experts who may be less invested and less knowledgeable about the long-term sustainability of the health system.

The issue of mistreatment of women is not simply an issue of producing reliable and valid evidence, but better conceptualised as a systems problem. Therefore, the solution requires coordinated action, movement building and accountability. Disrespectful and abusive care is a product of dysfunctional health and governmental systems and relates to the power imbalance between providers and patients. Mistreatment of women in birth facilities is worsened by lack of resources within the health system, by lack of recognition for human rights at all levels of society, and by gender inequality. The solution to this phenomenon can only be found in a comprehensive approach involving the community, providers and policy-makers, with a clear understanding that responsibility is borne not by any one actor, but by all. Similarly, any changes need to occur simultaneously at the community, facility and policy levels. This approach should make sure that women are at the centre and actively informing not only the way disrespect and abuse is defined, but also the possible solutions to achieve high-quality, respectful and dignified care in childbirth.

For example, in early 2017 White Ribbon Alliance India (WRA India) collected information from 143,556 women across India, asking them for just one request for when they access maternity care. The campaign was conducted across 24 states and Union Territories with the help of WRA India member organisations and volunteers. More than 23% of women answered that they were looking for services provided with dignity and respect, including no discrimination based on caste or religion. They also wished for privacy and confidentiality, having a single bed to a woman, and for the presence of a birth companion.[21] Results from the survey were shared with the Union Minister of Health and Family Welfare, and with representatives from the district level. As a result of the campaign the Government of India adopted respectful maternity care as one of the central pillars in a countrywide initiative to improve quality for maternal and newborn health.[20]

In Malawi, White Ribbon Alliance Malawi (WRA Malawi) employed a variety of advocacy techniques to bring attention to the fact that Malawi does not have enough midwives to provide critical life-saving maternal and newborn health services and the impact of this shortage on the quality of services currently provided. A WRA Malawi census-style count conducted in 2016 showed that an additional 20,217 midwives are needed.[22] Citizens' hearings, radio talk shows and media articles highlighted the consequences of low-quality care.[23,24] The issue garnered both public and political attention with the Minister of Health and the First Lady of Malawi, both of whom were driven by the campaign to recognise the need for more midwives and publicly commit to hiring an additional 800 midwives. Also, as a result of the campaign respectful maternity care has been included in the pre-service and in-service curricula for midwives, and has been incorporated into staff performance appraisals.

In Nepal, the Safe Motherhood Network Federation (SMNF) worked with the parliamentary committee on Women, Children, Senior Citizens and Social Welfare to advocate for the inclusion of respectful maternity care standards in the Safe Motherhood and New Born Health Care Bill (later renamed Safe Motherhood and Reproductive Health Rights Act). The meeting highlighted the fact that issues of disrespect and abuse cross all borders, including social status, as parliamentary members themselves were sharing stories of abuse and disrespect that they had experienced. This meeting was part of a comprehensive approach to RMC which included awareness-raising through the media, community dialogues and collection of evidence on disrespect and abuse, and engagement of all key stakeholders: government agencies, non-governmental organisations, international non-governmental organisations, professional associations and health workers.

In addition, SMNF brought the issues of respectful care to the attention of political parties' representatives and mobilised them to support the Bill and advocate to the Ministry and policy-makers to pass the Bill. To support health workers, SMNF produced a strategy paper that was ultimately presented to the Ministry of Health as a roadmap for instituting RMC training for health workers nationwide. It was only through these concerted efforts that the ultimate goal was achieved: RMC rights framework and language was included in the national Bill, thereby ensuring that RMC standards are incorporated into law and in-service curricula for all professional disciplines involved in providing maternal care.[25] The new law on Safe Motherhood and Reproductive Health Rights was passed in October 2018.

Global health metrics versus the imperative to care

Given the importance of good governance in furthering the RMC agenda, we want to explore another potential pitfall caused by the ways in which the demand for high-quality data becomes connected to foreign aid. The example of MDG5 to decrease the maternal mortality ratio is instructive here. Due to weak health systems struggling in the face of multiple challenges, measuring the maternal mortality ratio (MMR – the number of maternal deaths per 100,000 live births) presented significant challenges. Most deaths and births occurred outside the hospital, and both deaths and births were significantly underreported. As a result, epidemiologists developed population survey methods and used regression analytics to estimate MMRs. The World Bank-funded Demographic and Health Survey used household survey methods in many developing countries to provide estimates of maternal mortality. Once the MMR appeared as a number that could be compared across contexts it became thoroughly incorporated into foreign aid. Many countries rely heavily on this aid, and whether a country's MMR went up or down slowly became a sign of good or bad governance.[26]

Furthermore, hospitals became focused more and more on the bureaucratic function of counting and reviewing maternal deaths rather than providing care. Consider the example of a woman who presented to a Nigerian hospital with a life-threatening post-caesarean complication. This woman waited an exorbitant amount of time to be processed in her hospital because of a problem registering her into the hospital system to be counted; when this registration problem could not be rectified, no one took the time to examine the woman and lift up her clothing to find exposed intestines.[27] Her story demonstrates the irony of counting the MMR, which is tied to hospital failure or success, and by extrapolation, to government failure or success.

If metrics – including yet-to-be developed D&A metrics – cause hospitals to become more oriented toward bureaucratic rather than care functions, it becomes clear just how fragile the alignment between foreign aid, health and human rights really is. We use the above example of how not to implement measurements of D&A. Given that dysfunctional and underfunded health systems are drivers of D&A especially in low and middle-income countries, we believe that foreign aid to low and middle-income countries should not be tied to performance related to metrics. However, the subversion of care functions by bureaucratic and technological imperatives is endemic to health facilities everywhere. As Downe in a recent commentary argues, we must not only invest in metrics, machinery, and technology to diminish mistreatment, we must also invest everywhere in 'people, relationships, skills, and attitudes'.[28]

Conclusion: keeping the agenda broad

In this chapter we have called for multiple forms of evidence to address the mistreatment of women in birth facilities. In other arenas of global health an emphasis on 'gold standard' reliable and valid evidence to inform cross-country comparable metrics has made it difficult to maintain a broad human rights focus. The first publications on disrespect and abuse of pregnant women are only five years old, and no standardised metrics exist, and D&A metrics have not (yet) been incorporated into aid regimes. The lack of comparable metrics may actually be the greatest potential for broader change for Respectful Maternity Care. The concepts of RMC should *demand* adaptation and *limit* easy comparisons across birth systems and countries. This is a good thing. Privacy and dignity are highly contextual terms.

Time will tell whether the yet-to-be developed RMC metrics will be able to resist the same problems that befell the MMR. Given the clarity of hindsight, the lessons of the MMR should help us to proceed with cautious optimism and to remain closer to the experiences of women. We remain hopeful that the community of concern that has taken shape around RMC can navigate the pitfalls of 'development' and global aid. If there is any upside to the challenges of 'development', it is that 'development' brings people into contact to solve a problem. If RMC can stay near to the experiences of women and take a stance against imperialism, perhaps people working in diverse locales will more consciously address forms of disrespect and abuse facing many pregnant women in all countries, not just the poorest.[29]

Key points for consideration

- The mistreatment of women has risen to the top of the global health agenda thanks to the concerted efforts of researchers, advocates, clinicians, and women.

- Recent calls for standardising the quantitative measures of mistreatment may narrow the global conversation to a single question of study design. 'Study design' in global health often translates into complex and expensive designs, such as a randomised controlled trial.

- Simple interventions can raise political will and push solutions to mistreatment the top of the political agenda. We share three examples from India, Malawi and Nepal where women and civil society organisations played critical roles in identifying and promoting solutions to mistreatment.

- Furthermore, yet-to-be determined metrics to quantify mistreatment could orient care practices towards bureaucratic functions, like counting mistreatment, rather than taking care of actual women in a respectful manner.

- We challenge the global health community to approach measurement of mistreatment with methods that remain grounded in the experiences of women and communities.

References

1. Murphy-Lawless J. Reading Birth and Death: A history of obstetric thinking. Bloomington: Indiana University Press; 1998. 343 p.
2. Diniz SG, Salgado HDO, Aguiar Andrezzo HFd, Cardin de Carvalho PG, Albuquerque Carvalho PC, Azevedo Aguiar C, et al. Abuse and Disrespect in Childbirth Care as a Public Health Issue in Brazil: Origins, Definitions, Impacts on Maternal Health, and Proposals for Its Prevention. Journal of Human Growth and Development. 2015;25(3):377.
3. WHO. Raising the voices of pregnant women in Poland Accessed August 20, 2017 [Available from: http://www.who.int/features/2015/childbirth-dignity-poland/en/.
4. UNFPA. Carmen Barroso and Childbirth with Dignity Foundation win 2016 UN Population Award 2016 [Available from: http://www.unfpa.org/news/carmen-barroso-and-childbirth-dignity-foundation-win-2016-un-population-award
5. Rights CfR. Failure to Deliver: Violations of Women's Human Rights in Kenyan Health Facilities. United States; 2007 2007.
6. Secretariat AI. Deadly Delivery: The Maternal Health Care Crisis in the USA. London, United Kingdom; 2010 2010.
7. Bowser D, Hil K. Exploring Evidence for Disrespect and Abuse in Facility-Based Childbirth. Boston: Harvard School of Public Health; 2010 September 17, 2010.
8. Bohren MA, Vogel JP, Hunter EC, Lutsiv O, Makh SK, Souza JP, et al. The Mistreatment of Women during Childbirth in Health Facilities Globally. A Mixed-Methods Systematic Review. PLoS Med. 2015;12(6):1-32.
9. Miller S, Lalonde A. The global epidemic of abuse and disrespect during childbirth: History, evidence, interventions, and FIGO's mother-baby friendly birthing facilities initiative. Int J Gynaecol Obstet. Feb 2015;123(2):93-4.
10. Freedman LP, Ramsey K, Abuya T, Bellows B, Ndwiga C, Warren CE, et al. Defining disrespect and abuse of women in childbirth: a research, policy and rights agenda. Bull World Health Organ. 2014;92(12):915-7.
11. Council HR. Follow-up on the application of the technical guidance on the application of a human rights-based approach to the implementation of policies and programmes to reduce preventable maternal mortality and morbidity. New York: United Nations; 2016 19 July 2016.
12. Abuya T, Ndwiga C, Ritter J, Kanya L, Bellows B, Binkin N, et al. The effect of a multi-component intervention on disrespect and abuse during childbirth in Kenya. BMC Pregnancy Childbirth. 2015;15:224.

13. Tuncalp, Were WM, MacLennan C, Oladapo OT, Gulmezoglu AM, Bahl R, et al. Quality of care for pregnant women and newborns-the WHO vision. BJOG. 2015;122(8):1045-9.
14. Bohren MA, Vogel JP, Hunter EC, Lutsiv O, Makh SK, Souza JP, et al. The Mistreatment of Women during Childbirth in Health Facilities Globally: A Mixed-Methods Systematic Review. PLOS Med. Jun 2015;12(6).
15. Biehl J, Petryna A. When People Come First: Critical studies in global health. Princeton, New Jersey: Princeton University Press; 2013.
16. Hulley S, Cummings S, Browner W, Grady D, Newman T. Designing Clinical Research. Fourth ed. Philadelphia, PA: Lippincott Williams & Wilkins; 2013.
17. Barnes A, Parkhurst J. Can Global Health Policy be Depoliticized? A Critique of Global Calls for Evidence-Based Policy. In: Brown G, Yamey G, Wamala S, editors. The Handbook of Global Health Policy: John Wiley & Sons, Ltd; 2014.
18. Petticrew M, Roberts H. Evidence, hierarchies, and typologies: horses for courses. J Epidemiol Community Health. 2003;57(7):527-9.
19. Adams V. Evidence-Based Global Public Health: Subjects, profits, erasures. In: Biehl J, Petryna A, editors. When People Come First: Critical Studies in Global Health. Princeton, New Jersey: Princeton University Press; 2013.
20. Shiffman J, Smith S. Generation of political priority for global health initiatives: a framework and case study of maternal mortality. Lancet. 2007;370(9595):1370-9.
21. India D. 23% Indian women seek for dignity and respect in maternal healthcare. DNA India. 2016 July 26, 2017.
22. WRASM-Malawi. Health Policy Plus, Summary of a Count of Bedside Midwives in Malawi 2017 [Available from: http://www.healthpolicyplus.com/ns/pubs/7138-7249_WRAMalawiMidwivesBrief.pdf
23. Times N. Malawi needs more midwives amidst acute shortage Nyasa Times. 2017.
24. Times N. Cruelty in labour wards: Maternal health problems in Malawi. Nyasa Times. 2016.
25. Shrestha S. Force MHT, editor2015. Available from: https://www.mhtf.org/document/increasing-accountability-for-provision-of-respectful-maternity-care-in-nepal/.
26. Wendland C. Estimating Death: A close reading of maternal mortality metrics in Malawi. In: Adams V, editor. Metrics: What counts in global health. Durham, North Carolina: Duke University Press; 2016.
27. Oni-Orisan A. The Obligation to Count: The politics of monitoring maternal mortality in Nigeria. In: Adams V, editor. Metrics: What counts in global health. Durham, North Carolina: Duke Univeristy Press; 2016.
28. Downe S. Focusing on what works for person-centred maternity care. Lancet Glob Health. 2019(2214-109X (Electronic).).
29. Ferguson J. The Anti-Politics Machine: Development, Depoliticization, and Bureaucratic Power in Lesotho. Minneapolis, MN: University of Minnesota Press; 1994.

CHAPTER 25

Innovations around the world: case studies of change towards normal labour and positive childbirth

Lisa Bernstein, Tracey Cooper, Ramón Escuriet, Evita Fernandez, Tamsyn Green, Sandra Morano, Mary Newburn, Yoana Stancheva and Melanie Wendland

This chapter presents a series of case studies of activism, service user engagement and service development from around the world. Each section is written in the particular voice of the author, to capture their personal engagement with the topic, as well as the facts and outputs of the work they have done, and are still doing.

A paradigm shift to deliver healthier lives instead of preventing death – case study from Liberia

Lisa Bernstein

In Liberia pregnancy is idiomatically called 'big belly business' and it is the result, of course, of man-woman business. *Big Belly Business* is also the name of a joyous pregnancy book and multi-sectoral programme that plants its feet firmly and happily in an expecting Liberian woman's sandals and engages her partner, her family, her friends, her community – even her mother-in-law(!) to support and celebrate her journey towards motherhood. In a country identified with civil war, Ebola and maternal mortality, *Big Belly Business* is reimagining pregnancy and new parenthood as an opportunity, not just for a baby's birth, but also for a woman's personal rebirth and is working to organise systems and services around the needs of these two generations – helping parents and child thrive, not just survive.

Big Belly Business began by listening carefully to the story of pregnancy in Liberia. Those stories led to the creation of the *Big Belly Business* book which is a gift to every family. The book is a colourful, evidence-based pregnancy guide written in simple Liberian English, filled with stories, health information and wisdom collected from across the country. It is written from the perspective of parents, not experts. Created with Liberian writers, and joyously illustrated by a native artist, *Big Belly Business* is fun to look at and easy to read. Those who can't read can hear it read in the Big Belly Club, or download the audio version on their smartphone or hear it on the radio. A book, journal and pencil are also free for 'big belly women' who join the Club.

Big Belly Clubs are participatory groups that use the book to find evidence-based answers to health questions and the stories, art, and Club 'framework' to spark real conversations. Clubs are facilitated (not led) by trained and certified Big Belly Sisters or Brothers who know their community and personally invite each new 'big belly' to join. Big Belly Sisters are trained traditional midwives, health or literacy educators, community leaders and even two Big Belly Club graduates who run Clubs while attending college (a model we will hope to continue). Important health, family planning and safe delivery information is being discussed, always using the evidence-based information in the book, and contextualised to address the members' concerns. Clubs also address mental health issues, relationships; teaching reading, writing and numbers; creating a group savings club for delivery expenses; starting a vegetable garden, and cooking and recipe writing sessions – all mentioned in the book, and built by and with Club members or Sisters. The BB Sister's capacity expands with new training, partnerships, and program components they have requested (almost demanded!) when they meet to share best practices at BB Network meetings. Special club sessions that include husbands or partners and community members have addressed domestic violence, money (mis) management, men at ANC visits (and in the delivery room), endorsing staying at a maternal waiting home, and even a community discussion that led to a meeting with the closest hospital to plan a new triage strategy for emergencies.

All is not rosy in the *Big Belly Business* book or in Liberia. First person narratives address the powerful, traditional myths and practices of pregnancy that still influence a woman's access to medical care. These and stories of midwives as caring but overworked people, and crowded healthcare systems with limited capacity and compassion help Big Belly Sisters start difficult but very real and important conversations that do much more to encourage behaviour changes than any 'health message' to attend ANC or 'have a safe delivery' could ever accomplish. Big Belly Sisters have started to branch out – running Big Belly Clubs in clinic waiting rooms, accompanying women to ANC visits and even acting as doulas during delivery. The two-year pilot – with 50,000 books, reaching over 20,000 women, engaged 18 NGOs in 8 counties with over 138 trained Big Belly Sisters – has already amassed extraordinary anecdotes of changed behaviour, knowledge and attitudes.

The Clubs are just the first part of a reinterpretation of the pregnancy experience in Liberia. The Liberian Association of Nurses and Midwives has adopted *Big Belly Business* into their national training curriculum – to teach community health, health literacy, social determinants of health and respectful maternal care. Using a similar participatory learning and group discussion approach, the Big Belly philosophy plans to support the midwives, community health workers, clerks and guards who are trying to rebuild an overstressed system, giving them a chance to share their experience and identify their role in the story of pregnancy through group discussion and narrative. Quality Improvement strategies for healthcare systems is really about human development – and building opportunities for each of us to learn, find support and create change – truly making Big Belly Business Everybody's Business.

Simply Put Media is a non-profit that brings together the neuroscience of adult learning, with research on a myriad of social determinants of health from self-care and nurturing-care to respectful maternal care, the importance of fathers, the influence of adverse childhood experiences, and the role of language, gender, identity and power on the culture of pregnancy – all within a strength-based, joyful framework that develops the adult cortex and the associated skills of empathy, self-reflection and critical thinking that are the foundation of a civil society. Big Belly Business was funded by the US State Department Office of Global Women as the Women's Health Innovation Program (WHIP). The pilot was a partnership of the Open Society Initiative in West Africa (OSIWA) 18 NGOs and Simply Put the US and Liberian NGO that now leads the partnership and houses the Big Belly Business Network. The team also created Babu Barta in Bangladesh as part of WHIP. Simply Put is eager to partner in Liberia and is ready to replicate elsewhere. www.simplyputmedia.org

Key points for consideration

Here are questions and activities that will help put your mind into a Simply Put way of thinking:

1. We listen carefully to the story of pregnancy. What does that mean? Well first, to understand a story, you need to identify all of the characters. Perhaps gather together to answer these questions:

- Who are the important characters in the story of pregnancy in your country?
- If you brought together a group of parents and asked them who was important would their answers be different than if you asked a group of midwives and doctors?
- If you brought a group of religious leaders together or the clerical staff at a clinic – who would they think were important characters?

Writing a list of ALL of the people who have influence over the beliefs, understanding, and experiences of expecting women – the 'who' – is an important first step to seeing the bigger picture of the story of pregnancy in your country and culture and who has influence over making changes to that story.

2. Listening carefully to the story of pregnancy means listening to everyone on your list of characters in order to understand everyone's perspective. Here's a way to figure out what people know and believe to be true about pregnancy.

- Make a list of everything you believe pregnant women SHOULD do and yet, according to your research or studies, they just don't do.

- Turn that list into a question 'Why do you think pregnant women do (and don't) do this?' Ask and record your and your colleagues' answers.
- Ask all of the characters in the pregnancy story for their insights into this question. Do not explain, judge or tell them what you think. Simply ask with curiosity what they believe.

3. Be an actor. Imagine you are an expecting woman (or man) in your 'story of pregnancy'. Now act it out – in real life. Get in disguise and take a walk in a pregnant woman's sandals (or boots, or flip-flops) and experience ANC as they do. Be a 'secret shopper'. Through those eyes, notice what rules, services, health advice really work for 'your character's life', and what seems organised to work, instead, for the system's needs.

These are the first steps towards reimagining the story of pregnancy for your families.

Leading with compassion: making the impossible happen

Tracey Cooper

In 2012 I was working in a maternity service in the North of England, which had a freestanding birth centre that was under threat of closure through lack of use. Following the publication of the Birthplace study (Hollowell et al, 2011) the organisation wanted to develop plans for an alongside birth centre. Although some obstetricians and midwives were keen for the developments, there were some barriers to change. My strategy therefore was to ensure decision-makers understood the evidence for the proposed changes, and potential benefits the new service could bring for women and families, and the organisation as a whole. This included financial elements, in that the birth centres would result in financial savings. I collected qualitative data from women by attending service user groups and via a telephone survey. A successful bid for financial assistance from the Department of Health supported the creation of an alongside birth centre and refurbishment of the freestanding birth centre. The NICE guideline on intrapartum care for healthy women (2014) and the National Maternity Review (NHS England, 2016) have since been published and support the availability of midwifery-led settings for women with uncomplicated pregnancies.

Both birth centres were developed to ensure birth companions were involved as much as possible. Family rooms with double beds are provided for after the birth or drop-down double beds in the birthing rooms used for the rest of their stay. Bonding for the family is viewed as an essential part at this important time. Following the birth, partners are welcome to stay for up to 24 hours. Being active in labour and birth is encouraged using beanbags, birth balls, couches and pools.

Evidence on place of birth was and still is being used to maximum effect, changing the birth experiences of women and their families and improving the working lives of midwives. The freestanding birth centre is an integral part of the community. The impact is recognised nationally and internationally as an example of using evidence to change midwifery practice. Midwifery teams work in an integrated model between community and the birth centres. By providing this model it is improving continuity of care provided to women. The midwives and a maternity support worker work in small geographical teams providing birthing services at home and the two birth centres. They also provide antenatal and postnatal care in the community to all women throughout their childbirth experience. The teams have enthusiastically taken this way of working forward and are improving outcomes for women, improving the skills of midwives in normal birth, improving women's experiences, and enhancing job satisfaction.

The number of births at both establishments has continually increased, while the home birth rate remained unchanged. The increased use of water and reduced epidural rate has cut the expenditure for maternity services. Collaboration between the midwifery and obstetric teams, family doctors and commissioners helped to develop confidence throughout the process and as a result midwifery-led settings are promoted by all of these groups. The service supports the challenge of 'getting birth right first time', as the first birth will influence the next and subsequent births.

Key points for consideration

- Use the evidence to make your points. The NICE Intrapartum guideline provides tables of outcomes of each place of birth. These are extremely useful to discuss with women and their families and with other professionals.
- Keep 'chipping' away! Sit down with key people inside and outside the organisation, including service user groups and ensure they know the evidence. Ensure the multidisciplinary team know the evidence so they can discuss it with women and their families.
- Ensure you connect with others outside of the organisation who can support you.
- Be brave and courageous. Speak out when no one else will. Be a tall poppy.

Thank you to everyone at Lancashire Teaching Hospitals for your support and to the women and their families who have supported the journey (you know who you are ☺).

References

Cooper T (2013) Relaunch of a Freestanding Birth Centre to Promote Normal Birth. In: World Health Organization (WHO) Good practices in nursing and midwifery – from expert to expert: A manual for creating country case studies. WHO. Copenhagen

NHS England (2016) Better Births: A five Year Forward View for Maternity Care. https://www.england.nhs.uk/wp-content/uploads/2016/02/national-maternity-review-report.pdf (last accessed 20.1.17)

Hollowell J, Puddicombe D, Rowe R (2011). The Birthplace National Prospective Cohort Study: Perinatal and Maternal Outcomes by Planned Place of Birth. Birthplace in England Research Programme. Final Report Part 4. NIHR Service Delivery and Organisation prog http://www.sdo.nihr.ac.uk/projdetails.php?ref=08-1604-140

NICE (2014) Intrapartum Care for Women with Uncomplicated Pregnancies. CG190. https://www.nice.org.uk/guidance/cg190/resources/intrapartum-care-for-healthy-women-and-babies-35109866447557 (last accessed 20.1.17)

Changing the model of childbirth care through continuous assessment and participation: case study from Catalonia, Spain

Ramón Escuriet

Childbirth care in Catalonia has undergone important changes in recent years. Not only through improvements in clinical practice, but also by the adequacy of the spaces within some obstetric units. Many factors have contributed to these changes in childbirth care, from new evidence on best practice for optimal maternity care, to social and political changes that may have had an impact on health services' performance. Starting from the existing biomedical model, the changes have not been easy. The hierarchical organisation of the teams and the orientation of the care have had to adapt towards a model focused on the needs of women and their families. This has meant overcoming resistance on the part of the organisations themselves and of some health professionals.

Evaluation as a facilitator for change

In our case, it has been important to create adequate evaluation tools, and then to disseminate the results. The evaluation not only included aspects such as intervention rates, but also findings from surveys of women's satisfaction levels. This evaluation is continuous and dynamic, by incorporating new elements to provide information to those responsible for health policies. Up to now, and generally speaking, our evaluation has shown that hospitals with low intervention rates have improved maternal and newborn health, and promote women's participation and midwifery care. In our context, politicians are those who set the priorities of the health system and then hospital administrators are responsible for the implementing of such priorities and actions in each centre. But women and health professionals can also exert social pressure to create the optimum conditions for maternity care. It is for this reason that it is important to disseminate to all the results of the evaluation.

Best practice as change facilitators

Promoting and disseminating best practice carried out in a facility or by a group of health professionals can contribute to improve maternity care across the whole health system, but for this we must ensure that what works is transferred to, or replicated in, other centres. In our case, organising national workshops so that the professionals have the opportunity to present their work, has helped to extend good practice across the hospitals in our health system.

Showing variations

When evaluating maternity care performance in our context, we found important variations in intervention rates that are not justified by the clinical conditions of women, but that may be explained by the type of organisation of each centre. Increased rates of interventions have not been associated with better health outcomes for mothers or children, so it has been important to show these results and consider these findings for maternity health services planning and for the prioritisation of new health policy actions.

The involvement of women and professionals

In Catalonia there is an advisory committee for Sexual and Reproductive Health that independently assesses policies and proposes improvements. Institutions, women's representatives and health professional representatives form this committee. To promote a change in our model of care, it has been important to ensure that the committee has the results of the maternity care performance evaluation. Debating the results within the committee has made it possible to achieve consensus and propose improvements to policy-makers.

The proposed improvements have been included in the Catalonia health policy framework for the 2016–20 period. The Catalonia Health Plan for 2016–20 includes a compulsory action, which is to review the normal childbirth model of care in public hospitals. This fact gives the opportunity to create midwife-led units and also to promote women's decision-making regarding childbirth care. The fact that this action is included in the Health Plan means that hospital managers feel involved and facilitate such improvements. Also, the official protocols of the Ministry of Health for normal pregnancy and intrapartum care are now including the option for MLU to be chosen by women.

Key points for consideration

- Involvement of health services personnel who are responsible for planning maternity care is important for to ensure the way maternity services is evaluated is effective. This should also include continuous evaluation and benchmarking among health services providers.
- Variations: use the current maternity care indicators for the evaluation (those commonly used in your context), then show the variations among different hospitals or settings to policy-makers and stakeholders.
- Explore clinical practice and service organisation in those settings (hospitals) with best results. Write a report and show it to policy-makers!
- Disseminate results among the population and health professionals. Let people know what works and give power to those who can exert social and political pressure.
- For policy-makers: include improvement actions among priority political actions and maintain a continuous and fluid communication system between politicians and all stakeholders.

Promoting normal birth through developing midwives: an example from India

Evita Fernandez

I was one of those very fortunate young doctors to have inherited a hospital, which was painstakingly put together by my parents. Given a head start, I quickly worked on developing a perinatal tertiary referral unit with the hope of providing comprehensive care for women and their babies. The most challenging and heartbreaking moments occurred when young mothers referred to us with multi-organ failure died without giving us a chance to attempt treatment. This led me to read all I could on maternal mortality and I discovered that countries with low maternal and newborn mortality were those who had invested in professional midwives. India did not establish this unique cadre. I felt compelled to pilot a two-year in-house Professional Midwifery Education and Training (PMET) programme with the objective of understanding the essence of midwifery care and hopefully utilising human resources more effectively. I felt if we could produce professional midwives and have them in the community we could perhaps aim to reduce maternal morbidity and mortality. Coupled with this was the realisation that we as a tertiary referral perinatal centre had grown horribly interventional and birth was looked upon as a potential life-threatening emergency.

A lot to unlearn, and much more to learn

Thanks to the generosity, leadership and interest of senior midwives from the UK who volunteered time to teach and train, today we have 35 qualified midwives and 13 trainees in the wings. Many vital lessons were learnt – the topmost being the understanding and appreciation of woman-centred care, the importance of mobility and freedom to birth in positions of choice, the efficacy and safety of non-pharmacological options of pain relief, the magical beauty of birthing in water and the humbling acceptance of the reality that emerged – low-risk pregnant women preferred midwifery care and did not need us obstetricians.

There was a lot I had to unlearn and much more to learn. It was exciting, challenging but worth every moment. From an interventional perspective, I switched to a non-interventional approach. The 20-member obstetric consultant team joined me in introspecting and reviewing every intervention we 'offered' virtually by default!

I was in awe of women who birthed naturally. I regained my lost sense of wonder and belief in a woman's ability to birth and THAT called for a whole new understanding of the physiology of birth. I began to read everything I could on natural birth and realised this had opened up a whole new world, which demanded new thinking.

PROMISE of a brighter future

The midwifery programme has multiple positive impacts and influenced the quality of our care. A feedback survey introduced in 2014 (still running) to understand birthing women's views on midwifery support and care convinced me to launch the campaign PROMISE (PROfessional MIdwifery SErvices) with four objectives:

- Making pregnancy and childbirth safe
- To humanise birth

- Train a workforce of professional midwives
- Promote professional midwifery

The PROMISE campaign was strengthened by the presence of Ms Inderjeet Kaur, a consultant midwife from London, who took several years sabbatical to help teach/train/mentor midwives in the in-house programme. She was instrumental in establishing a confident team of midwives to support women who wished to birth in water. She also ensured the midwives were confident to train and run 'hands-on' workshops for nurses and doctors across the state and neighbouring states of India.

In November 2017, the Government of Telangana State invited us to run a midwifery-training programme for a cohort of 30 registered nurses with varying years of experience in maternity services. UNICEF facilitated the private-public partnership and ensured the unique tripartite venture of introducing professional midwifery into public hospitals would be a success.

It has been soul satisfying to work with this diverse group of experienced obstetric nurses who in the first six weeks of the 18-month course were encouraged to focus on respectful maternity care. Using different techniques, which included role-play, reflective discussions, videos and interactive talks, the trainees began to introspect on the topic. This led to an open sharing of experiences, which in turn motivated the trainees to believe they were now 'agents of change', who will firmly embed respectful care into their individual practice as midwives. The training programme was completed with the first cohort of trainees graduating and receiving their certificates on 5 May 2019, the International Day of the Midwife.

As a seasoned obstetrician (three decades) I am today convinced that India needs professional midwives forming the foundation of maternity services. It has been a privilege to contribute towards this goal.

The Government of India, in December 2018, announced its commitment to promote and establish professional midwifery as a vital component of the country's maternity services. This decision provides a channel to help establish woman-centred respectful maternity care.

Key points for consideration

- The training curriculum for obstetricians must include a full understanding of natural birth and woman-centred care. Only then will obstetricians see another way.
- Midwives and obstetricians must learn to work together with mutual respect and trust – to offer the collaborative model of care, where the midwife is the primary carer for low-risk pregnancies and birth.
- In low-income, high-population settings like India, midwives meeting global standards of skill and competence are vitally and urgently needed.

Eve's Mama: a beacon of hope for positive birth in Kenya

Tamsyn Green

When I travelled to Kenya in spring 2017 public hospitals and health centres were in turmoil following a strike, which was the result of doctors exasperated by low pay, unpaid overtime, inadequate resources and suspected embezzlement of the national health budget. Women that can afford health insurance will usually have obstetric-led care in private hospitals, where caesarean-section rates are high, but the majority of women in Kenya give birth without a skilled health professional (World Health Organization, 2016).The picture of maternity care is therefore one of extremes – under-resourced government services and obstetric-led private healthcare. The result: a persistently high morbidity and mortality rate alongside an increasing number of caesarean sections. Initiatives to promote normal birth are therefore challenging to set up but desperately needed.

In Kenya everyone has a side hustle: nannies make soap to sell at weekends and taxi drivers grow maize up country. Lucy Muchiri is a midwife, a doula, a childbirth educator and a businesswoman with an inspiring model of maternity care. Predominantly working in hospitals, Lucy became frustrated by the lack of information given to women, the high levels of intervention and the subsequent physical and emotional trauma that she witnessed. Her own birth experiences consolidated her belief that birth is a unique event in a woman's life that requires individualised, holistic care. This led her to become a doula and antenatal teacher. The first home birth she attended was as a favour for a friend, but in less than a year she'd established herself as an independent midwife. Shortly after, Lucy founded Nairobi's first birth centre, Eve's Mama.

Lucy's small team share a caseload of about 80 women, almost a quarter of whom have a home birth. Meeting Quinn and Cecilia revealed the extent to which Lucy's practice differs from the norm – both midwives had previously worked in hospitals and felt that the care they were now able to give was revolutionary: 'In hospitals women don't have a chance to labour normally'; 'lots of interventions are carried out unnecessarily'. It's not uncommon for doulas to refuse to support women at home births, which illustrates the systemic medicalisation of birth and the pioneering work that Lucy and her team have undertaken.

The midwives at Eve's Mama run antenatal classes for women in their third trimester. Many couples plan to have their baby at hospital with doula support. However, towards the end of pregnancy, what they have learnt about the labour process and the finely balanced cocktail of hormones that it depends on, leads most women to choose midwife-led care. The antenatal classes include exercises to encourage optimum pelvic alignment and foetal positioning, information about the labour process and how to prepare for birth, as well as a chance for couples to share fears and anxieties. The valuable information is reinforced through freely available videos that Lucy has made to answer questions that she is regularly asked as a midwife.

A significant number of women in their caseload have had previous ceasarean sections, most never fully understanding the indication. For many of these women opting for a vaginal birth is a brave decision because it is widely believed that obstetric-led care is the safest choice. Medicalised birth is also idealised because it represents modernity and progress. Couples at Eve's Mama often make good friends, which is important because they may not be supported in their choices by other friends and family. One woman I met cried as she told us how alone she felt simply because she wanted to give birth at home, and was later ridiculed when things hadn't gone to plan.

The positive correlation between for-profit healthcare and caesarean section rates has recently been highlighted in a study by Hoxha et al (2017).[*] Fortunately, the continuity of care provided by the midwives at Eve's Mama is a beacon of hope for women seeking a positive and safe birth experience in Nairobi.

Key points for consideration

- Improve your knowledge and skills by accessing online resources.
- Share your knowledge, skills and initiatives through online resources.
- Set up forums and spaces for women to be able to support one another in their birth choices and experiences.
- Eve's Mama website evesmama.com and videos on YouTube: @evesmama

Building midwifery: facts and considerations from an obstetrician's perspective

Sandra Morano

In 2000 a group of women clinicians, an obstetrician and some midwives were able to open the first Italian alongside birth centre. It was not a gift, but the last step of a long stressful and thrilling process towards a women-centered birth setting. They all sensed how essential it was to change the organisation and structure of birth places, or the principles of care so that they could enable normal birth. The opening of the new site happened in Genoa, in a large old hospital. This is the story of its beginnings, a story about the tenacity of the women involved, and their dignity, compassionate care, and solidarity. It shows the importance of working for the same aim, with all involved sharing lives, battles, defeats and authority. It is told from an obstetrician's point of view, showing all the barriers I met in working on this agenda without any allies among my obstetric colleagues, and all the stages of a progressive shift from a traditional medical perspective towards midwifery as a new conceptual framework. Building a new culture for all professionals involved in childbirth is the biggest challenge for the future. It needs vision, humility, heart, sensible choices and also facts and the development of practices suitable to be transferred to young professionals, women, and society.

---

[*] Hoxha I, Syrogiannouli L, Luta X, et al. Caesarean sections and for-profit status of hospitals: systematic review and metaanalysis. *BMJ Open* 2017;7: e013670. doi:10.1136/bmjopen-2016-013670

Getting official authorisation can change your life and mark a point of no return in your work: both your workplace and your professional and personal life will never be the same again. You're free to introduce important little changes. In our case, this started with colour. When the hospital decorators first saw their orange brushstrokes in the corridors of the new birth centre, and their colour tests on the walls, that made us all feel like we were in an Almodovar film, or a Mexican village, they looked at each other in astonishment and then started to enjoy it. They called us in to look at each new experiment, starting off with the few colours available to us, to see what we thought of it. And the same thing happened with all the other workmen and tradesmen, the carpenters, the electricians and so on, who responded to ever more unusual requests from this new hospital ward.

It didn't take much, with IKEA furnishings, to replace the useless, antiquated hospital equipment, to turn a sad, anaemic-looking ward into the first alongside birth centre in Italy, with five ensuite bedrooms on a single floor comprising a beautiful terrace, a room for water births, and an outpatient clinic which could also be used for meetings with the women visiting the centre; together with all this, we opened a door whose reach and repercussions we could only begin to imagine at the time. Up until then we had been squeezed into the cramped space of the delivery room, in constant conflict with our midwife, paediatrician and nurse colleagues; now this self-managed space, separate from the official wards, was ours to define, and ultimately, to defend. Those first years were terrible and, at the same time, exhilarating. On the one hand, women appreciated this new model of care, and on the other, we still had the obstetricians, my colleagues, in their typical peculiar way, looking on their patients as their property, to butter up or terrorise as they pleased, a sport begun last century for this specialisation and which still goes on today. Checking up on, quoting or denigrating clinical studies depending on the situation, in contrast with the quiet fascination of hospital procedures, so reassuring and undisputed. Not to mention the war on anything which is different, mistrust of anything new, seen at best as a source of problems, in a job which is already difficult enough.

And so, as a result of this change, my professional life was lived from the midwife's perspective. It was actually midwives who had studied and demonstrated that the best outcomes of birth practice came from non-specialists; they were the ones, together with epidemiologists, and (the few) enlightened obstetricians, who had shown that most routine procedures were in fact useless, or even harmful; they were the ones who had set up the first birth centres in Europe and Australia. They were the ones who reported the effects of interference on the part of specialists on the progress and outcome of labour. I had no doubt about whose side I was on. I felt uncomfortable in the world of 'Medicine for Women', while I'd like rather to teach and practice a 'Medicine of Women'. So from then on I was with my midwife colleagues, some of whom were streets ahead and well prepared to face the challenge together, and to try out new ways of working which would free them up to humanise their relationships with women.

I now had a centre which I could manage independently, where I could at last bring together all the characteristics I had previously judged to be positive. The moment had come to put them into practice. But the price to pay was my separation from what, up until that time, had been my professional community. A colleague said to me: '*But why?*

From now on you'll be only involved in the physiological side of things …think carefully about it'. He was expressing, for me, a regret which I myself did not feel, as I was already leaning in that direction. Throughout these last, long years, I have lived among midwives, I've seen their world of tried and tested traditional practices, I've suffered for the limitations placed on their profession by specialists in labour wards, but also for their inability to stay united and, more recently, for their tendency towards imitating medicalised procedures and even, alas, teaching methods.

I watched from afar the world which was mine, and which I still belong to, suspended in a sort of limbo. I don't like its standards, its lack of balance with regard to patients, keystone of the paternalism present in treatment 'for women'. I dislike the total lack of any kind of educational project, as everything, from prevention to freedom of choice is ruled by the market. Over the years, from my somewhat detached observation post, and in part due to the financial crisis, I have seen an upsurge in the debate around private patients; I've seen suspicion of midwife-led normal birth as dangerous, and I've noticed a certain self-referentiality, all of which are contributing to the end of obstetrics, in my view. I am not comfortable with this situation. I'm searching for outside alliances and new eyes to cure the short-sighted thinking afflicting the dissatisfied. I've taken note of the bewilderment of new graduates, despite the fact that they are for the most part women; so young and so frustrated, women with male minds lining up for a piece of the power over female bodies. My colleague was wrong about one thing, though; to paraphrase a Bertold Brecht quote *'it's simplicity/which is difficult/to achieve'*, it's normality which is the most difficult thing to cultivate in this context.

But who cares about normality? Not the specialist, who delegates it to the midwife, who is taught according to medical canons. Who researches it, or considers it a precious gift? Who promotes it? And who should receive it? I have learned through humility over the years that normality is the fruit of so many competencies, and many different abilities found in various fields, and is the most difficult thing of all to define, the most complex to maintain. Helping women to discover and understand the strongest and strangest of abilities, the transformation of body and mind, a form of pure creativity, not just physical, but an extraordinary 'natural laboratory of molecular biology' as scientists put it – our training makes us incapable of studying the capacity for adaptation involved.

We are always ready to step in, to turn normality into pathology, to build new parameters of 'physiology': curves, ranges, cut off points, to be calculated continuously in the search for figures/criteria and abilities to hone to perfection: age, BMI, weight in pregnancy, and then BP and AFI and so on and so on … all in the search for the indentikit of Miss Birth, the only one that can guarantee relative calm. I'm happy to have been involved in all of this, even though I am on the margins of the scientific community I belong to. A community which reigns supreme over the entire, and generally healthy, female population; which cannot seem to offer ways to achieve global wellbeing, or integrity in giving birth, which does not prioritise these goals, and which has still not managed to objectively analyse the reasons for the rapid rise in the number of caesarean sections, which nowadays in Italy is mainly attributed to hospital logistics, or, rather, to the continuing existence of too many facilities with less than 500 births a year.

Pending an unlikely overhaul of the hospital system, somewhat difficult to achieve in a time of dramatic restrictions in health services, and given the current political vision, we need to address without delay the redefining of the aims of midwifery both for students and professionals. In an ever fiercer and more powerful reproduction market, and in the face of uncertainty due to the fear of medical liability, it is probably inconceivable to imagine reducing the number of operative births simply by rethinking the mission. Who will be able to reconcile the thousand-year history of midwifery with the day-to-day stories of these last few decades, in order to try to redefine its purpose and restore trust between the players? This is not the stuff of specialists, as recent times have proved.

And yet... Participating in Optibirth, an interdisciplinary European study whose aim was to reduce the number of C-sections through increasing VBAC (www.Optibirth.eu), I had the opportunity to hear both what women really want, and also how midwives and obstetricians think nowadays. Some of them remember a time when they worked towards the same goals to care for women during labour, each using their particular skills at the right moment. What surprised me about clinicians who still remember the old ways was their willingness to take part in a study which aimed to encourage vaginal delivery, to share other women's positive experiences and to support the health professionals: the power of ideas, the power of words. I'm taking the apparently disarming anachronism of this challenge as a (post)modern opportunity: and who knows? Maybe we can start up all together a new educational project using the power of words, the strength of equity, and trust in women's competence to safely and joyfully give birth to the future of humanity.

Key points for consideration

- Standard birthplaces can change.
- Everyone is able to achieve, it doesn't need heroes/heroines.
- If you feel uncomfortable in your workplace, you have to try to change it. Either as a pregnant woman or as a clinician working there, don't hesitate, don't postpone, don't give up.
- Seek out alliances, look for other women, mothers, associations.
- Don't get tired to knock on doors, speak, explain, listen.
- If you're pregnant, remember that birth is (one of) the most important experiences in your life.
- If you're a clinician (in particular a young female obstetrician) remember that you'll spend most of your life in birthplaces.
- Changing places of birth means building new spaces in which empathy and confidence can be normally expressed.
- There's no change without supporting an appropriate education able to reverse the fear-risk duo recently raised in childbirth, and finally, in our lives.
- Changing structures means having in mind different childbirth care models, requires attitude, study and courage as well, to deal with difficulties, battles, ridicule. However it means building salutogenesis, equality, gratitude, love.

Childbirth activism in the UK

Mary Newburn

I got involved with other women and made tentative steps towards influencing local maternity services at the end of the 1970s, when my first two sons were young, with an NCT branch in Grange-over-Sands, England.

I had wanted to give birth using relaxation and breathing. I'd read Sheila Kitzinger's *Some women's experiences of childbirth* and my mum had had four homebirths. It just seemed the right thing for me. In my first pregnancy, I was transferred from a midwifery/GP unit to an obstetric unit as my baby was occipito-posterior at 39 weeks. The environment was brutal, all hard white tiles and duckboards on the floor. Many of the staff were grumbling and chilly towards me (a frightened 18-year-old). However, one midwife made a real connection when I so badly needed kindness. She believed in me and gave me encouragement. I learned so powerfully what a difference the attitudes and behaviour of staff make to a woman's experience. Now, decades later and those two sons both fathers, I am still motivated to work for change.

In the UK, there is a rich history of childbirth activism and voluntary sector influence on maternity policies, on services, research and evidence reviews, and on guidance to the NHS. Influence varies from low-key input to more overt 'activism'. Activism can be defined as 'vigorous campaigning to bring about political or social change' or simply 'activities undertaken to create positive change', as Karen Spring explores in her Communication4health blog (2013).

The National Childbirth Trust (NCT)

After graduating from university as a mature student and working in research, I joined the NCT staff in 1988. NCT involvement provides informal network support as well as formal influencing opportunities. After attending a brilliant NCT antenatal course, I had trained as an antenatal teacher in 1980. NCT's training courses for its practitioners raised awareness about physiological birth and breastfeeding. Talking and reflecting with well-read, networked women raised my awareness about issues of gender and power. Many NCT practitioners, as well as providing support and information to expectant and new parents, also worked to influence NHS maternity services. Their interests were very varied, and included extending choice of place of birth; improving the birth environment, e.g. getting birthing pools installed; supporting home birth services and birth centres; and promoting continuity of midwifery care. As with so many voluntary organisations, great innovations were forged through new relationships and shared interests.

I was involved in some of NCT's key influencing work in the 1990s and 2000s. NCT set up the Maternity Care Working Party in 1999 and organised conferences with the Royal College of Midwives (RCM) and the Royal College of Obstetricians and Gynaecologists (RCOG) on The rising caesarean rate: a public health issue and The rising caesarean rate: from audit to action. The charity worked with members of parliament to establish the All Party Parliamentary Group on Maternity (APPGM) in 2000, providing the secretariat, suggesting speakers and briefing politicians. A consensus statement on normal labour and birth, Making normal birth a reality, was developed collaboratively through the Maternity Care Working Party with multiple stakeholders including the RCM, the RCOG and BirthChoiceUK (see below). The statement was launched at an APPGM meeting (Maternity Care Working Party, 2007; Werkmeister et al, 2008). During the Working Party's most active period, working closely with BirthchoiceUK, the decline in the normal birth rate in England was stopped and even briefly reversed. But when the campaigning work ceased the normal birth rates continued to decline. We cannot be sure that this change in recorded rates was the result of the Maternity Care Working Party and related activities at that time, but I believe that without continuing active leadership, the tide of medicalisation continues to rise, pulled by desire to reduce stillbirths, lack of knowledge and experience of physiological labour and birth, particular perceptions of risk, and changing demographics (women having babies when they are older, more first-time babies, more primary caesareans and higher levels of obesity, to name a few). We were pleased to be able to work with the Albany Midwives, pioneers in delivering woman-centred care to women in an area of high deprivation and ethnic diversity. Their model of care included continuity of midwifery care and offering home birth. Becky Reed, and the parents she worked with, provided photographic images we could use in publications, to show what physiological birth looks like.

In 2018, the NCT had around 46,000 members across the UK and parents in 90,000 households attended an NCT course. This means that around 13–14% of families having a baby attended an NCT course, indicating the extent of the charity's local networks. Recent NCT campaigns have centred around maternal mental health and consistent provision of 6–8 week postnatal health appointments.

BirthChoiceUK

In 2001, a new organisation, BirthChoiceUK, launched a website to help women choose where to give birth. Miranda Scanlon (then Dodwell) and Rod Gibson were two parents with a strong commitment and the skills to provide women with accessible, epidemiological data about different places for birth. Their pioneering work changed the way women could access information about their birth options and related maternity data. They later collaborated with the trusted consumer association Which? to provide a really useful interactive 'where to give birth' guide. The original comprehensive Which Birth Choice website with detailed birth data for each NHS trust is no longer available, but legacy information on their main site still serves to raise awareness about birth choices. In 2021, BirthChoiceUK worked with Best Beginnings on their updated, accessible, interactive, highly visual app, Baby Buddy 2.0, to provide direct links to birth options pages on NHS trust websites

National Maternity Voices and National Maternity Partnerships

Activists have worked to create structural changes, so that parents can have a voice within every local maternity service. In the UK, maternity service liaison committees (MSLCs), multi-disciplinary planning and monitoring groups usually chaired by a service user or 'lay person', have been functioning for over 30 years, but they have had varying degrees of political and professional support and funding. Without the infrastructure of budgets, NHS Executive guidance, marketing, etc, MSLCs varied widely from active to atrophied (Calvert, 2016, Newburn et al 2017). Then, in 2016, MSLCs had an overhaul in England, becoming maternity voices partnerships (Newburn, 2016; NHS England, 2017) with an explicit commitment to co-production (Coalition for Collaborative Care and NHS England, 2016; Newburn and Fletcher, 2015). See some case studies at 'NCT', in References below.

National Maternity Voices, the MVP coordinating body, is now established, with elected representatives and part-time staff, funded by NHS England (see links below), providing toolkits, a lively discussion forum for sharing good practice and problem-solving, and mentoring support for MVP chairs, with priority for Black, Asian and minority ethnic women.

People who are involved in working for change over decades can be described as persistent maternity activists, a phrase coined by Eugene Declercq at the Normal Birth Research conference in Sydney in 2016. I really like this positive affirmation for those who make a difference through long-term commitment. There are many individuals who fit this description, among them midwives, researchers, doctors, policymakers, and people working from a service user perspective). But, lobbying has become polarised, with some groups focusing more on outcomes for babies and others on birth from a woman's perspective. It is important to find common ground and to avoid separating into adversarial factions. We should have a both/ and approach.

We need to think about labour and birth in an historical and cultural context. And, as Chimamanda Ngozi Adichie says, 'we should all be feminists'! We need to ensure that both women and their babies have the best opportunity to give birth safely and joyfully. We need to support pregnant women and new mothers to speak and be heard. We need a strong movement of activists with knowledge, insights and commitment to keep plugging away for change. All woman need to be well informed, well supported and competently cared for with kindness and respect for their personal autonomy.

Mary Newburn, Patient and Public Involvement Lead for Maternity and Perinatal Mental Health Theme, ARC South London, King's College London. Issues discussed here are explored in greater depth in Newburn M. MIDIRS Midwifery Digest, vol 27, no 1, March 2017, pp5-10 www.midirs.org/women-maternity-services-user-involvement-uk

References

BirthChoiceUK see https://bit.ly/3n8BVsS

Calvert H, (2016). Why your MSLC matters. https://bit.ly/2YqUVJ5

Coalition for Collaborative Care and NHS England (2016). A Co-production Model; Five values and seven steps to make this happen in reality.

Maternity Care Working Party (2007). Making normal birth a reality. Consensus statement from the Maternity Care Working Party: our shared views about the need to recognise, facilitate and audit normal birth. London: NCT/RCM/RCOG.

National Maternity Voices http://nationalmaternityvoices.org.uk/, https://bit.ly/MVPDiversity

NCT case studies: https://www.nct.org.uk/professional/mslcs, https://bit.ly/LewishamMSLC2015, https://bit.ly/CaldedaleBirth

Newburn M, (2016). Maternity Voices Partnership the new MSLC. Practising Midwife 19(10):8-12.

Newburn M, Easter A, Fletcher G et al (2017). Maternity partnership working - mapping MSLCs in England. The Practising Midwife 20(1):26.

Newburn M, Fletcher G (2015). Running your Maternity Services Liaison Committee: a practical guide from good practice to troubleshooting. London: NCT. http://bit.ly/2j6r13L

Ngozi Adichie, C. We should all be feminists. Fourth Estate. First presented as a TED talk given in the United Kingdom at TEDxEuston, 2012.

NHS England (2017) Implementing Better Births; A resource pack for Local Maternity Systems. NHS England.

Spring K (2013) Advocacy versus Activism: What is the difference? https://bit.ly/2YqUVJ5

Werkmeister G, Jokinen M, Mahmood T, Newburn M. Making normal labour and birth a reality – developing a multi-disciplinary consensus. Midwifery 2008;24(3):256-9.

Which? Where to give birth 12 July 2021 https://bit.ly/3tfSOCZ

Zebra Midwives striping the circle in Bulgaria

Yoana Stancheva

This section describes the process of moving from Bulgarian maternity services that had no space for autonomous midwifery, to care provision that now offers increasing access to midwifery care. Somewhere amid all the hard work, despair blossomed into a beautiful network of mentorship, lifelong friendships and, ultimately, genuine hope. The feeling that the struggle for improving maternity services in Bulgaria is a lost cause may still be lurking sometimes, but it is no longer everything that we feel. We are now part of a transnational circle of trust and support which cannot be manipulated or overruled by local sentiments. We now know that we belong to a global community which will always back us up in our struggles, or at least hold our coats while we fight for evidence-based, respectful care in Bulgaria.

No trodden path that we could follow

It all started with the dream for establishing the first autonomous midwifery practice, Zebra Midwives. Being a midwife and a primary caregiver in Bulgaria is about as foreign as a zebra strolling about in Eastern Europe. Still in midwifery school, we were far from obtaining our diplomas and ever further away from providing midwifery-led care on our own. However, we were determined to create a positive space for women to receive childbirth education, prenatal and intrapartum care like never before. No one before had tried offering evidence-based midwifery or continuity of care, and there was no trodden path that we could follow. Just the opposite, the organisation of maternity services in the country and the culture of birth were going to be our greatest hurdles to overcome. After much brainstorming and deliberation for a general strategy, two things emerged for us as must-haves for our dream to come true. One, we had to be so proactive and motivated to an extent that would feel exhausting and uncomfortable throughout. Two, we needed solid international support.

International support

Having embraced the level of 'crazy' that we would have to maintain, we sought the international allies that would help us make a case for midwifery and women. We used every opportunity to attend conferences where we could speak about a feasible plan that would be achieved if we had international support. Professor Soo Downe, UK, has been instrumental in connecting us to a rich network of midwives and obstetricians who listened to our plan and took our plan to heart. Obstetrician Professor Sandra Morano from Italy shared her birth centre, her expertise and time to serve as an example for how we can make the first steps. Dr Tracey Cooper, UK, has literally held our hands through the beginning stages of Zebra and has made us feel much more confident in our clinical skills and rapport with women. Dr Sheena Byrom, UK, has also physically been with us in the setting up of the first attempt for a midwife-led birth centre that we have run for two years.

These excellent professionals and women with so much compassion have to be mentioned because they form the backbone of a larger circle of trust that we could not have made it without. They have shared their space with us very generously and are always available for us for guidance. This is our first experience with professionals in the fields of midwifery and obstetrics who have so much passion for justice, women and birth that we strive to work harder and emulate the brilliance of their work in order to brighten up the path to dignified birth for our communities.

Key points for consideration

- Read the evidence
- Listen to women
- Be brave
- Seek out support
- Believe in yourself

Better Beginnings: a connected service journey with a positive message to increase demand and provision of quality of care in Uganda and Nigeria

Melanie Wendland

In the world of consumer goods and services, customers have long become accustomed to demand not only high-quality services but also premium experiences from their service providers. In industries such as airline travel, hospitality, entertainment and consumer goods, providers need to innovate in order to stay competitive on the market. Service experience and service quality have become the key differentiators in service provision and providers have long harnessed the power of branding and customer-centred service design in binding their customers to their services and products. In healthcare however the thought of health service provision as a service experience is fairly new and the need for innovation for the sake of competitive advantage rather obsolete.

Service design approach

The WHO Better Outcomes in Labour Difficulty project (BOLD) (Olufemi et al, 2015) took on a service design approach to create a set of innovative tools to strengthen the linkages between communities and facilities in low-resource settings in order to increase the demand and provision of quality of care at the time of childbirth. The so called Passport to Safer Birth objective of the BOLD project applied a service design process with facilities and communities in Uganda and Nigeria between 2014 and 2016 to design a service journey that would allow women and their families to gain a deeper understanding of pregnancy related topics and facility-based childbirth, as well as provide healthcare providers with tools to deliver more customised woman-centred care.

Fragmented services

During pregnancy, a woman has many encounters with touchpoints of maternal health related service provision, for example through community health worker visits, antenatal care (ANC) visits, pharmacy visits or discussions with friends or family members about past experiences. As of now in many settings, these touchpoints where women, often with low literacy, access services related to maternal health are dispersed, fragmented and inconsistent in the way content and messages are provided and communicated. In addition in many facilities in low-resource settings, care at the point of childbirth is provided as a series of technical protocol steps rather than as a customer-centred service. Overcrowding of wards, lack of skills and training, low pay and difficult work environment are only a few of the challenges healthcare providers face. This fragmentation, lack of information and empathic customised care leaves women vulnerable, fearful, uninformed and unprepared at the moment of childbirth.

Optimising touchpoints

'Better Beginnings' has therefore been designed as a service to support women at the most important touchpoints of her journey through pregnancy and childbirth and to provide information and tools for both the woman, her family members and the healthcare provider to gain a better understanding of needs, preferences and expectations. See Figure 1. The service has been conceived and designed together with women, their male partners and healthcare providers in Uganda and Nigeria, ensuring their needs and preferences are reflected in the solutions.

Figure 1
Service design model

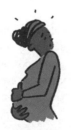
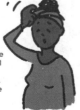
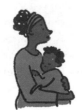
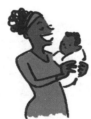

VULNERABLE
She worries about pregnancy and needs emotional support. She wants the best for the baby but avoids busy hospitals and turns away because of the fear of bad care, discrimination or lack of privacy. She values soft approach and traditional care.

EMPOWERED
She values medical care and emotional support. She actively selects the best option accessible and has a holistic view about pregnancy and delivery. She knows partly about risks. She prepares and plans for the delivery and has a positive attitude towards family-planning. She wants to be in control and demands.

PASSIVE
Pregnancy and childbirth needs no special attention. Only god has the power to give life. Facility has no meaningful role, and other stakeholders make decisions on her behalf. Facility/ANC visits only in case of an emergency.

ACCEPTER
She believes in the need for medical care but doesn't know much. She wants the best outcome for her delivery but she can be passive and postpones critical decisions. She shows weak demand for quality, and other stakeholders have a strong effect on her decisions.

'Better Beginnings' is designed to be introduced to the pregnant woman at her first ANC visit with the 'Pregnancy Purse'. The midwife or nurse hands out the 'Pregnancy Purse', a paper-based folder that contains important material for her and her supporter to foster curiosity about pregnancy and childbirth and develop an understanding of the upcoming journey and milestones throughout her pregnancy. See Figure 2.

Figure 2
Pregnancy purse

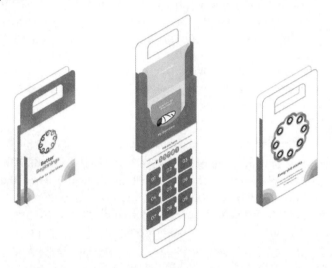

While maternal and infant mortality rates have dropped significantly in the last 20 years, complications during pregnancy and childbirth claim the lives of thousands of mothers and newborns each year. Every two minutes, a woman dies from causes related to pregnancy or childbirth, and each year more than one million children die on the day they are born.

As the number of births taking place in health facilities around the world continues to rise, maternity wards must be adequately prepared to deliver high-quality care to women and newborns everywhere. Overcrowding, poor infection prevention and control and the lack of essential health infrastructure mean that for many women, the experience of birth is neither safe nor comfortable.

Holistic experience

A woman's physical surroundings during childbirth can affect her perception of how easy or difficult it is to give birth. Focusing on a woman's holistic experience of childbirth, including the services, products and surrounding spaces available to her at health facilities, has the potential to improve maternal and newborn health outcomes. The Lab.our Ward Innovation Project* looks at both existing and new ways to deliver improved quality of care based on evidence and inspired through a human-centered

---

* labourward.org

design process. The project brings together expertise from the fields of product, service and architectural design, in collaboration with maternal and newborn health experts, to improve the birth experience in low-resource settings. Through innovations and tools applied to new and existing health facilities, the Lab.our Ward project aims to improve quality of care from the perspectives of both women and care providers. Ultimately, the Labour Ward innovation project seeks a positive impact on health outcomes for mothers and newborns worldwide.

The project has been developed through a collaborative process, bringing together partners at global and national levels. By employing a human-centered design approach, the project has rethought the birth experience through service, product and space innovations tailored for maternity wards in resource-constrained settings.

In doing so, the Lab.our Ward has focused on the woman's journey of care and has sought to improve health outcomes by practical application of and alignment to WHO's Quality of Care framework. The design proposals and concepts, presented in summarised form here, are thus rooted in clinical evidence, combined with user insights gathered through field research in India, Kenya, Uganda and Nigeria. By focusing on a woman's holistic experience of childbirth, supporting facilities to find solutions most fitting for their needs and by forging collaborative partnerships, we seek to make a safe and dignified childbirth experience a reality for all.

Key points for consideration

- In healthcare service interactions, it is important to map out how value is created between the provider and the service recipient. When we can design around this value, interactions are more meaningful, efficient and effective.
- Listen to healthcare providers and service users and how they make sense of their interactions.
- Testing and failing and improving: iterating new concepts and ideas with real users in real settings as early as possible to get feedback and shape tools and services around the needs of those who will use them.

References

Oladapo OT, Souza JP, Bohren MA, Tuncalp O, Vogel JP, Fawole B, Mugerwa K, Gulmezoglu AM (2015) WHO Better Outcomes in Labour Difficulty (BOLD) project: innovating to improve quality of care around the time of childbirth Reproductive Health Vol 12, Issue 46

Illustrations

Fig1: International Journal of Gynecology & Obstetrics, Volume: 139, Issue: S1, Pages: 56-66, First published: 07 December 2017, DOI: (10.1002/ijgo.12381)

Fig 2: International Journal of Gynecology & Obstetrics, Volume: 139, Issue: S1, Pages: 67-73, First published: 07 December 2017, DOI: (10.1002/ijgo.12381)

CHAPTER 26

Improvements in maternity services through birth activism

Daniela Drandić, Milli Hill and Duncan Fisher

Introduction

Parents are the largest and most motivated stakeholders in maternity care. As a group, they hold immense power to effect local, national and international changes in maternity care, and in Europe, parents advocating for improvements in maternity services has a long history. The development of the Internet, and social media especially, has amplified parents' voices and increased general awareness about problems in maternity care.

This chapter will discuss the work of contemporary parents' advocacy groups. It includes brief personal accounts from those who have worked within, and/or set up such groups. It is mainly focused on the European region; despite linguistic diversity, countries in this region share common maternity care and legislative frameworks, which allow for more accurate comparisons.[1] However, many of the issues raised can also be applied to countries outside Europe, and one of the personal accounts relates to a family advocacy group that has global reach. The chapter ends with a series of insights for action in this area, based on the experiences of childbirth advocates from around the world.

A brief history of parents' advocacy

The first modern parents' groups advocating for changes in maternity care were formed in the United Kingdom in the 1950s and 1960s, at a time when the majority of births in that country were already taking place in hospital.[2] Groups then, as now, took approaches that included providing education for parents (in the case of the National Childbirth Trust, formed in 1956)[3] and advocating for improvements and changes in services, as is the case of the Association for Improvements in Maternity Services (formed in 1960).[4] These organisations managed to take the issue of childbearing from the privacy of the family and turn it into a public issue.[5] This advocacy ultimately resulted in changes to maternity care in the UK, including having fathers present in the birthing room.[6] A few years later, in 1977, behind the Iron Curtain in then-communist Hungary, obstetrician-gynaecologist Agnes Gereb began secretly allowing fathers into the birthing room, a practice she would later lose her job for.[7]

Discourse on the need to reform the culture and delivery of modern maternity services began to appear in professional literature in 1982, when researchers wrote about how much of what happened during birth had more to do with policies and unwritten rules than with evidence-based care.[8] Later, in 1988, the then-European Commission was presented with a draft Resolution on a Charter of the Rights of Women in Childbirth, which unfortunately did not go far through the policy process.[9] The issues parents raise about failings of maternity care have remained very similar from the 1960s all the way to the present day.

Parents' advocacy associations we see today in other parts of Europe began to form in a similar way as UK organisations had, with grassroots support. The European Network of Childbirth Associations (1993) brought together representatives from grassroots organisations from throughout the continent.[10] Contemporary, active organisations continued to form afterwards, and a short list of active ones can include countries like Poland Fundacja Rodzić po Ludzku (Childbirth With Dignity, 1994),[11] Croatia Roditelji u akciji – Roda (Parents in Action, 2001),[12] and Spain El Parto es Nuestro (Birth is Ours, 2003).[13] Networking among parent-groups and other stakeholders, including human rights lawyers, culminated at the first Human Rights in Childbirth Conference in The Hague, Netherlands, in 2012.[14]

Using modern communications technology for advocacy

The dawn of social media has further amplified parents' concerns, providing them a platform to communicate their experiences in maternity care, both positive and negative, to a much wider and more diverse audience. Obstetric violence has been an issue particularly discussed on this platform, with grassroots organisations calling women to share their stories under a common name (also known as a hashtag). Campaigns that have garnered national and international attention over the past five years have included #genoeggezwegen in the Netherlands,[15] #BastaTacere in Italy,[16] #StopViolenciaObstetrica in Spain,[17] #PrekinimoSutnju in Croatia and throughout the former Yugoslavia[18] and others. The Italian campaign has led to proposals for legislation,[19] while the Croatian campaign culminated in a pilot program of the Mother-Friendly Hospital Initiative in four hospitals.[20]

Parents have also taken their concerns to national and global professional organisations, international watchdogs, UNICEF, the World Health Organization and others, resulting in changes in discourse. Over the past few years, the WHO has, for example, expanded its definition of good maternity care to include a life-course approach to health, emphasising surviving but also thriving in the childbearing year and beyond,[21] the importance of a positive experience[22] and has addressed the problem of disrespect and abuse in maternity care.[23]

Parents are also taking maternity care to human rights bodies, evident in European Court of Human Rights judgements addressing lack of access to out-of-hospital birth[24] and having medical students present during childbirth against a woman's wishes.[25] However, not all such cases have been successful, demonstrated by Dubská and Krejzová v. the Czech Republic.[26]

Thanks to advocacy and collaboration with national NGOs, problems in maternity care are also being included in concluding country reports of human rights committees such as the UN Committee for the Elimination of All Forms of Discrimination Against Women (CEDAW), which has warned Greece to lower its caesarean section rate,[27] and told countries like Croatia to deal with problems of lack of access to midwives and obstetric violence.[28] Some national organisations have also made presentations to the UN Special Rapporteur on the Right to Health[29] and petitioned the European Parliament regarding lack of access to midwifery care.[30,31]

Parents' expectations of maternity services

A recent systematic qualitative review looking at studies from 1996–2006 in 19 countries concluded that women hoped for a maternity care experience that 'enables them to use their inherent physical and psychosocial capacities to labour and give birth to a healthy baby in a clinically, culturally, and psychologically safe environment with continuity of practical and emotional support from a birth companion(s), and with kind, sensitive clinical staff, who provide reassurance and technical competency.'[32] These findings are in line with the advocacy work that has been taking place in Europe over the same period, in which women have been campaigning for services that would allow them to use their own power to give birth with emotional support in a setting they feel safe in.

Moving away from the disease mentality of childbearing and increasing public awareness about the value of optimising normal pregnancy and childbirth processes, and of being realistic about risks in the childbearing period, would also contribute to an increasing emphasis on social support systems for expectant parents in addition to the usual almost exclusive focus on clinical tests, screening, and treatments. Case study one describes how Milli Hill's personal engagement with this need for support led unexpectedly to a global online movement.

CASE STUDY ONE : the unexpected Positive Birth Movement

Milli Hill

People often ask me why I set up the Positive Birth Movement (PBM), and of course, I have to remind them that, when I set it up, I never expected it to snowball into the huge global organisation it is today! I just wanted to have a few women round my house to drink tea, eat cake, and talk about birth! Then I wondered if other people held similar groups, and we all linked up via social media, could this work? And the world responded with an 'enormous yes' – applications to run groups flooded my inbox, and we now have over 250 groups in the UK, and another 200 or so more across literally every corner of the globe – and these numbers continue to rise.

At the time the whole thing started, which was 2012, I was at the tail end of a 10-

year career as a group therapist, and I think this background strongly influenced my thinking, although I perhaps didn't realise it at the time. In group therapy – in which I had participated both as the therapist and as the 'therapee' – the transformative power comes from the group, not from the leader. Healing and change happens when people listen to each other, and perhaps more so, when they feel they are truly being heard themselves. An atmosphere of non-judgement and acceptance is fostered, in which people can feel safe to admit to their diversity while at the same time often realising the many ways in which they are not alone. Belonging to the group is in itself also a vital factor – bringing both an identity and a new sense of purpose, responsibility and self confidence.

How does this translate to birth? Well, looking at the formation of the PBM retrospectively I can also tell you that another main driving factor was the way that the huge *imbalance of power in the birth room* seemed to be going completely unnoticed. As a feminist I could never quite believe my ears when I heard women of my own generation talk about their birth experiences in terms of what they were allowed or not allowed to do. Every birth story I heard seemed to be peppered with this language, and often, but not always, ended badly for the woman, but with the 'healthy baby' that she would then be repeatedly told was 'all that mattered'.

I wanted to change this, and my therapeutic work had taught me that healing and change was often a grass-roots, people's movement, rather than coming from the top down. Women coming together in groups where they were encouraged to see everyone else in the room as 'the expert', including themselves, might just chip gently away at the existing dynamic, where 'doctor knew best', and permission had to be sought even for the finer details, 'Is it ok if I get on/off the bed?', 'Am I allowed a drink?', and so on.

And so, whether or not I consciously thought all of this, the Positive Birth Movement was born out of a melting pot of these and many other thoughts and ideas, and the coming together of women in groups to listen to and learn from each other, and empower each other with confidence regardless of their birth choices, became a way to potentially transform birth for the better.

The Positive Birth Movement: www.positivebirthmovement.org

More similar than we are different

Identifying the needs parents have expressed and improvements they have identified as necessary, both regionally and locally, provides an excellent framework for the actions of parents' advocacy groups. Even across countries that are members of the European Union, cultural and system differences are associated with considerable differences in the way maternity services are planned and delivered, even at the level of professional guidelines, which should all be based on the same evidence. At the extreme, a small number of expectant parents who feel their options in certain settings are not sufficient sometimes have the means and/or motivation to seek out care in a neighbouring jurisdiction, or to ask healthcare providers to cross borders and attend home births in countries where these services are not available. Information about this comes mostly by word of mouth in community and online groups, which unfortunately leads to a 'no statistics means no problems' data vacuum.

In reality, despite the variations in the funding and provision and outcomes of maternity care around the world, most parents' experience of maternity care in Europe and elsewhere is more similar than it is different at certain levels.

Underpinning what parents, especially mothers, want from maternity care is, of course, the utmost regard for the safety of mothers and babies, and this is particularly relevant in countries with high levels of adverse outcomes. However, as experience has shown, safety alone does not provide an adequate foundation for the design and provision of a humane maternity system, as women experience it, in any economic setting. Treating the majority of normal pregnancies and births as abnormal or high-risk 'just in case', with consequent violations of maternal human rights in some cases, has little effect on improving outcomes for mothers and babies, and may be harmful for some healthy women and babies.[33] Case study two, presented by Duncan Fisher, provides an account of how particular events experienced by an individual were the catalyst for the formation of an activist group that has developed into a global campaign that balances both safety and wellbeing for women, fathers, babies, parents, partners and families around the world.

CASE STUDY TWO: the inspiration for 'Family Included'

Duncan Fisher

When our first baby was born, our family encountered maternity services in the UK for the first time. They did not fit the way we wanted to share our roles and responsibilities. The assumption was that mothers do babies and fathers help out, probably rather cluelessly. Sheila Kitzinger referred to the father as the mother's second baby. This single comment galvanised me into action, spurred on by my wife. For 10 years I campaigned in the UK for maternity services that engaged fathers more effectively as partners with equal responsibilities for the health of the mother and baby. I ended up on the Government's *Maternity Matters* working group. I launched an information service for new fathers, *Dad. Info*, and another service inclusive of mothers and family members in Liverpool, *Maternity Assist*. I drafted guidelines for maternity services, which culminated in the Royal College of Midwives guidelines, *Reaching out: Involving Fathers in Maternity Care*. Now that my children are growing up and leaving home, I am returning to the international work I gave up for them, taking the same campaign globally.

Over the years I feel I have made little progress. I have learned that the changes I seek will be measured in generations, not years. What are the barriers?

A key problem is the idea that the interests of women and men are considered at some fundamental level to be in competition. That means that, as a man campaigning in this area, I can be perceived as advocating 'for men' in competition with the fundamental purpose of maternity care.

But this perception is wrong. Engaging fathers in maternity care is not actually about men at all: it is about the health of mothers and babies. If men are equally responsible for the health of mothers and babies then my presence in this field is as it should be.

The evidence base, which I have started building on a website, FamilyIncluded.com, is strong: when those closest to the mother are engaged effectively, health outcomes improve. This is not surprising when one considers the degree to which humans are related to and interdependent with each other. Ultimately families influence the health of mothers and babies more than health professionals do and so families have to be brought on board in a 'partnership of care'. The evidence does not support the idea that the only important person to engage with is the father; the important thing for the mother is to be surrounded by informed and confident support from close loved ones, no matter who they happen to be. Hence the name of the new site is 'Family Included'.

A second key problem is the structure of maternal health. Birth has been taken into a medical setting where there are three categories of people: the patient, the professional, and the visitor. But the father doesn't fit into this picture – he is the other parent of the baby. In 2012, Mary Steen published an article in *Midwifery*, 'Not-patient and not-visitor', describing the indeterminate position of the father. Birth as a family event mixes with birth as a medical event like oil and water.

The other area of health where this phenomenon presents challenges is at the other end of life: death. The hospice movement has pioneered family-inclusive care and is now an inspiration for the design of some of the best maternity units in the world, for example, the Serenity Suite at Salford Hospital, a beacon of family-inclusive maternal healthcare.

A third problem globally is patriarchal structures that separate mothers and fathers into very different roles. Patriarchy not only disempowers women and consigns them to economically weak roles, it also separates men from caring roles.

This is important because recent research on the biology and neurobiology of fatherhood has shown that human fathers have profound caring instincts, but these are only triggered by close contact with the infant. I have been inviting the world's leading researchers in this field to write about their work on the website, Fatherhood. Global. Hormonal changes take place in men in similar ways to women and, also like women, their plastic brains change through the act of caring for a baby, sensitising them to the infant's needs. With this comes a decrease in aggression and competition in men. In remarkable research from Israel, the researchers found that the brain patterns of fathers become more and more similar to mothers the more they care, with sole care fathers in gay father-father couples undergoing the most profound changes. All this fits exactly with the study of anthropology, which demonstrates that the fundamental characteristic of human parenting is immensely flexible collaboration within a group of carers, starting from the hour the baby is born.

But if, as a result of social structures, men are never allowed to be close to their babies, then these changes are never triggered and fathers remain unchanged and external to the world of intimate care. This perpetuates inequality globally. This driver of inequality, however, is hardly ever discussed: the idea of caring men attracts minimal interest. In 2016 I attended the huge global equality conference, Women Deliver. The session on 'powerful men' attracted about 2,000 delegates. The session on 'caring men' (at which I spoke) attracted 40.

But there is hope. The fact is that human parenting is fundamentally collaborative and the fact is that men can care. This applies to all human families everywhere in the world. Social media is spreading new aspirations about fatherhood like wildfire: when men see other men being close to their babies it triggers strong feelings. Videos of active fatherhood regularly clock up tens of millions of views. During the Women Deliver conference, while about 100 delegates discussed 'kangaroo mother care', 7 million people watched the Groovaroo video on Facebook portraying kangaroo father care (since then the video has attracted a further 5 million views).

A mistake I made in the last 10 years has been to depend entirely on trying to influence the supply side of delivery, working just with professionals. Equally important is to change the expectations of maternal healthcare of women and their families, so that they become more confident in demanding family inclusive care if they want it. And with digital communications spreading to every corner of the globe, that now becomes a potent force for change.

Family Included: familyincluded.com

Discussion: making advocacy sustainable

'If you want to go fast, go alone. If you want to go far, go together.'

The final section of this chapter sets out some suggestions for those who want to advocate for improvements in maternity care. Parents advocating for improvements to maternity services across the world are facing similar challenges, and can learn much from each other's experiences. Since 2001, Roda – Parents in Action, a group based in Croatia, has overcome many crises in a country that does not provide a very supportive framework for non-profits or advocates. This experience is a valuable resource that can help advocacy groups that are just starting out on their journey to advocating improvements in maternity services. In making these suggestions, we are building on our experience, and that of other organisations such as those described in the boxes in this chapter.

Assembling a team

You may start out as a group of new parents just interested in learning more about their own options in maternity care, but over time you will become a local resource and repository of information. Organise regular child-friendly meet-ups and invite new people to attend, start up a closed Facebook group and start building your virtual community. You can also consider joining an existing local group, such as a breastfeeding support group, or perhaps starting up the first community Positive Birth Movement group. Networking with other local organisations, immediately related to maternity care or not, is always beneficial.

Identify allies in your community, region and nation – these may be individuals that work in hospitals, professional organisations, local governments, ministries or agencies, other non-profits, especially those that discuss gender or women's issues, academic departments or international NGOs like UNICEF or UN Women: depending on your location different options will be available. Tell them about the work you are doing, offer to work with them on some of their projects or events, and invite them to yours. When it comes to working with your allies, much of the work is done by replying to emails in a timely manner, encouraging collaboration and sometimes, simply showing up. The more you show you are invested in your work, the more others will try to understand and assist you in attaining your goals.

Decide on your values and make a plan of action

Expectant families are a very valuable target group for marketers, and for this reason it is imperative to decide what types of companies and organisations you will and will not work with. Committing to uphold the WHO Code on the Marketing of Breastmilk Substitutes[34] is a great place to start. Having a clear but flexible code of ethics will help guide your work and increase your credibility as an organisation. Finally, it is important to note the importance of intersectionality in maternity care, and problems are exacerbated by racial, sexual, cultural, ability and other forms of discrimination. The needs faced by vulnerable groups in our communities must be sought out and addressed, and seeking out these communities is vital.

Once you have a set of values in place, it is useful to make a plan of action with attainable goals for a manageable period of time. One or three years is a good place to start. Then it's time to get to work!

Increase your capacities

Although your attention is mostly focused on achieving your goals, it is always important to find time to increase the capacities and knowledge of all your team members. Quality communication is key, so it is helpful to find a psychologist willing to volunteer a few hours and hold communications training for your team early on. This person may also be willing to mediate when communications problems arise. This can mean the difference between an organisation working well together for a long period of time or dissipating after only a few months.

Not-for-profit organisations usually run project management or grant-making trainings a few times per year. Join a few local mailing lists and keep an eye out for these types of events. They are invaluable for increasing your group's capacities to run your own projects, but also in helping you to apply for funding in the future.

Networking is also very important. Consider joining local and national coalitions, but also regional groups; some will have social media groups or mailing lists you can join too. If time and financing allow, attend conferences organised by advocacy organisations. Often the best ideas come from these opportunities to learn about each other's work and experiences.

Know your stuff

Learn all you can about the maternity services, local hospital statistics and practices in your area, as well as where people can find more information. If the information is not available, start collecting it. Read up on evidence-based maternity care and use social media to follow new developments, people and organisations active in the field. Attend conferences in your community or virtually by reading the live tweets posted by audience members. Prepare reports and publish them online. Over time you can participate in shadow-reporting processes with other organisations, working together to put maternity issues on the agenda.[35] Consider joining local coalitions and advisory groups.

Conclusion

Advocating for improvements in maternity services can be a process that seems to take forever with little or no progress – and then, over a short period of time, change occurs rapidly. This does not happen by chance: it is the culmination of years of consistent and constant advocacy efforts by many stakeholders. For those involved in contributing to this chapter, experience has shown that advocacy groups can never be complacent in advocating for improvements to maternity services. Persistence is key, as it only takes a short time for new leadership to make changes that restrict or degrade maternity services. Conversely, building positive relationships over time with up and coming leaders can lead to sudden and unexpected change in the right direction.

From rallies to conferences, meetings to radio shows, much of the work is done just by consistently showing up and reminding others that parents must be a stakeholder at the table: decisions about us, cannot be made without us.

A third case-study by Mary Newburn is included in Chapter 25.

Key points for consideration

- *Assemble a team:* People from a certain community or region with different types of skills and backgrounds. Seek out vulnerable groups in your community and see how you can include them. Develop effective communications that work for you.
- *Decide on values and make a plan of action:* Decide what your group stands for and who you will work with. Have a strategy – who do you want to engage and why, and how will you answer to their needs best? Make a plan of action with clear goals and activities for one to three years. Every few months, revisit your action plan and see how far you've got.
- *Increase capacity:* Take courses on grant-writing and project administration. Invest in your online presence – websites and social media are key to your image and engagement. Learn from groups from other regions and countries; join alliances.
- *Be knowledgeable:* Get to know stakeholders in your community – researchers, healthcare providers, policy-makers. Take time to do research and keep up with new developments. Know your limits, you cannot know everything and shouldn't pretend you do.

References

Association for Improvements in Maternity Services. "About AIMS | AIMS". 2018. Aims.Org.Uk. https://www.aims. org.uk/about-aims. Accessed 29 May 2018.

Blondel B, Alexander S, Bjarnadottir RI, Gissler M, Langhoff-Roos J, Novak-Antolic Z, et al. Variations in rates of severe perineal tears and episiotomies in 20 European countries: a study based on routine national data in Euro-Peristat Project. Acta Obstet Gynecol Scand 2016; 95:746–754.

Betrán AP, Ye J, Moller A-B, Zhang J, Gülmezoglu AM, Torloni MR (2016) The Increasing Trend in Caesarean Section Rates: Global, Regional and National Estimates: 1990-2014. PLoS ONE 11(2): e0148343.

Case of *Dubská and Krejzová v. the Czech Republic, 2017, 28859/11 and 28473/12. European Court of Human Rights. Available at:* http://www.globalhealthrights.org/wp-content/uploads/2018/03/CASE-OF-DUBSKA-AND-KREJZOVA-v.-THE-CZECH-REPUBLIC.pdf

Case of Konvalova v. Russia. 2015, 37873/04. European Court of Human Rights. Available at: http://hudoc.echr.coe. int/app/conversion/pdf/?Library=ECHR&id=001-146773&filename=001-146773.pdf

Case of Ternovszky v. Hungary. 2010, 67545/09. European Court of Human Rights. Available at: https://hudoc.echr.coe.int/ eng#{%22dmdocnumber%22:[%22878621%22],%22itemid%22:[%22001-102254%22]}

Committee on the Elimination of Discrimination against Women. 2013. "Concluding Observations On The Seventh Periodic Report Of Greece Adopted By The Committee At Its Fifty Fourth Session (11 February – 1 March 2013)". Geneva: CEDAW. http://www2.ohchr.org/english/bodies/cedaw/docs/co/CEDAW.C.GRC.CO.7.doc.

Committee on the Elimination of Discrimination against Women. 2015." Concluding observations on the combined fourth and fifth periodic reports of Croatia". Geneva: CEDAW. https://digitallibrary.un.org/record/805691/files/ CEDAW_C_HRV_CO_4-5-EN.pdf

Davis, Angela. 2013. "Choice, Policy And Practice In Maternity Care Since 1948". History & Policy. http://www. historyandpolicy.org/policy-papers/papers/choice-policy-and-practice-in-maternity-care-since-1948.

Drandić, Daniela. 2017. "Pilot Program Rodilišta Prijatelji Majki I Djece U RH". Rodilišta.Roda.Hr. http://rodilista.roda. hr/rodilista-prijatelji-majki/pilot-program-rodilista-prijatelji-majki-i-djece-u-rh.html.

Downe, Soo, Kenneth Finlayson, Olufemi Oladapo, Mercedes Bonet, and A. Metin Gülmezoglu. 2018."What Matters To Women During Childbirth: A Systematic Qualitative Review". PLOS ONE 13 (4): e0194906. doi:10.1371/ journal.pone.0194906.

El parto es nuestro. "Que somos." 2018. Elpartoesnuestro.es. https://www.elpartoesnuestro.es/pagina/que-somos

Emma Egyesulet. "Oral Hearing At The European Parliament Petition Committee". 2013. Emmaegyesulet.Hu. http://www. emmaegyesulet.hu/en/european-parlaiment-petition-committee/. Accessed 29 May 2018.

European Parliament Committee on Petitions. "Petition 1954/2012 By Fazakas Palma (Hungarian) And Two Other Signatories, On Behalf Of The Birth House Association, On Alleged Breach By Hungary Of The Directive On The Recognition Of Professional Qualifications". 2014. Committee On Petitions. http://www.europarl.europa.eu/ meetdocs/2014_2019/documents/peti/cm/1032/1032484/1032484en.pdf.

Euro-Peristat project with SCPE and Eurocat. European Perinatal health report. The health of pregnant women and babies in Europe in 2010. May 2013. Available: www.europeristat.com. Accessed 20 April 2017.

European Network of Childbirth Associations. "About The European Network of Childbirth Associations". 2018. Enca.Info. http://enca.info/.

Fawsitt, Christopher Godfrey et al. What women want: Exploring pregnant women's preferences for alternative models of maternity care. Health Policy, Volume 121, Issue 1, 66 – 74. October 2016.

Fundacija Rodzic po ludzku. "About Us". 2018. http://www.rodzicpoludzku.pl/About-us/Who-we-are.html

Human Rights Council of the United Nations. Report of the Special Rapporteur on the right of everyone to the enjoyment of the highest attainable standard of physical and mental health on his visit to Croatia, March 2017. Available: http://www.roda.hr/media/attachments/udruga/dokumenti/reakcije/342567581-Izjava-posebnog-izvjestitelja-UN-a-o-Hrvatskoj.pdf.

Human Rights in Childbirth. "Hague Conference 2012". 2013. Human Rights In Childbirth. http://www. humanrightsinchildbirth.org/event/hague-2012. Accessed 29 May 2018.

MacFarlane, A.J., Blondel, B., Mohangoo, A.D., Cuttini, M., Nijhuis, J., Novak, Z., Olafsd ottir, H.S., Zeitlin, J. & the Euro-Peristat Scientific Committee (2015). Wide differences in mode of delivery within Europe: risk-stratified analyses of aggregated routine data from the Euro-Peristat study. *BJOG: an International Journal of Obstetrics and Gynaecology*, 123(4), pp. 559-568.

Midwives for Choice (Ireland). Submission to the Committee on the Elimination of Discrimination Against Women (CEDAW) for its consideration in the context of examining Ireland's sixth and seventh period reports on compliance with the Convention on the Elimination of Discrimination Against Women, January 2017. Available: http://midwivesforchoice.ie/wp-content/uploads/2017/01/MfC-Submission-to-CEDAW-FINAL.pdf. Accessed 10 April 2017.

National Childbirth Trust. "History". 2018. Nct.Org.Uk. https://www.nct.org.uk/about-nct/history.

Nove, Andrea, Berrington, Ann and Matthews, Zoe. 2008."Home Births In The UK, 1955 To 2006". Population Trends 133. London: Office for National Statistics. https://www.ons.gov.uk/ons/rel/.../home-births-in-the-uk--1955-to-2006.pdf.

Lazdane, Gunta, ed. A Life-Course Approach to Sexual and Reproductive Health. Entre-Nous, the European Magazine for Sexual and Reproductive Health, no. 82, 2015. Available: http://www.euro.who.int/__data/assets/pdf_file/0019/292204/Entre-Nous-82.pdf.

Papp, Reka Kinga. 2017. "Decriminalizing Childbirth: Power Dynamics In Hungarian Birthing Care". Eurozine. https://www.eurozine.com/decriminalising-childbirth-power-dynamics-in-hungarian-birthing-care/.

Proposta Di Legge: BINETTI E CESA: "Norme Per La Promozione Del Parto Fisiologico E La Salvaguardia Della Salute Della Partoriente E Del Neonato" (93). n.d. http://www.camera.it/leg17/126?tab=4&leg=17&idDocumento=93&sede=ac&tipo=: Camera dei Deputati, Italia.

Plotkin, Lisa. Support Overdue: Women's experiences of maternity services 2017. National Federation of Women's Institutes and the National Childbirth Trust. Available: https://www.nct.org.uk/sites/default/files/related_documents/Support_Overdue_2017.pdf Accessed 20 April 2017.

Official Journal of the European Communities. RESOLUTION on a Charter on the rights of women in childbirth. No. C 235/183, Doc. A2-38/88. 8 July 1988.

Official Journal of the European Union. DIRECTIVE 2011/24/EU of the European Parliament and of the Council of 9 March 2011 on the application of patients' rights in cross-border healthcare. No. L 88/45, 4.4.2011. Available: http://eur-lex.europa.eu/LexUriServ/LexUriServ.do?uri=OJ:L:2011:088:0045:0065:en:PDF.

Richards, M. P. M. The Trouble with "Choice" in Childbirth. Birth, 9: 253–260. December 1982.

Roda – Parents in Action. Committee on the Elimination of Discrimination Against Women's 61st session Periodic review of Croatia July 2015 Joint submission by the Center for Reproductive Rights, Centar za edukaciju, savjetovanje i istraživanje (Center for Education, Counselling and Research - CESI) and Roditelji u akciji (Parents in Action - RODA). Available: http://tbinternet.ohchr.org/Treaties/CEDAW/Shared%20Documents/CRO/INT_CEDAW_NGO_CRO_20902_E.pdf. Accessed 10 April 2017.

Roda – Parents in Action. Eastern Europe and Central Asia Caucus Consensus Statement. Women Deliver Conference, Copenhagen, 2016. Available: http://www.roda.hr/udruga/projekti/women-deliver/reproductive-health-issues-that-impact-women-during-pregnancy-childbirth-and-postpartum.html. Accessed 15 April 2017.

Roda – parents in Action. "Roda's Vital Statistics." 2016. Roda – Parents in Action. http://www.roda.hr/en/about-us/rodas-vital-statistics.html

World Health Organization. WHO recommendations: intrapartum care for a positive childbirth experience. Geneva: World Health Organization; 2018. Licence: CC BY-NC-SA 3.0 IGO.

World Health Association. 2015. "The Prevention and Elimination Of Disrespect And Abuse During Facility-Based Childbirth". WHO Statement. Geneva: WHO. http://apps.who.int/iris/bitstream/handle/10665/134588/WHO_RHR_14.23_eng.pdf?sequence=1.

World Health Association. Code on the Marketing of Breastmilk Substitutes. Geneva: World Health Association, 1981. http://www.who.int/nutrition/publications/code_english.pdf

Endnotes

1   Roda – Parents in Action, 2016.
2   Nove, Berrington and Matthews, 2008.
3   National Childbirth Trust, 2018.
4   Association for Improvements in Maternity Services, 2018.
5   Davis, Angela. 2013. "Choice, Policy and Practice In Maternity Care Since 1948". History & Policy. http://www.historyandpolicy.org/policy-papers/papers/choice-policy-and-practice-in-maternity-care-since-1948.
6   Davis, 2013.
7   Papp, 2017.
8   Richards, M., 1982.
9   Official Journal of the European Communities, 1988.
10 European Network of Childbirth Associations, 2018.
11 Fundacija Rodzic po ludzku, 2018.
12 Roda – Parents in Action, 2016.
13 El parto es nuestro, 2018.
14 Human Rights in Childbirth. "Hague Conference 2012". 2013. Human Rights In Childbirth. http://www.humanrightsinchildbirth.org/event/hague-2012. Accessed 29 May 2018.
15 The campaign is available here: https://www.facebook.com/GeboorteBeweging/photos/a.452440388127211.95184.431092006928716/1164654606905782/?type=3&theater
16 The campaign is available here: https://www.facebook.com/bastatacere/?ref=br_rs
17 The campaign is available here: https://www.facebook.com/pg/elpartoesnuestro/photos/?tab=album&album_id=1759814414084522
18 The campaign is available here: https://www.facebook.com/pg/udrugaroda/photos/?tab=album&album_id=10152423832752051

19 Proposta Di Legge: BINETTI E CESA.
20 Drandić, Daniela. 2017. "Pilot Program Rodilišta Prijatelji Majki I Djece U RH". Rodilišta.Roda. Hr. http://rodilista.roda.hr/rodilista-prijatelji-majki/pilot-program-rodilista-prijatelji-majki-i-djece-u-rh.html.
21 Lazdane, 2015.
22 WHO, 2018.
23 WHO, 2015.
24 CASE OF TERNOVSZKY v. HUNGARY, 2010.
25 CASE OF KONVALOVA v. RUSSIA, 2015.
26 Case of *Dubská and Krejzová v. the Czech Republic, 2017*.
27 CEDAW, 2013.
28 CEDAW, 2015
29 Emma Egyesulet, 2013.
30 European Parliament Committee on Petitions, 2014.
31 Roda – Parents in Action. "Petition to European Parliament on Access to Midwifery". 2014. Roda.hr, http://www.roda.hr/en/reports/petition-to-the-european-parliament-on-access-to- midwifery.htm'
32 Downe et al., 2018.
33 Richards, 1982.
34 WHO, 1981.
35 CEDAW concluding observations for Greece (2013), Slovakia (2014), Croatia (2015), Ireland (2017) have included references to the need to improve maternity services, thanks in part to input from parents' advocates who collaborated with others to put these issues on the agenda.

CHAPTER 27

Between the circle and the square

Sheena Byrom and *Soo Downe*

Introduction

The dilemma at the centre of this book is the difficulty of understanding and supporting normal physiological birth when it is rapidly vanishing, particularly in institutional settings around the world. The following email, sent to one of us in 2014, is one of many similar communications we have received over the past few years:

> *'I became very disheartened and concerned about my own experiences. As a student midwife, I completed my second year of training after having witnessed and participated in 52 caesarean sections, 16 instrumental deliveries and very sadly, only 11 normal deliveries. I can vouch for the fact this story is not unique and many students are having a chronic lack of exposure to normality. In fact what the professional organisations seem to call 'normal', to me seemed like a fantasy, not the world in which I was training and learning'.* Sophie

If this is true for many student and qualified midwives, how much more must it be the case for obstetricians and other doctors who work in maternity care, especially when there seems to be an unwritten rule or belief often shared in practice and on social media that doctors should be 'kept out of the normal birth room'. Midwives witness the broad spectrum of maternity care, that is, all types of pregnancies and birth. But if doctors don't regularly see or even facilitate physiological birth, how can they trust the process, especially when they are regularly exposed to emergencies or pathologies? As with other maternity care workers, and women who never experience or hear about physiological labour and birth, they 'don't know what they don't know' (Lokumage and Bourne, 2014).

There is also a safety issue implicit in the overextension of risk-aversion. If most or all women and babies are considered as, and treated as, high risk, care providers become less and less sensitive to those who are exhibiting true pathology. As labour rooms become crowded with women who are subject to labour induction 'just in case', those who need close watching and intervention are more and more likely to be missed.

The authors in this book have each addressed this issue from their particular perspective. In the process, they have advanced understanding of how to build on the figure we presented in the introduction chapter. The next section summarises the key issues they have raised.

The circle, squared

In the first section of the book the authors explore the nature and context of normal birth. They highlight the biological and physiological reasons for understanding and respecting birth physiology, including the influence on mother-infant transition. While acknowledging that many aspects of physiological labour and birth are not fully understood, the authors suggest that there is enough evidence to promote a shift in maternity care services towards protecting, supporting and promoting physiological childbirth, and safeguarding healthy mothers and babies from unnecessary interventions.

The concept of 'unique normality' of labouring women is considered in Part 2, in addition to the suggestion that salutogenic or wellbeing approaches to maternity care provision should be balanced with reducing risk and improving safety. Some authors challenge readers to apply the 'technologies of risk' with caution and to promote a culture of trust, properly balanced with safety. This incorporates the importance of engendering compassionate relationships with both women and families and work colleagues. In addition, the human rights in childbirth movement provides a mechanism for ensuring a culture of safe, respectful and individualised maternity care. The section debates the evidence on external influences on the childbirth agenda, such as the media, and suggests strategies for change.

Overall, the chapters in this section articulate the compelling need for maternity services to provide services based on positive authentic relationships, and to utilise the overwhelming evidence that continuity of care offers choice and control to childbearing women, and that it is sustainable, woman-centred and midwife-friendly.

Parts 3 and 4 investigate the interconnectivity of psychological, emotional, and physiological states, and the impact on birth outcomes. The growing body of evidence demonstrating potential harm caused from current practices in maternity care systems is highlighted, and that more research into potential epigenetic consequences of labour and birth in the short, medium and longer term is needed. Two authors propose a model for improvements by understanding of the interconnectedness of the birth place, which incorporates spatial, behavioural, neurobiological and cultural influences on caregivers and labouring women. The design of the physical space where women give birth, and the attitudes of maternity care workers to the approach to labour pain and potential impact on birth outcomes are explored in depth, with evidence-based suggestions for positive change. Providing the tools and sharing examples of how to shift the status quo that exists is important to us as editors of this book. The final section therefore suggests that we engage in positive change through the use of Big Data and implementation science, while asking different kinds of research questions in all areas of research in maternity care in the future.

We were keen to demonstrate the importance of supporting psychological processes for women with complex needs, and to provide evidence of where, throughout the world, individuals have influenced and effected innovative programmes of work to support normal birth, enhance childbirth experience and improve maternal morbidity and mortality. Various authors have proposed the Quality Maternal and Newborn Care (QMNC) framework that is presented in The *Lancet* Midwifery Series (Renfrew et al, 2014) as part of the solution to achieve optimal health for mothers and babies. Others have highlighted the essential importance of the eradication of the disrespect and abuse that continues to infiltrate and affect both the experience of childbirth and physical outcomes. The crucial role of parents, including fathers, and childbirth activists is also presented as a solution by a range of authors, including activists themselves.

Conclusion

It is imperative that, in collaboration with women and their families, those researching, funding and providing maternity care square the circle between understanding and recognition of physiological processes, especially where they are unusual, and appropriate identification and treatment of pathology. Respect for these processes, and for the individual women who experience them, is paramount. Designing models of care and places of birth that support both physiology, and proper identification of and intervention for true pathology, will ensure an equal balance between safety and positive wellbeing for mothers, babies and families. The research, practice examples, debates, and points for consideration in this book are offered as the basis for moving maternity care around the world back towards optimum physical, psychological, emotional and spiritual health, and long-term human flourishing.

References:

International Confederation of Midwives (2017) Scope of Practice of the Midwife Available from https://www.internationalmidwives.org/our-work/policy-and-practice/icm-definitions.html Accessed on 3.1.19

Lokumage A, Bourne T (2015) 'They don't know what they don't know' In (Eds) Byrom S, Downe S, *The Roar Behind the Silence: why kindness, compassion and respect matter in maternity care* Pinter and Martin: London

Renfrew M, McFadden A, Bastos M, Campbell J, Channon A, Cheung N et al (2014) Midwifery and quality care: findings from a new evidence-informed framework for maternal and newborn care. The Lancet. 2014;384(9948):1129-1145.

Contributor Biographies

Neal M. Ashkanasy OAM, PhD is Professor of Management at the UQ Business School (University of Queensland, Australia). He studies emotion, leadership, culture, and ethical behaviour.

Elena Ateva is a Human Rights Attorney and an activist for women's rights in childbirth. She currently works with the White Ribbon Alliance and focuses on advocacy in Africa, Asia, Europe and Latin America.

Lisa Bernstein is the founder of Simply Put, a non-profit media and programming organisation that reaches neglected audiences in the US and around the world with information, art and stories that are created for (and with) expecting and new parents, and support 'Engaged Learning Experiences' for families as well as health and social service providers.

Martin Brown is a UK based sustainability provocateur and improvement consultant, working with a diverse range of organisations through his Fairsnape support business. He is passionate about a regenerative sustainability that is ecologically, socially and culturally sound, where we see ourselves as part of nature, rather than apart from nature.

Dr **Sarah Buckley** is a GP (family physician) and in GP obstetrics. She has a special interest in the hormones of labour and birth and is the author of the report *Hormonal Physiology of Childbearing*.

Sheena Byrom OBE is a consultant midwife and director of All4Maternity. Sheena has a long midwifery career of more than 40 years, received an OBE for services to midwifery, and two honorary doctorates. She is an Honorary Fellow of the Royal College of Midwives.

Helen Cheyne is Professor of Maternal and Child Health and RCM Professor of Midwifery Research (Scotland) at the University of Stirling. Her research interests include early labour, models of midwifery care and clinical decision making.

Melissa Cheyney is Associate Professor of Clinical Medical Anthropology at Oregon State University (OSU) and a Licensed Midwife in home birth practice. She also directs the International Reproductive Health Laboratory at Oregon State University.

Professor Sir **Cary L. Cooper** CBE is the 50th Anniversary Professor of Organisational Psychology and Health at the ALLIANCE Manchester Business School, University of Manchester and President of the Chartered Institute of Personnel and Development.

Dr **Tracey Cooper** MBE is Head of Midwifery at Warrington and Halton Hospitals NHS Foundation Trust. She was awarded an MBE in the 2018 New Year's Honours list for her contribution to midwifery. Tracey also received an Outstanding Contribution Award for Midwifery and Maternity Services in 2018 from the Midwifery Forum and became a Fellow of the RCM in 2017.

Jeffrey Craig is an Associate Professor at Deakin University, Australia. He studies the role of epigenetics in mediating the effects of early life environment on chronic disease risk. His expertise also includes twin studies and birth cohorts.

Susan Crowther is a Visiting Professor of Midwifery, Robert Gordon University, Aberdeen, Scotland. Working between New Zealand and the United Kingdom. Midwife, researcher, author and educator.

Hannah Dahlen is a Professor of Midwifery in the School of Nursing and Midwifery at Western Sydney University and is the Higher Degree Research Director.

Lorna Davies PhD is a UK midwife, educator and researcher now based in Christchurch, New Zealand. She has been researching midwifery through the lens of sustainability for over a decade.

Kate Dawson is a Clinical Educator and midwife at Northern Health in Melbourne. She is currently a PhD candidate with the Judith Lumley Centre at Latrobe University, researching the sustainability of caseload midwifery care in Australia.

Ank de Jonge currently works as an Associate Professor at the Department of Midwifery Science, VU University Medical Center, Amsterdam in the Netherlands. Ank does research in quality of midwifery care, organisation of care, place of birth and birthing positions.

Mark Dooris is Professor in Health & Sustainability and Director of the Healthy & Sustainable Settings Unit at the University of Central Lancashire. Mark is Chair of the International Health Promoting Universities & Colleges Steering Group and Co-Chair/Co-ordinator of the UK Healthy Universities Network.

Professor **Soo Downe** is a Professor of Midwifery Studies at the University of Central Lancashire. Her main research focus is the nature of, and cultures around, normal birth. She is currently working with the WHO on a range of maternity care guidelines, and has been a co-editor on three *Lancet* Series (Midwifery, Stillbirth, and Reducing Caesarean Section).

Daniela Drandić has been head of the Reproductive Rights Program at RODA – Parents in Action, the largest parents' advocacy group in Croatia and the region since 2012. Daniela is currently studying for a Master's Degree from the University of Dundee (UK) in Maternal and Infant Health and holds a bachelor's degree from the University of Toronto (Canada).

Margaret Duff is a midwife and Adjunct Fellow with the School of Nursing and Midwifery at Western Sydney. She has worked in Australia, New Zealand and China developing curriculums for midwifery education and other short courses.

Ramón Escuriet RM, MSc, PhD is currently working at Catalan Health Service as Health Commissioner responsible for Sexual and Reproductive Health. He is a lecturer at Faculty of Health Sciences Blanquerna-University Ramon Llull, and collaborator of the Research Centre in Economics and Health. He was coordinator of the Normal Birth Care Program at the Catalan Ministry of health from 2008 to 2017. He has also participated in different national and international funded research projects about maternity care. His research interest is focused on health services organisation and reproductive health rights.

Claire Feeley qualified as a midwife in 2011 at Oxford Brookes University, graduating with a Master's degree at the University of Central Lancashire in 2015. She has recently submitted her PhD with the University of Central Lancashire.

Evita Fernandez FRCOG is a consultant obstetrician, who has committed her professional life to promoting professional midwifery in India via PROMISE (PROfessional MIdwifery SErvices campaign) which teaches, trains nurses in midwifery, humanises birth and helps to make pregnancy safe.

Duncan Fisher is working to help health and family services engage better with the wider family group, fathers in particular, and has recently taken this work onto the international level. His website, FamilyIncluded.com, has reported on 250 pieces of research on the topic of family engagement in maternal health since 2015. In the UK he co-founded the Fatherhood Institute.

Maralyn Foureur is Professor of Nursing and Midwifery Research at Hunter New England Local Health District and the University of Newcastle in New South Wales, Australia. Maralyn is an experienced midwifery clinician, academic and researcher.

Tamsyn Green is a midwife based in London working in a continuity team built on a philosophy of compassionate, relationship-based care. She is also interested in how we can reconcile the often polarised worlds of midwifery and obstetrics to ensure women, not professional agendas, are at the centre of all our care.

Athena Hammond is an Australian midwife and has worked with innovative qualitative methods in midwifery and primary health research for the last ten years. She completed her doctorate in 2017 and has a particular interest in the design of spaces that enhance the wellbeing of women and midwives.

James Harris PhD RM is a Senior Clinical Lecturer for UCLH, splitting his time between clinical work and research. His research interests concentrate on implementing improvements in maternity, with a focus on patient-safety and implementing continuity of midwifery carer.

Milli Hill is a writer, mum of three and founder of the global Positive Birth Movement. Her first book, *The Positive Birth Book*, is a bestseller. Her second book, *Give Birth like a Feminist*, was published in 2019.

Vanora Hundley is Professor of Midwifery in the Centre for Midwifery, Maternal and Perinatal Health at Bournemouth University. She is an internationally recognised midwifery researcher, having written over 100 peer-reviewed research articles on pregnancy, maternity care and midwifery. She is co-editor of the book *Midwifery, Childbirth and the Media*.

Matthew Hyde is a researcher in neonatal medicine at Imperial College London. He holds a PhD in Animal Physiology (University of London/Imperial College London) and his research is focused on the long-term outcomes for the offspring of the mode of delivery.

Holly Jenkins is a researcher at King's College London. She has a background in microbiology and public health and has held research posts at Imperial College London and University of Queensland, Australia. Her research has focused on the microbiome of mother and infant (particularly preterm infants) around birth, with more recent work focusing on the role of exosomes in preterm birth.

Sigfridur Inga Karlsdottir is an Associate Professor at the School of Health Sciences, University of Akureyri, Iceland.

Dr **Lesley Kay** is an Associate Professor in Midwifery at the Faculty of Health, Education and Social Care, a joint venture between Kingston University and St. George's University of London.

Nicky Leap is a Professor of Midwifery with over 40 years experience of midwifery practice, research, education and maternity service reform. Her extensive publications focus on the art and philosophy of woman centred midwifery practice, and the social support of women through pregnancy, labour and birth, and new motherhood.

Fran McConville qualified as a midwife and a nurse, has a BSc in Zoology and an MSc in Health Economics. After being a VSO midwife in Bangladesh in the mid-1980s, Fran spent much of her career in sexual, reproductive, maternal and newborn health and gender in South East Asia, Africa and the Middle East, working with a range of NGOs and UN agencies and as a Health Adviser to the UK department of international development (DFID). Fran is currently the Midwifery Adviser to the World Health Organization, based in Geneva, providing technical and policy support to the 194 Member States.

Christine McCourt is Professor of Maternal and Child Health at City, University of London, where she leads the Centre for Maternal and Child Health Research. Her key interests are in applying anthropological theory and methods to childbirth and maternal health, with particular interests in institutions and service change and reform, on women's experiences of childbirth and maternity care and in the culture and organisation of maternity care.

Fiona Meechan is Wellbeing Lead at the UK College of Policing and Associate Lecturer at the Alliance Manchester Business School, University of Manchester.

Sandra Morano is an Italian obstetrician and researcher at Genoa University, where she created the first Italian Birth Centre, aiming to promote continuity of care, women-centred and satisfaction birthplaces, and to reduce intervention rate. She currently teaches Obstetrics and Gynaecology at the Medical School of Genoa University.

Mary Newburn is a service user researcher and activist. She has worked with the NCT (National Childbirth Trust), Midwifery Unit Network, Maternity Voices Partnerships and the Positive Birth Movement. She is Patient and Public Involvement Lead for CLAHRC maternity at Kings College London, on the Stakeholder Council for the implementation of *Better Births* and was a co-investigator on Birthplace in England, and the INFANT trial.

Elizabeth Newnham PhD is a midwife academic whose research interests centre on cultural and political analysis of birthing practice, and the role of midwives in promoting physiological and humanised birth. She is a passionate midwifery advocate, and has held leadership roles in the Australian College of Midwives, including state Committee Chair, and was also active within the Midwives Association of Ireland while working at Trinity College Dublin. She is currently Lecturer in Midwifery at Griffith University, Brisbane.

Michelle Newton is a Senior Lecturer in Midwifery and Director of Learning and Teaching in the School of Nursing and Midwifery at La Trobe University (Melbourne, Australia). Michelle's PhD explored the implementation of caseload midwifery models of care, and current research focuses on the growth and sustainability of caseload models from a workforce and implementation perspective.

Lesley Page CBE is a well-known international midwifery leader developing and promoting the humanisation of birth. Lesley has been deeply involved in the development of woman centred maternity care in the UK and around the world. Her work has involved leadership, national policy development, management of large services, hands on practice and academic work.

Mercedes Perez-Botella is a Senior Midwifery Lecturer and member of the Research in Childbirth and Health unit (ReaCH), at the University of Central Lancashire, England. She is currently undertaking a PhD, studying the routine use of labour interventions in Spanish maternity care contexts.

Lilian Peters PhD is an epidemiologist who conducts research in the area of Women's Health Epidemiology. She examines the effect of (lifestyle) behaviour, pregnancy and birth events on maternal and child health. Dr Peters is affiliated at the department of Midwifery Science located in Amsterdam (Amsterdam UMC) and Groningen (University Medical Center Groningen). As an adjunct Fellow at Western Sydney University in Australia she is examining the long-term health effects for mothers and babies following intervention in childbirth.

Nicola Philbin is a British lawyer, doula and childbirth educator who has lived and worked around the world, gaining wide experience of maternity care in different countries and systems. She was a founding board member of Human Rights in Childbirth and is currently a PhD research student at the University of Southampton in the UK, investigating the role of the Human Right to Health in addressing medicalisation of maternity care.

Holly Powell Kennedy, is the inaugural *Helen Varney Professor of Midwifery* at the Yale University School of Nursing and past President of the American College of Nurse-Midwives. She received her midwifery education from the Frontier School of Midwifery & Family Nursing, her masters and family nurse practitioner education from Georgia Regent's University, and her doctorate from the University of Rhode Island. She completed a Fulbright Distinguished Fellowship at King's College London in 2008. Her programme of research is focused on a greater understanding of the effectiveness of specific models of care during the childbearing year.

Mary Renfrew is Professor of Mother and Infant Health at the University of Dundee, Scotland. A health researcher, midwife, educator, and writer for over 40 years, her research has informed maternity and public health policy and practice internationally. She was Principal Investigator for the *Lancet* Series on Midwifery, and is currently working with the World Health Organization to advise on midwifery education and quality of care.

Lucia Rocca-Ihenacho PhD works at City University of London as a midwifery lecturer and researcher. Lucia is one of the co-founders and CEO of the Midwifery Unit Network.

Nicholas Rubashkin is an obstetrician/gynaecologist at the University of California San Francisco where he is also a PhD student in Global Health.

Jane Sandall is a midwife and NIHR senior investigator. She is a Professor of Social Science and Women's Health and leads the Maternal Health Systems and Implementation Research Group in the Department of Women and Children's Health, King's College, London. She is also an Adjunct Professor at University of Technology, Sydney.

Mandie Scamell is a Senior Midwifery Lecturer, postgraduate programme director and senior tutor for research at the Maternal and Child Health Research Centre at City, University of London.

Rebecca Schiller is co-founder and Trustee of the human rights in childbirth charity Birthrights. She's an experienced birth doula, a journalist and an author specialising in women's rights, pregnancy, birth and parenting.

Nicoletta Setola is an architect, PhD in Architectural Technology and Design (2009), Assistant Professor at the School of Architecture at University of Florence and member of the TESIS Centre, Department of Architecture.

Neel Shah is an Assistant Professor of Obstetrics, Gynecology and Reproductive Biology at Harvard Medical School, and Director of the Delivery Decisions Initiative at Harvard's Ariadne Labs.

Yoana Stancheva is a midwife and co-founder of the first autonomous midwifery practice in Bulgaria, Zebra Midwives. Yoana has participated in numerous international platforms for raising awareness about the state of midwifery in Eastern Europe.

Nancy Stone is a birth centre midwife in Berlin, Germany. She recently completed her doctoral studies exploring how midwives and women perceive and create risk and safety at birth centre births.

Petra ten Hoope-Bender is the Technical Adviser for Sexual and Reproductive Health and Rights at the UNFPA Office of Geneva. She is a Dutch midwife and worked in a group midwifery practice in the migrant quarters of Rotterdam from 1987 to 1998.

Gillian Thomson is a Reader (Associate Professor) in Perinatal Health at the University of Central Lancashire, Preston. Gill's research interests relate to psychosocial influences and implications of perinatal care, with a particular focus on factors that impact upon maternal mental health.

Anastasia Topalidou PhD is a Research Associate, Research in Childbirth and Health Unit, School of Community Health and Midwifery, Faculty of Health and Wellbeing, UCLan. She specialises in the fields of clinical biomechanics, musculoskeletal biomechanics and clinical measurements, with extensive experience in non-invasive techniques, thermal imaging applications and sensors for use in medicine and clinical research, in a range of context. Anastasia has received several fellowships, awards and honours and she is an active member of scientific and academic societies.

Sally Tracy is Professor of Midwifery at the University of Sydney and conjoint Professor of Midwifery, School of Women's and Children's Health, Faculty of Medicine, UNSW. She has published widely on the epidemiology of preterm birth; birth centre care; admission to neonatal care and the safety of midwifery group practice and stand-alone maternity units.

Nadezhda Tsekulova is a Bulgarian journalist and human rights activist. Her professional activities and personal interests focus on causes which directly influence the health, welfare and the best interests of women and children. In 2016 Nadezhda was awarded "Human of the year" the annual award recognising contributions to human rights in Bulgaria.

Kerstin Uvnäs Moberg is a specialist in women's health and female physiology and has worked within these fields for more than 30 years. She is a pioneer in research about oxytocin 'the hormone of love and wellbeing' and was one of first researchers to point out the behavioural, psychological and physiological effects of oxytocin during birth, breastfeeding and menopause.

Logan van Lessen is a Consultant Midwife (Public Health) based at Whittington Health NHS Trust. Her role is to promote, teach, support and lead on improving maternity care for women and babies locally and strategically.

Shawn Walker PhD is a Midwifery Lecturer at King's College London and Consultant Breech Specialist Midwife at St Thomas' Hospital. Her research focuses on the development of competence and expertise to facilitate breech births (breechbirth.org.uk).

Melanie Wendland is a designer for social innovation and co-founder of Sonder Collective. Melanie currently leads design projects around health system design and detecting social vulnerability in health service delivery across Sub Saharan Africa and India. Her expertise is in using service and system design to facilitate collaborative design processes across organisations. More information at www.sonderdesign.org.

Index